Recent Advances in Child and Adolescent Psychiatry

Recent Advances in Child and Adolescent Psychiatry

Editor

Matteo Chiappedi

MDPI • Basel • Beijing • Wuhan • Barcelona • Belgrade • Manchester • Tokyo • Cluj • Tianjin

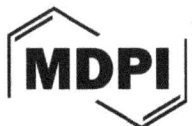

Editor
Matteo Chiappedi
Child Neurology
and Psychiatry
Unit–Vigevano–ASST Pavia
University of Pavia
Pavia
Italy

Editorial Office
MDPI
St. Alban-Anlage 66
4052 Basel, Switzerland

This is a reprint of articles from the Special Issue published online in the open access journal *Children* (ISSN 2227-9067) (available at: www.mdpi.com/journal/children/special_issues/Child_Adolescent_Psychiatry).

For citation purposes, cite each article independently as indicated on the article page online and as indicated below:

LastName, A.A.; LastName, B.B.; LastName, C.C. Article Title. *Journal Name* **Year**, *Volume Number*, Page Range.

ISBN 978-3-0365-6873-7 (Hbk)
ISBN 978-3-0365-6872-0 (PDF)

© 2023 by the authors. Articles in this book are Open Access and distributed under the Creative Commons Attribution (CC BY) license, which allows users to download, copy and build upon published articles, as long as the author and publisher are properly credited, which ensures maximum dissemination and a wider impact of our publications.

The book as a whole is distributed by MDPI under the terms and conditions of the Creative Commons license CC BY-NC-ND.

Contents

About the Editor ix

Preface to "Recent Advances in Child and Adolescent Psychiatry" xi

Matteo Chiappedi and Martina Maria Mensi
Recent Advances in Child and Adolescent Psychiatry
Reprinted from: *Children* 2022, 9, 489, doi:10.3390/children9040489 1

Matteo Chiappedi
Conclusive Thoughts for a New Beginning
Reprinted from: *Children* 2022, 10, 60, doi:10.3390/children10010060 3

Anna Malerba, Sara Iannattone, Giorgia Casano, Marco Lauriola and Gioia Bottesi
The Trap of the COVID-19 Pandemic: Italian Adolescents Fare Well at First, Maybe Thanks to Protective Trait Expression
Reprinted from: *Children* 2022, 9, 1631, doi:10.3390/children9111631 7

Cinzia Correale, Chiara Falamesca, Ilaria Tondo, Marta Borgi, Francesca Cirulli and Mauro Truglio et al.
Depressive Anxiety Symptoms in Hospitalized Children with Chronic Illness during the First Italian COVID-19 Lockdown
Reprinted from: *Children* 2022, 9, 1156, doi:10.3390/children9081156 25

Raúl Vigil-Dopico, Laura Delgado-Lobete, Rebeca Montes-Montes and José Antonio Prieto-Saborit
A Comprehensive Analysis of the Relationship between Play Performance and Psychosocial Problems in School-Aged Children
Reprinted from: *Children* 2022, 9, 1110, doi:10.3390/children9081110 37

Chiara Coci, Livio Provenzi, Valentina De Giorgis, Renato Borgatti, Matteo Chiappedi and Martina Maria Mensi et al.
Family Dysfunctional Interactive Patterns and Alexithymia in Adolescent Patients with Restrictive Eating Disorders
Reprinted from: *Children* 2022, 9, 1038, doi:10.3390/children9071038 49

Hao-Chuan Liu, Chung-Hsien Chaou, Chiao-Wei Lo, Hung-Tao Chung and Mao-Sheng Hwang
Factors Affecting Psychological and Health-Related Quality-of-Life Status in Children and Adolescents with Congenital Heart Diseases
Reprinted from: *Children* 2022, 9, 578, doi:10.3390/children9040578 59

Xin Chen, Kaixin Liang, Liuyue Huang, Wenlong Mu, Wenjing Dong and Shiyun Chen et al.
The Psychometric Properties and Cutoff Score of the Child and Adolescent Mindfulness Measure (CAMM) in Chinese Primary School Students
Reprinted from: *Children* 2022, 9, 499, doi:10.3390/children9040499 73

Saray Bonete, Clara Molinero and Adrián Garrido-Zurita
Generalization Task for Developing Social Problem-Solving Skills among Young People with Autism Spectrum Disorder
Reprinted from: *Children* 2022, 9, 166, doi:10.3390/children9020166 85

Leonhard Thun-Hohenstein, Franka Weltjen, Beatrix Kunas, Roman Winkler and Corinna Fritz
Outcome Quality of Inpatient and Day-Clinic Treatment in Child and Adolescent Psychiatry—A Naturalistic Study
Reprinted from: *Children* **2021**, *8*, 1175, doi:10.3390/children8121175 . . . . **99**

Susan Muriel Schwarz, Mersiha Feike and Ulrich Stangier
Mental Imagery and Social Pain in Adolescents—Analysis of Imagery Characteristics and Perspective—A Pilot Study
Reprinted from: *Children* **2021**, *8*, 1160, doi:10.3390/children8121160 . . . . **113**

Marco Esposito, Laura Pignotti, Federica Mondani, Martina D'Errico, Orlando Ricciardi and Paolo Mirizzi et al.
Stimulus Control Procedure for Reducing Vocal Stereotypies in an Autistic Child
Reprinted from: *Children* **2021**, *8*, 1107, doi:10.3390/children8121107 . . . . **127**

Marco Colizzi, Giulia Antolini, Laura Passarella, Valentina Rizzo, Elena Puttini and Leonardo Zoccante
Additional Evidence for Neuropsychiatric Manifestations in Mosaic Trisomy 20: A Case Report and Brief Review
Reprinted from: *Children* **2021**, *8*, 1030, doi:10.3390/children8111030 . . . . **139**

Pietro Muratori, Carlo Buonanno, Anna Gallani, Giuseppe Grossi, Valentina Levantini and Annarita Milone et al.
Validation of the Proposed Specifiers for Conduct Disorder (PSCD) Scale in a Sample of Italian Students
Reprinted from: *Children* **2021**, *8*, 1020, doi:10.3390/children8111020 . . . . **151**

Claudia Calvano, Elena Murray, Lea Bentz, Sascha Bos, Kathrin Reiter and Loretta Ihme et al.
Evaluation of an Early Intervention Model for Child and Adolescent Victims of Interpersonal Violence
Reprinted from: *Children* **2021**, *8*, 941, doi:10.3390/children8100941 . . . . **163**

Barbara Forresi, Marcella Caputi, Simona Scaini, Ernesto Caffo, Gabriella Aggazzotti and Elena Righi
Parental Internalizing Psychopathology and PTSD in Offspring after the 2012 Earthquake in Italy
Reprinted from: *Children* **2021**, *8*, 930, doi:10.3390/children8100930 . . . . **175**

Alexandra Brecht, Sascha Bos, Laura Ries, Sibylle M. Winter and Claudia Calvano
Assessment of Psychological Distress and Peer Relations among Trans Adolescents—An Examination of the Use of Gender Norms and Parent–Child Congruence of the YSR-R/CBCL-R among a Treatment-Seeking Sample
Reprinted from: *Children* **2021**, *8*, 864, doi:10.3390/children8100864 . . . . **189**

Maurizio Bonati, Francesca Scarpellini, Massimo Cartabia, Michele Zanetti and on behalf of the Lombardy ADHD Group
Ten Years (2011–2021) of the Italian Lombardy ADHD Register for the Diagnosis and Treatment of Children and Adolescents with ADHD
Reprinted from: *Children* **2021**, *8*, 598, doi:10.3390/children8070598 . . . . **207**

Ilaria Maria Carlotta Baschenis, Laura Farinotti, Elena Zavani, Serena Grumi, Patrizia Bernasconi and Enrica Rosso et al.
Reading Skills of Children with Dyslexia Improved Less Than Expected during the COVID-19 Lockdown in Italy
Reprinted from: *Children* **2021**, *8*, 560, doi:10.3390/children8070560 . . . . **221**

Ina Nehring, Heribert Sattel, Maesa Al-Hallak, Martin Sack, Peter Henningsen and Volker Mall et al.
The Child Behavior Checklist as a Screening Instrument for PTSD in Refugee Children
Reprinted from: *Children* **2021**, *8*, 521, doi:10.3390/children8060521 . . . . **229**

Concetta De Pasquale, Matteo Chiappedi, Federica Sciacca, Valentina Martinelli and Zira Hichy
Online Videogames Use and Anxiety in Children during the COVID-19 Pandemic
Reprinted from: *Children* **2021**, *8*, 205, doi:10.3390/children8030205 . . . . **239**

Sara Iannattone, Marina Miscioscia, Alessia Raffagnato and Michela Gatta
The Role of Alexithymia in Social Withdrawal during Adolescence: A Case–Control Study
Reprinted from: *Children* **2021**, *8*, 165, doi:10.3390/children8020165 . . . . **247**

About the Editor

Matteo Chiappedi

Dr Matteo Alessio Chiappedi is a child neuropsychiatrist working in the Child Neurology and Psychiatry Unit of Vigevano (ASST Pavia). He also has a specialization in Psychodynamic Psychotherapy, a Master in Diagnosis and Treatment of Learning Disabilities and a Ph.D. in Physiology and Neuroscience.

He was Adjunct Professor for the F. Bonaccorsi Foundation, for the Catholic University of Brescia, for the University of Milan and for the University of Pavia; he lectured on different aspects of child and adolescent neurology and psychiatry.

He has published in international indexed journals a number of papers, concerning mostly child and adolescent psychiatry (but also neurological and rehabilitative aspects of neuropsychiatric disorders in all life ages).

His main research interests are the understanding of psychiatric disorders, especially in children and adolescents, and the possible treatment options to lower their effect on patients' and caregivers' life quality.

Preface to "Recent Advances in Child and Adolescent Psychiatry"

Psychiatric disorders in children and adolescents are relevant both in terms of their prevalence (they are roughly estimated to affect about 20% of school-aged children and adolescents) and of their impact on the quality of life of the child/adolescent and their family, but also on the society as a whole. Disorders affecting children and adolescents are increasingly seen as having highly specific features, and, therefore, require an equally specific approach despite the coexisting need to integrate contributions from other professions (e.g., pediatricians, psychiatrists, psychologists, and therapists of different sorts). However, the available data are still insufficient, especially for treatment options and too often therapeutic choices are still made based on studies conducted in adults. Even more important, the existence itself of some disorders is questioned especially outside the scientific field (e.g., ADHD).

This Special Issue provided cutting edge data on different aspects of child and adolescent psychiatry, including etiopatogenesis, clinical characteristics and diagnosis, medical and neurological comorbidities (and psychiatric comorbidities of medical and neurological disorders), impact on patients/families/society (including school and other social groups), prognosis, and treatment options of the different disorders.

Matteo Chiappedi
Editor

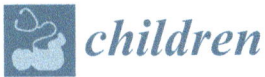

Editorial

Recent Advances in Child and Adolescent Psychiatry

Matteo Chiappedi * and Martina Maria Mensi

Child Neuropsychiatry Unit, IRCCS Mondino Foundation, 27100 Pavia, Italy; martina.mensi@mondino.it
* Correspondence: matteo.chiappedi@mondino.it

The field of child and adolescent psychiatry is receiving growing attention, although a number of local differences still exist in terms of academic curricula, board certifications and even definitions of what is to be considered part of this field or not. An Italian study showed that approximately 1 out of 10 children showed significant psychopathological problems [1]; this study was conducted before the COVID-19 pandemic, and it is plausible (and seems to be confirmed both by clinical observation and literature findings [2]) that these figures are going to increase significantly in the next few months and years.

The main goal of this Special Issue is therefore to provide cutting-edge data regarding all aspects of child and adolescent psychiatry, including (but not limited to) the etiopathogenesis and presentation of the different disorders, treatment options and management of comorbidities. This is important because the peculiarities of the psychopathological manifestations in different age groups are increasingly recognized in classification systems, when a developmental perspective is applied [3].

Two papers in this Special Issue are case reports. Colizzi et al. provide a detailed description of a case of mosaic trisomy 20, analyzing the neuropsychiatric aspects in the light of a careful analysis of the existing literature [4]. Esposito et al. described the successful application of a stimulus discrimination training to reduce vocal stereotypies in an autistic child, offering an interesting background for future controlled studies [5].

Three more papers focused on different psychopathological sequelae of traumatic experiences. Calvano et al. provide evidence of the utility of a highly specialized approach in the form of an outpatient trauma clinic to start the therapeutic process and increase victims' motivation towards a more prolonged intervention [6]. Forresi et al. described the effect of the exposure to an earthquake in a large sample of Italian families, showing the existing bidirectional correlation between parental and children internalizing symptoms and post-traumatic stress disorder [7]. Nehring et al. reported the utility of the Child Behavior Checklist Post-Traumatic Stress Disorder Scale and of an alternative scale (developed using a psychometrically guided item selection) as screening tools for post-traumatic stress disorder in a population of Syrian refugee children [8].

Two papers focused on the consequences of the COVID-19 pandemic. De Pasquale et al. studied the prevalence of online videogaming during the so-called "lockdown" in Italy, with anxiety (and especially state anxiety) being a relevant predictor of videogame use and addiction [9]. Baschenis et al. documented that children with dyslexia saw a reduction in their potential for reading evolution during school closure due to the COVID-19 pandemic, a fact that was coupled with greater social isolation and fewer worries about the pandemic and school closure [10].

The other papers testify the variety of subjects and approaches in child and adolescent psychiatry. Thun-Hohenstein et al. applied a naturalistic approach to assess the outcome of a group of adolescents consecutively admitted to an inpatient and day-clinic treatment [11]; they also showed that psychopathological severity at diagnosis and the relationship with the therapist were significantly related to the prognosis. Schwarz et al. provide initial findings regarding the understudied topic of the correlation between mental imagery and social pain, distinguishing its unique contribution not present in other anxiety-related disorders or in mood disorders [12]. Muratori et al. explored the utility of the Proposed Specifiers Conduct

Citation: Chiappedi, M.; Mensi, M.M. Recent Advances in Child and Adolescent Psychiatry. *Children* 2022, 9, 489. https://doi.org/10.3390/children9040489

Received: 24 December 2021
Accepted: 23 March 2022
Published: 1 April 2022

Publisher's Note: MDPI stays neutral with regard to jurisdictional claims in published maps and institutional affiliations.

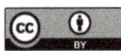

Copyright: © 2022 by the authors. Licensee MDPI, Basel, Switzerland. This article is an open access article distributed under the terms and conditions of the Creative Commons Attribution (CC BY) license (https://creativecommons.org/licenses/by/4.0/).

Disorder scale, and their findings support its use as a reliable, easy-to-use tool for measuring psychopathic traits in Italian children and young adolescents [13]. Brecht et al. studied a group of trans adolescents and evidenced a high level of psychopathological and especially internalizing problems, largely predicted by a reduced concordance between parental and subjects' reports and by poor peer relations [14]. Iannattone et al. studied the role of alexithymia as a predictor of social withdrawal, especially when coupled with internalizing problems [15]. Last but not least, Bonati et al. provide the 10-year experience of the Lombardy ADHD Registry, offering many valuable insights concerning diagnosis and treatment emerging from this unmet experience [16], together with a description of unmet needs of these children and adolescents.

These contributions, with their variety in terms of explored topics and used methods, provide a mirror of the complexity of the topic of this Special Issue; hopefully, they will be thought- and action-stimulating reading for all those willing to pay comprehensive attention to children and adolescents.

Author Contributions: M.C. and M.M.M. equally contributed to all aspects of the manuscript. All authors have read and agreed to the published version of the manuscript.

Funding: This research was supported by the Italian Health Ministry (Ricerca Corrente 2021).

Conflicts of Interest: The authors declare no conflict of interest.

References

1. Frigerio, A.; Rucci, P.; Goodman, R.; Ammaniti, M.; Carlet, O.; Cavolina, P.; De Girolamo, G.; Lenti, C.; Lucarelli, L.; Mani, E.; et al. Prevalence and correlates of mental disorders among adolescents in Italy: The PrISMA study. *Eur. Child Adolesc. Psychiatry* **2009**, *18*, 217–226. [CrossRef] [PubMed]
2. Mensi, M.M.; Capone, L.; Rogantini, C.; Orlandi, M.; Ballante, E.; Borgatti, R. COVID-19-related psychiatric impact on Italian adolescent population: A cross-sectional cohort study. *J. Community Psychol.* **2021**, *49*, 1457–1469. [CrossRef] [PubMed]
3. American Psychiatric Association. *Diagnostic and Statistical Manual of Mental Disorders*, 5th ed.; APA Publisher: Washington, DC, USA, 2013.
4. Colizzi, M.; Antolini, G.; Passarella, L.; Rizzo, V.; Puttini, E.; Zoccante, L. Additional Evidence for Neuropsychiatric Manifestations in Mosaic Trisomy 20: A Case Report and Brief Review. *Children* **2021**, *8*, 1030. [CrossRef] [PubMed]
5. Esposito, M.; Pignotti, L.; Mondani, F.; D'Errico, M.; Ricciardi, O.; Mirizzi, P.; Mazza, M.; Valenti, M. Stimulus Control Procedure for Reducing Vocal Stereotypies in an Autistic Child. *Children* **2021**, *8*, 1107. [CrossRef] [PubMed]
6. Calvano, C.; Murray, E.; Bentz, L.; Bos, S.; Reiter, K.; Ihme, L.; Winter, S.M. Evaluation of an Early Intervention Model for Child and Adolescent Victims of Interpersonal Violence. *Children* **2021**, *8*, 941. [CrossRef] [PubMed]
7. Forresi, B.; Caputi, M.; Scaini, S.; Caffo, E.; Aggazzotti, G.; Righi, E. Parental Internalizing Psychopathology and PTSD in Offspring after the 2012 Earthquake in Italy. *Children* **2021**, *8*, 930. [CrossRef] [PubMed]
8. Nehring, I.; Sattel, H.; Al-Hallak, M.; Sack, M.; Henningsen, P.; Mall, V.; Aberl, S. The Child Behavior Checklist as a Screening Instrument for PTSD in Refugee Children. *Children* **2021**, *8*, 521. [CrossRef] [PubMed]
9. De Pasquale, C.; Chiappedi, M.; Sciacca, F.; Martinelli, V.; Hichy, Z. Online Videogames Use and Anxiety in Children during the COVID-19 Pandemic. *Children* **2021**, *8*, 205. [CrossRef] [PubMed]
10. Baschenis, I.M.C.; Farinotti, L.; Zavani, E.; Grumi, S.; Bernasconi, P.; Rosso, E.; Provenzi, L.; Borgatti, R.; Termine, C.; Chiappedi, M. Reading Skills of Children with Dyslexia Improved Less Than Expected during the COVID-19 Lockdown in Italy. *Children* **2021**, *8*, 560. [CrossRef] [PubMed]
11. Thun-Hohenstein, L.; Weltjen, F.; Kunas, B.; Winkler, R.; Fritz, C. Outcome Quality of Inpatient and Day-Clinic Treatment in Child and Adolescent Psychiatry—A Naturalistic Study. *Children* **2021**, *8*, 1175. [CrossRef] [PubMed]
12. Schwarz, S.M.; Feike, M.; Stangier, U. Mental Imagery and Social Pain in Adolescents—Analysis of Imagery Characteristics and Perspective—A Pilot Study. *Children* **2021**, *8*, 1160. [CrossRef] [PubMed]
13. Muratori, P.; Buonanno, C.; Gallani, A.; Grossi, G.; Levantini, V.; Milone, A.; Pisano, S.; Salekin, R.T.; Sesso, G.; Masi, G.; et al. Validation of the Proposed Specifiers for Conduct Disorder (PSCD) Scale in a Sample of Italian Students. *Children* **2021**, *8*, 1020. [CrossRef] [PubMed]
14. Brecht, A.; Bos, S.; Ries, L.; Winter, S.M.; Calvano, C. Assessment of Psychological Distress and Peer Relations among Trans Adolescents—An Examination of the Use of Gender Norms and Parent–Child Congruence of the YSR-R/CBCL-R among a Treatment-Seeking Sample. *Children* **2021**, *8*, 864. [CrossRef] [PubMed]
15. Iannattone, S.; Miscioscia, M.; Raffagnato, A.; Gatta, M. The Role of Alexithymia in Social Withdrawal during Adolescence: A Case–Control Study. *Children* **2021**, *8*, 165. [CrossRef] [PubMed]
16. Bonati, M.; Scarpellini, F.; Cartabia, M.; Zanetti, M.; on behalf of the Lombardy ADHD Group. Ten Years (2011–2021) of the Italian Lombardy ADHD Register for the Diagnosis and Treatment of Children and Adolescents with ADHD. *Children* **2021**, *8*, 598. [CrossRef] [PubMed]

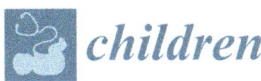

Editorial

Conclusive Thoughts for a New Beginning

Matteo Chiappedi

Vigevano Child Neurology and Psychiatry Unit, ASST Pavia, 27100 Pavia, Italy; matteo_chiappedi@asst-pavia.it

When I was asked to name this Special Issue, I was both honored and worried, as being appointed the Guest Editor was a significant achievement and honor. Although I had been trained as a child neuropsychiatrist (as in Italy, pediatric psychiatry and neurology are still joined in one discipline), my main interest has always been child psychiatry. Thus, I was worried that relatively few papers concerning child and adolescent psychiatry had previously been published in *Children*. However, many things have changed since this Special Issue was created under the Child Neurology Section (which was, at that time, the best fit available) and now, a Child and Adolescent Psychiatry Section exists as a part of *Children*.

Since the previous Editorial concerning this Special Issue [1], many interesting manuscripts have been submitted. This was surprising, since a number of other Special Issue had been opened and some of them potentially overlap with this wide topic I had chosen ("Recent Advances in Child and Adolescent Psychiatry"). When the Special Issue was closed, 33 manuscripts had been submitted and 20 had been accepted (this does not include the above mentioned Editorial [1]). As the Guest Editor, I am privileged to have the opportunity to read these interesting contributions and to choose those that I (and the wonderful colleagues that provided their service as reviewers) believed were not only scientifically sound (which was true for all submitted manuscripts), but also of a high interest for the wide readership of *Children*.

Dr. Bonete and coworkers provided data concerning the development of the Interpersonal Problem-Solving Skills Program [2]. They discussed the use of a task meant to increase the generalization of interpersonal problem-solving skills in adolescents and young adults with autism spectrum disorder who showed a reduced ability to imagine different possible scenarios. Their findings showed that this improved after treatment.

Dr. Chen and coworkers studied the psychometric properties of the Child and Adolescent Mindfulness Measure (CAMM) in Chinese primary school students [3]. Mindfulness has become a trending topic in psychiatry over the last 10 years, and this study combined a description of its role in physical and mental health with a rigorous psychometric analysis. Although conducted in a rather specific population, this was a good example of what is expected to happen before a tool is used in psychiatry (and in medicine in general).

The interaction between a physical disease, psychological factors and health-related quality of life (HRQoL) was the focus of the paper by Dr. Liu and coworkers [4]. They studied children with congenital heart disease to show that there was a higher impact on patients' psychological adjustment and HRQoL in those with cyanotic heart disease, although the need for invasive treatments was another relevant factor.

The Mondino Foundation Eating Disorders Clinical and Research Group contributed a manuscript concerning the interactive patterns in families of patients with restrictive eating disorders [5]. They used the clinical version of the Lausanne Triadic Play to assess family functioning and confirmed the presence of a collusive alliance in these families, but expanded the existing literature on this topic by showing a correlation between this interactive pattern and a higher global score for alexithymia in the patient, according to the Toronto Alexithymia Scale.

The paper written by Dr. Vigil-Dopico and coworkers [6] deals with a highly relevant topic for child psychiatry, i.e., play. The authors studied a significant number of children to assess play performance and compared their performance with internalizing and externalizing problems that were reported by their parents through the Strengths and Difficulties Questionnaire. A relationship was found between reduced play performance and higher psychosocial problems. The authors provide a tentative explanation, assuming that executive functions could have a role in self-regulation (in particular, during play performance) and in social cognition.

A cross-sectional study conducted in some of the most important pediatric departments in Italy during the so-called "first lockdown" (i.e., the first application of the stay-at-home order) was presented by Dr. Correale and coworkers [7]. They evaluated pediatric patients with different forms of chronic illness hospitalized from March to May 2021 and found a high proportion of significant depressive and anxious symptoms (reported by roughly two out of three children). This highlighted the need to study the effect of the COVID-19 pandemic (and of the related preventive measures) in the most vulnerable subjects.

A more positive view of the effects of the first phase of the COVID-19 pandemic on adolescents was provided by Malerba and coworkers [8]. In their longitudinal study on a sample of Italian adolescents, they found, on average, a good adjustment, which seemed to be mainly associated with a high degree of positivity as a trait, a factor that could have somehow overweighted the difficulties caused by the many uncertainties that emerged in those months.

It is rather evident that the COVID-19 pandemic had a significant influence on this Special Issue, not only because it was started in 2020, but also because 4 research papers [7–10] out of the 20 published explored aspects connected with it. Since the epidemiologic situation seems to be evolving favorably, although some concerns are still present, one could begin to conduct research on the factors that acted as facilitators or as barriers, on the new models of intervention (exploiting technology to vehiculate treatments and support) and on the psychic scars left from these years. However, the fact that 16 research papers, even in such unprecedented times, addressed relevant aspects of child and adolescent psychiatry independent from the COVID-19 pandemic shows that there is a lot more to yet explore. Maybe, in a relatively short time, a new Special Issue will be needed.

Funding: This research received no external funding.

Conflicts of Interest: The author declares no conflict of interest.

References

1. Chiappedi, M.; Mensi, M.M. Recent Advances in Child and Adolescent Psychiatry. *Children* **2022**, *9*, 489. [CrossRef] [PubMed]
2. Bonete, S.; Molinero, C.; Garrido-Zurita, A. Generalization Task for Developing Social Problem-Solving Skills among Young People with Autism Spectrum Disorder. *Children* **2022**, *9*, 166. [CrossRef] [PubMed]
3. Chen, X.; Liang, K.; Huang, L.; Mu, W.; Dong, W.; Chen, S.; Chen, S.; Chix, X. The Psychometric Properties and Cutoff Score of the Child and Adolescent Mindfulness Measure (CAMM) in Chinese Primary School Students. *Children* **2022**, *9*, 499. [CrossRef] [PubMed]
4. Liu, H.-C.; Chaou, C.-H.; Lo, C.-W.; Chung, H.-T.; Hwang, M.-S. Factors Affecting Psychological and Health-Related Quality-of-Life Status in Children and Adolescents with Congenital Heart Disease. *Children* **2022**, *9*, 578. [CrossRef] [PubMed]
5. Coci, C.; Provenzi, L.; De Giorgis, V.; Borgatti, R.; Chiappedi, M.; Mensi, M.M.; on behalf of the Mondino Foundation Eating Disorders Clinical and Research Group. Family Dysfunctional Interactive Patterns and Alexithymia in Adolescent Patients with Restrictive Eating Disorders. *Children* **2002**, *9*, 1038. [CrossRef] [PubMed]
6. Vigil-Dopico, R.; Delgado-Lobete, L.; Montes-Montes, R.; Prieto-Saborit, J.A. A Comprehensive Analysis of the Relationship between Play Performance and Psychosocial Problems in School-Aged Children. *Children* **2022**, *9*, 1110. [CrossRef] [PubMed]
7. Correale, C.; Falamesca, C.; Tondo, I.; Borgi, M.; Cirulli, F.; Truglio, M.; Papa, O.; Vagnoli, L.; Arzilli, C.; Venturino, C.; et al. Depressive Anxiety Symptoms in Hospitalized Children with Chronic Illness during the First Italian COVID-19 Lockdown. *Children* **2022**, *9*, 1156. [CrossRef] [PubMed]
8. Malerba, A.; Iannattone, S.; Casano, G.; Lauriola, M.; Bottesi, G. The Trap of the COVID-19 Pandemic: Italian Adolescents Fare Well at First, Maybe Thanks to Protective Trait Expression. *Children* **2022**, *9*, 1631. [CrossRef] [PubMed]

9. De Pasquale, C.; Chiappedi, M.; Sciacca, F.; Martinelli, V.; Hichy, Z. Online Videogames Use and Anxiety in Children during the COVID-19 Pandemic. *Children* **2021**, *8*, 205. [CrossRef] [PubMed]
10. Baschenis, I.M.C.; Farinotti, L.; Zavani, E.; Grumi, S.; Bernasconi, P.; Rosso, E.; Provenzi, L.; Borgatti, R.; Termine, C.; Chiappedi, M. Reading Skills of Children with Dyslexia Improved Less than Expected during the COVID-19 Lockdown in Italy. *Children* **2021**, *8*, 560. [CrossRef] [PubMed]

Disclaimer/Publisher's Note: The statements, opinions and data contained in all publications are solely those of the individual author(s) and contributor(s) and not of MDPI and/or the editor(s). MDPI and/or the editor(s) disclaim responsibility for any injury to people or property resulting from any ideas, methods, instructions or products referred to in the content.

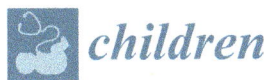

Article

The Trap of the COVID-19 Pandemic: Italian Adolescents Fare Well at First, Maybe Thanks to Protective Trait Expression

Anna Malerba [1], Sara Iannattone [1,*], Giorgia Casano [1], Marco Lauriola [2] and Gioia Bottesi [1]

1. Department of General Psychology, University of Padova, 35131 Padova, Italy
2. Department of Developmental and Social Psychology, Sapienza University of Rome, 00185 Rome, Italy
* Correspondence: sara.iannattone@phd.unipd.it

Abstract: Abundant research indicates that the COVID-19 pandemic has been negatively affecting mental health in adolescence. Few works, however, benefit from data from the same sample before and after the onset of the pandemic. The present longitudinal study involved a non-clinical group of 136 Italian adolescents (M_{age} = 16.3 years ± 1.08, 67% girls) to investigate their psychological response to the first lockdown and explore the role of a protective trait (i.e., Positivity) in moderating the effect of Intolerance of Uncertainty (IU) on internalizing symptoms before and during the COVID-19 outbreak. Participants completed self-report questionnaires assessing psychopathological symptoms, psychological well-being, IU, and Positivity on three separate occasions: October 2019 (T1), January 2020 (T2), and April 2020 (T3). The results showed that internalizing and externalizing symptoms as well as psychological well-being did not vary significantly over time. Positivity was found to significantly moderate the relationship between IU and internalizing symptoms at T3 (i.e., during the COVID-19 lockdown) only. Overall, our findings suggest that the teenagers' good adjustment to the initial phase of the pandemic might have been associated with the enhanced weight of the Positivity trait, which may have encouraged a positive attitude towards self, life, and the future.

Keywords: COVID-19; positivity; intolerance of uncertainty; psychopathological symptoms; psychological adjustment; adolescence; longitudinal study

Citation: Malerba, A.; Iannattone, S.; Casano, G.; Lauriola, M.; Bottesi, G. The Trap of the COVID-19 Pandemic: Italian Adolescents Fare Well at First, Maybe Thanks to Protective Trait Expression. *Children* **2022**, *9*, 1631. https://doi.org/10.3390/children9111631

Academic Editor: Matteo Alessio Chiappedi

Received: 1 October 2022
Accepted: 24 October 2022
Published: 26 October 2022

Publisher's Note: MDPI stays neutral with regard to jurisdictional claims in published maps and institutional affiliations.

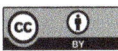

Copyright: © 2022 by the authors. Licensee MDPI, Basel, Switzerland. This article is an open access article distributed under the terms and conditions of the Creative Commons Attribution (CC BY) license (https://creativecommons.org/licenses/by/4.0/).

1. Introduction

In February 2020, Italy was struck by the spread of a new strain of coronavirus, the SARS-CoV-2, which caused the COVID-19 infectious disease pandemic in the following months. The need to limit the contagion warranted prompt action by the national administration resulting in a total lockdown, whereby the entire population was conditioned to restrictive physical and social distancing measures, substantially limiting their movements and their engagement in social activities. Restrictions became effective as early as the 11th of March and lasted until the 3rd of May 2020 (so-called "phase 1") [1]. Generally speaking, the COVID-19 outbreak had severe repercussions on mental health and well-being worldwide, leading to a sharp increase in cases of major depressive disorder and anxiety disorders in the adult population [2]. The greatest increases were found in places highly affected by the pandemic, i.e., places with the highest daily COVID-19 infection rates and the greatest reductions in human mobility. Indeed, Italy experienced a 21 to 25% change in prevalence rates of anxiety disorders and major depressive disorder in the first year of the pandemic outbreak [3].

In this scenario, people in developmental age should be carefully taken into consideration. The COVID-19 lockdown was characterized by the mandatory closure of schools. As a consequence, youth were subject to a major and long-lasting disruption in their daily lives: a structured program of at-home remote classes was put into place for all students, setting off widespread uncertainty around their immediate and mid-term future [4]. A new set of challenges emerged: exposure to physical social spaces was drastically reduced and virtual ones became prominent to many [5], learning modalities changed radically, and exposure to the family environment suddenly increased [6]. Moreover, exposure to once pleasurable activities (e.g., physical activity, social engagements, travelling) decreased, while fear of contagion was being encouraged both by government agencies and media outlets [7]. The exposure to such environmental changes together with major reductions in regulatory and coping mechanisms to face them [4] was expected to have substantial effects especially on internalizing symptoms in children and adolescents [8]. Importantly, adolescence is known as a developmental period marked by rapid biological and social changes [9]. It is connected to specific developmental tasks such as the definition of personal identity through the development of autonomy and bonds with peers [10,11]. The risk of interference of the described pandemic-related factors with developmental trajectories led authors to speculate that youth might be at an even greater risk of adverse mental health outcomes from infectious outbreaks [12,13], also considering that adolescence is *per se* characterized by a high psychopathological vulnerability, especially in terms of internalizing problems [14].

Nonetheless, estimates seem rather inconclusive in evaluating early internalizing outcomes for the adolescent population [2]. The World Health Organization (WHO) indicates that a major limitation of existing estimates comes from the scarcity of baseline pre-pandemic comparison data to match measurements collected during the first months of this unanticipated event. A systematic review and meta-analysis of longitudinal cohort studies examining changes in mental health among the same group of children and adolescents ($n = 38$) before vs. during the pandemic in 2020 found no significant differences [15]. Two meta-analyses of pooled prevalence rates (from 2020), on the other hand, were convergent in reporting increased rates of depression and anxiety during COVID-19, particularly for older adolescents, especially girls, with increasing estimates over time [16,17].

To date, published literature on mental health outcomes of adolescents during the pandemic is wanting, especially in the Italian context [18]. In this regard, two well-known risk and protective factors of internalizing outcomes worthy of further attention are, respectively, Intolerance of Uncertainty (IU) and Positivity [19–21].

1.1. Intolerance of Uncertainty

Uncertainty was plainly described as 'the psychological state of "not knowing"' [22] (p. 199), and, more specifically, as the perceived lack of sufficient or salient information in a given situation [23]. It is a characteristically unpleasant state that can arise in several circumstances. IU, distinctively, is the stable disposition not to tolerate the aversive reactions elicited by uncertainty, maintained by the perception of uncertainty itself [23].

Originally conceptualized as the key cognitive vulnerability factor for worry [24], IU is now established as a trans-diagnostic risk factor across internalizing disorders, putatively underlying neuroticism [23,25]. Indeed, Carleton has described IU as a transdiagnostic dispositional risk factor for clinically relevant anxiety and depression. Consistently, IU has been shown to account for statistically significant amounts of variance in symptoms of several anxiety disorders and to be strongly associated with depression (for a review see Carleton and colleagues [23]) [26].

To date, few studies have investigated IU in adolescent samples, although this developmental stage seems per se characterized by elevated uncertainty, thus exposing teenagers to a higher risk of developing psychopathological symptoms [27]. Some studies have uncovered the role played by IU in several disorders in adolescence [14], although research in this field is still in its infancy. Research on worry in adolescence showed that around this age concerns grow increasingly abstract, detailed, and related to temporally distant factors, thus proving that adolescents, much like adults, can suffer from concerns surrounding the future in general, in addition to those surrounding social evaluation or academic performance [14,28].

A 5-year, ten-wave longitudinal study of 338 high school adolescents provided enticing insight into the evolution of IU in this population. Despite observing relative stability of change trajectories in IU, the main findings showed that the highest levels of IU were observed at the beginning and end of secondary school (i.e., time points 1 and 10). The authors argued these to be transition periods, marked by significant and simultaneous changes in both internal and external domains of adolescent life, explaining temporary yet meaningful inflations in IU. This evidence seems to support the idea that IU is also a malleable construct, since prolonged periods during which adolescents are challenged by uncertainty can cause alterations in this usually stable disposition [28].

According to the WHO [29], extended school closures have left young people "vulnerable to social isolation and disconnectedness which can fuel feelings of anxiety, uncertainty, and loneliness and lead to affective and behavioral problems" (p. 20). Indeed, uncertainty has afflicted youth during the COVID-19 pandemic, as young people have experienced it from when evaluating the probability of infecting family members to when anticipating educational and employment outcomes in the future, following several months of school closure [4]. When adolescents catastrophically misinterpret uncertainties such as those naturally occurring within a pandemic [30,31], IU is likely to grow, and this represents a breeding ground for adverse outcomes such as anxiety and depression [32]. Extant research has chiefly examined the role of IU in buffering health-related anxiety in adults during COVID-19 [32], while, to our knowledge, no study has yet tapped into the relationship between adolescent IU and internalizing symptoms during this pandemic.

1.2. Positivity

In 2004, the WHO published an influential report addressing the promotion of mental health and redefined it as: not merely the absence of illness, but the presence of "a state of well-being in which the individual realizes his or her abilities, can cope with the normal stresses of life, can work productively and fruitfully, and is able to make a contribution to his or her community" [33] (p. 12). This contribution brought about the rejection of the traditional conceptualization of well-being and ill-being as two extremes of a continuum, thus allowing for the recognition of mental health as a unique set of "symptoms of positive functioning", as opposed to the constellation of symptoms of bad functioning involved in mental illness [34].

Building upon the call for research on adequate indicators of positive mental functioning or flourishing [35], Caprara and colleagues developed a conceptualization of the cognitive component to well-being encompassing self-esteem [36], life satisfaction [37], and dispositional optimism [38]. These dimensions represent phenomenological expressions of the latent construct named Positivity [39]. Positivity is described as a "pervasive mode of appraising, viewing, and perceiving life from a positive stance" [40] (p. 353), a process closely associated with the management and consequences of positive affect. Positivity predisposes people to "recruit, amplify and benefit from it through the promotion of experiences that carry positive feelings and by enhancing and prolonging their savoring" [41] (p. 4).

Extant literature underscores the heritable mechanism behind individual positive orientation [39], while also revealing a meaningful susceptibility of this disposition to environmental influence [42]. A significant component linked to experience speaks to its moderate malleability: life experiences play a role in the different forms that self-esteem, life satisfaction and optimism may take and in their combinations [41]. For example, a daily study on an adolescent sample has expounded on the genetic evidence, showing a significant variation of Positivity from one day to the next [43], while evidence from a longitudinal study showed a high degree of consistency of positive orientation over adolescents' developmental trajectory [44].

Several studies have provided evidence supporting the role of Positivity as an individual's resource sustaining optimal functioning in several domains (e.g., [45,46]) and empirical studies have found significant positive links between Positivity and different indices of well-being in adolescents and young adults (e.g., [34,40,47]). Notably, two studies have pointed out its key contribution to predicting adolescent and adult resilience, which is the ability to adapt successfully to changing and stressful environmental challenges and life events [48,49]. Specifically, Milioni and colleagues [48] provided longitudinal evidence for the predictive effect of Positivity on later adolescent ego-resiliency over 10 years, while the contrary was not found, and a study [49] conducted during the COVID-19 pandemic corroborated the protective role of Positivity in reducing adults' anxiety and depressive symptoms.

Finally, Positivity is consistently linked to lower levels of internalizing and externalizing symptoms in early adolescents [19,50]. Extant literature emphasizes the possibility that Positivity might constitute a "syndrome of optimal functioning", acting as a protective factor in general against mental illness and specifically against depression [39]. This beneficial effect is posited in accordance with cognitive theories that see negative views of the self, the world, and the future as the basis of depression [39,51].

1.3. The Present Study

The COVID-19 pandemic has acted as a major stressor on adolescents' psychological well-being [2], requiring them to tolerate an uncertain future drawing upon personal resources to face a pervasive uneasy mental state [4,52]. However, research addressing this issue is constrained by the limited number of studies providing same-sample data on mental health both pre- and during the COVID-19 pandemic [2,15]. Furthermore, to our knowledge, only one international study [53] has navigated the role played by stable, trait-like dispositions in moderating mental health outcomes during such uncertain and unsettling times for youth [49]. However, such an attempt is yet to be made in Italy.

Extant literature holds Positivity and IU as key cognitive precursors to internalizing problems (i.e., anxiety and depressive symptoms) [19,23], the former acting as a protective factor providing the dispositional base to experience happiness in life and the latter hindering adolescents' capacity to endure uncertainty, thus promoting emotional distress (e.g., [54]). Although both constructs have been defined as stable dispositions, some studies highlighted their malleability under the influence of (stressful) environmental factors [28,39]. Nevertheless, to the best of our knowledge, no study has yet examined IU in an adolescent sample during the COVID-19 pandemic. Given the established and strong link between IU and anxiety and depressive symptoms [23], an important step is to investigate its role in adolescence during the COVID-19 pandemic, in light of the aforementioned factors: pandemics in general are ridden with uncertainty [30], adolescence is itself characterized by elevated uncertainty [27], and internalizing problems often emerge in adolescence [14]. Furthermore, no study has yet investigated the relationship between IU and Positivity in affecting internalizing symptoms during any time. The relevance of providing further evidence on protective and risk factors to adolescent mental health in trying times lies in the opportunity to identify useful indicators of resilience or, conversely, vulnerability, thus contributing to the implementation of broad-spectrum and trait-specific intervention programs [39].

Aims and Hypotheses

In light of the aforementioned considerations, we involved an Italian non-clinical adolescent sample with the twofold aim of:

1. Describing what changes, if any, have occurred in internalizing and externalizing symptoms, and psychological well-being with the first COVID-19 lockdown. We were particularly interested in investigating those psychopathological dimensions that are chiefly associated with the social and scholastic environment (i.e., attention problems, social, scholastic and separation anxiety).

    According to the previous literature, we hypothesized to observe a substantial stagnation in internalizing (H1a), externalizing (H1b), and attention problems (H1c), social anxiety (H1d), and generalized anxiety (H1e) [15,55]. No studies conducted on non-clinical adolescent samples explored these issues in relation to separation anxiety, school anxiety, and psychological well-being, thus we did not make specific predictions.

2. Exploring whether Positivity moderated the relationship between IU and internalizing symptoms before and during the COVID-19 lockdown. We chose to focus on internalizing symptoms in light of the literature supporting their association with both IU and Positivity [19,23,26].

In particular, we hypothesized that IU would positively predict internalizing symptoms at both times (H2) [23,26], and Positivity would negatively predict internalizing symptoms at both times (H3) [19]. Moreover, we also expected sex (H4) [56,57] and age (H5) [58,59] to significantly predict internalizing symptoms at both times, with higher levels more likely in girls and older adolescents.

We chose to test the same model twice, including the same variables but at different time points, because we had the unique opportunity of comparing the moderating effect of a trait-like disposition before and during the lockdown to observe the lockdown's effect on trait-like dispositions' interactions; this enabled us to scrutinize whether and how a simple cognitive and psychopathological system reacts to a major stressor, capitalizing on cognitive resources to produce resilience. This condition offered a unique standpoint that enabled us to investigate the effect of the environment on two cognitive factors that, albeit dispositional, can take different forms and express differently under certain circumstances [28,39,41]. No previous research has focused on this issue, so we did not formulate any specific hypothesis.

2. Materials and Methods

2.1. Participants and Procedure

The present work stems from a larger longitudinal study originally designed to investigate the role of protective factors for psychopathology in nonclinical adolescents across six months. Participants were recruited at high schools in Veneto (one of the most severely affected regions of Italy from COVID-19-related mortality [60]). After obtaining the approval of the school directors, a written informed consent form was collected from parents or legal guardians of minor students, whereas 18 years old students provided their own consent. The study was conducted in accordance with the Declaration of Helsinki and approved by the local Ethical Committee.

An online survey was developed in the Google Modules platform. It included a battery of self-report questionnaires measuring several constructs (e.g., happiness, mindfulness, broadband symptomatology) and a socio-demographic survey, soliciting information on sex, age, school year, and presence of psychological difficulties. Given the aims of the current study, we only considered the questionnaires described in Section 2.2. The first two administrations took place in October 2019 (T1) and January 2020 (T2) at the school's computer room. Completion required 45–50 min on average and occurred during school hours. The third administration (T3) occurred during the national lockdown (i.e., April 2020), when schools were closed to prevent contagion. Consequently, the form was delivered to participants through the school's web platform and completed outside the school building. Data collected at each time point were paired through alphanumeric codes, assigned to each participant.

The final sample consisted of 136 Italian adolescents (M_{age} = 16.3 years, SD = 1.08), including 44 boys (32.4%) and 92 girls (67.6%) aged 14 to 18. 2.9% of the sample was 14 years old, 22.8% was 15, 32.4% was 16, 25.7% was 17 and 16.2% was 18 years old. 9.6% of participants answered yes to a question addressing having had, either currently or in the past, psychological difficulties that warranted professional help (e.g., problems with anxiety and depressive symptoms).

2.2. Measures

The Positivity scale (P Scale; [19]) evaluates the respondents' dispositional tendency to have a positive attitude towards themselves, their lives, and their future. The scale is composed of 8 items rated on a 5-point Likert scale ranging from 1 (strongly disagree) to 5 (strongly agree). The P Scale operationalizes Positivity in three aspects (i.e., self-esteem, life satisfaction, and optimism); however, there is consensus that these facets can be traced to a single, general self-evaluative latent construct. Higher scores reflect greater Positivity. The unidimensionality of the questionnaire was confirmed both in adult and adolescent samples [19,50,61]. The P Scale showed high reliability coefficients in secondary school students (ω = 0.84) [19].

The Intolerance of Uncertainty Scale-Revised (IUS-R; [27]) is a 12-item self-report questionnaire assessing the disposition not to tolerate the aversive reactions elicited by uncertainty. Each item is rated on a 5-point Likert scale (1 = Not at all like me, 5 = Entirely like me). The Italian version of this measure showed excellent internal consistency in a large adolescent sample (Cronbach's α = 0.90, McDonald's ω = 0.90) and a good one-month test-retest reliability (r = 0.74) in undergraduate and adult samples [62]. Higher scores reflect higher levels of IU.

The Youth Self-Report 11–18 (YSR; [63,64]) is a self-report questionnaire consisting of 113 items that examine social competencies and psychopathological behavior. The latter includes 9 syndrome scales: anxious/depressed; withdrawn/depressed; somatic complaints; social problems; thought disorders; attention disorders; deviant behavior; aggressive behavior and other problems. These subscales are then grouped to obtain three global scales for internalizing problems, externalizing problems, and total problems. In our study, we considered two global scales (internalizing problems and externalizing problems), and one syndrome scale (i.e., attention problems). Items of the internalizing problems global scale reflect anxiety and depression symptoms (e.g., fears, worries, isolation, sadness, crying a lot). The externalizing problems global scale refers to aggressive and rule-breaking behavior (e.g., lack of guilt, substance use, mean and disobedient behavior). The internalizing problems scale includes the social withdrawal, somatic complaints, and anxiety–depression scales. The externalizing problems scale includes the deviant behavior and aggressive behavior scales. Higher scores on each scale reflect higher levels of the measured syndrome or syndromes. This tool has good reliability, with Cronbach's alpha ranging from 0.71 to 0.95.

The Self Administrated Psychiatric Scales for Children and Adolescents-Anxiety evaluation scale (SAFA-A; [65]) is an Italian self-report questionnaire for the evaluation of anxiety symptomatology in the adolescent population ranging between 11 and 18 years old. This tool measures generalized anxiety, social anxiety, separation anxiety, and school-related anxiety. Respondents provide answers to 50 items, among three alternatives: true, partly true, and false. This tool showed a good test-retest reliability in its original validation (r > 0.75), and a very good internal consistency (Cronbach's α coefficient > 0.85) [65].

The Psychological Well-Being Scales (PWB; [66,67]) is an 18-item self-report questionnaire that evaluates six dimensions of psychological well-being, by Ryff's and Keyes' theoretical model: self-acceptance, autonomy, environmental mastery, personal growth, purpose in life, and positive relations. Participants provide their responses on a six-point Likert scale (1 = strongly disagree, 6 = strongly agree). The factorial structure of the PWB has been also supported among Italian adolescents and showed adequate psychometric properties (Cronbach's α ranging from 0.60 to 0.70) [68,69]. For the present study, we only considered the PWB total score, which showed a good internal consistency (Cronbach's α = 0.86).

2.3. Data Analysis

First, we calculated descriptive statistics to highlight the main features of the population under study.

Then, a series of 1 × 3 repeated measures analyses of covariance (ANCOVAs) were performed to examine changes over time (T1 vs. T2 vs. T3) in the following variables: YSR externalizing problems, internalizing problems, and attention problems scales; SAFA-A generalized anxiety, school-related anxiety, social anxiety, and separation anxiety scales; PWB total score. In all analyses, age and sex (male = 1, female = 2) were included as covariates since, in light of existing literature [56–59], they were expected to have an important influence on the primary variables.

Subsequently, Pearson's bivariate correlations between the YSR internalizing problems scale (i.e., outcome variable of the following analysis), and the scales assessing transdiagnostic risk and protective factors (i.e., IUS-R and P Scale) at T1 (i.e., pre-COVID-19) and at T3 (i.e., during COVID-19) were preliminarily run.

Finally, two moderation models were tested (see Figure 1). In the first model, the YSR internalizing problems scale (T1) was included as the dependent variable, and the IUS-R (T1) and P Scale (T1) were included as predictors. The second model was the same but included scores on these three questionnaires (e.g., IUS-R, P Scale, and YSR internalizing problems) administered at T3. In both models, age and sex were included as covariates. In the first step of each model, the IUS-R was entered as a predictor of the YSR internalizing problems scale; the P Scale was then entered as an additional predictor in the second step, and finally, to test the interaction between the two predictors, the product of centered IUS-R and centered P Scale scores was entered as an additional predictor in the third step. Finally, to further describe the quality of significant interactions, we employed the Johnson-Neymann (JN) technique [70]. The JN technique is a tool for probing significant interactions, identifying values in the range of the moderator variable where the conditional effect of the predictor on the outcome transitions between statistical significance and non-significance. In this way, one can find the value of the moderator for which the ratio of the conditional effect (of the predictor) to its standard error is equal to the critical t score. Effectively, it identifies a "region of significance" of the effect of the predictor on the outcome, that being the range of values where the moderator acts as such on the predictor-outcome relationship. A bias-corrected bootstrapping method was applied for testing significant effects with 5000 bootstrap samples and 95% confidence intervals.

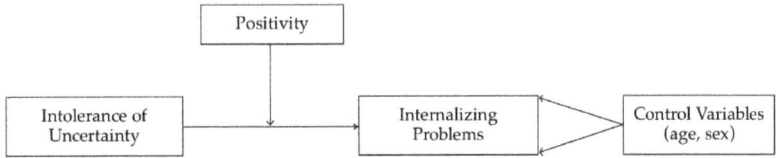

Figure 1. Proposed theoretical model.

The statistical software JASP 0.16.3 [71] was used to run the ANCOVAs and bivariate correlations, while Model 1 of the SPSS PROCESS macro [70] was adopted to conduct moderation analyses. Statistical significance was set at $p < 0.05$.

3. Results

3.1. Changes in Psychopathological Symptoms and Psychological Well-Being over Time

When repeated measures ANCOVAs were computed, no change over time came to light in any of the considered scales (Table 1). No significant effects of time by sex or age emerged for these analyses (all p-values > 0.05).

Table 1. Mean values, standard deviations (SD), F, and p-values for the 8 outcome variables (N = 136).

	T1 (SD)	T2 (SD)	T3 (SD)	F	p
YSR Internalizing problems	19.37 (9.23)	18.89 (9.13)	17.54 (9.06)	1.95 (2, 266)	0.145
YSR Externalizing problems	12.76 (7.63)	11.99 (7.05)	11.07 (7.12)	1.87 (2, 266)	0.156
YSR Attention problems	7.18 (3.40)	7.01 (3.38)	6.59 (3.33)	0.87 (2, 266)	0.42
SAFA Generalized anxiety	12.04 (6.49)	11.61 (6.11)	10.99 (5.19)	0.24 (2, 266)	0.78
SAFA Social anxiety	8.92 (4.45)	8.88 (4.97)	8.75 (4.73)	0.122 (2, 266)	0.88
SAFA Separation anxiety	6.71 (4.40)	5.98 (4.45)	6.03 (4.40)	0.39 (2, 266)	0.67
SAFA School anxiety	8.74 (5.27)	8.29 (5.40)	8.26 (5.40)	0.51 (2, 266)	0.60
PWB	52.74 (11.97)	53.79 (13.51)	54.21 (17.40)	0.20 (2, 266)	0.81

Note. YSR: Youth Self-Report; SAFA: Self Administrated Psychiatric Scales for Children and Adolescents-Anxiety evaluation scale; PWB: Psychological Well-Being Scale.

3.2. Moderation by Positivity on the Relationship between IU and Internalizing Problems Pre and during COVID-19

Zero-order correlations (Table A1) showed that the IUS-R was positively associated with the internalizing problems scale of the YSR at both T1 and T3 (T1: $r = 0.519$, $p < 0.001$; T3: $r = 0.408$, $p < 0.001$). Along the same line, the P Scale was negatively correlated with the YSR internalizing problems scale at both time points (T1: $r = -0.479$, $p < 0.001$; T3: $r = -0.295$, $p < 0.001$).

The results of the first moderation model (T1, October 2019) are reported in Table 2. Entering the IUS-R in the first step as predictor of the YSR internalizing problems scale yielded a significant positive effect ($t = 6.698$, $p < 0.001$, $\beta = 0.495$, Adjusted $R^2 = 0.280$ $f^2 = 0.42$). When the P Scale score was entered as an additional predictor in the second step, it showed a significant negative effect over and above the effects of the IUS-R ($t = -5.903$, $p < 0.001$, $\beta = -0.396$, Adjusted $R^2 = 0.427$, $f^2 = 0.17$). Finally, no significant interaction between centered IUS-R and centered P Scale scores emerged, whereas for this step a significant effect for sex emerged ($t = 2.311$, $p = 0.022$, $B = 3.014$, Adjusted $R^2 = 0.424$).

Table 2. Results of hierarchical linear regression model examining the main and interactive effects of the IUS-R and P Scale on the YSR internalizing problems scale at T1 (N = 136).

	β	SE	p	95% CI Lower	95% CI Upper	ΔR²
Model 1			<0.001			
Age	0.016	0.623	0.825	−1.094	1.37	
Sex	3.194	1.452	0.03	0.321	6.067	
IUS-R	0.495	0.07	<0.001	0.33	0.606	
Model 2			<0.001			0.148
Age	0.066	0.56	0.32	−0.549	1.668	
Sex	2.959	1.296	0.024	0.395	5.524	
IUS-R	0.420	0.063	<0.001	0.271	0.522	
P Scale	−0.396	0.098	<0.001	−0.774	−0.386	
Model 3			<0.001			0.001
Age	0.56	0.562	0.321	−0.551	1.671	
Sex	3.014	1.304	0.022	0.434	5.593	
IUS-R	0.396	0.064	<0.001	0.27	0.522	
P Scale	−0.584	0.099	<0.001	−0.779	−0.388	
IUS-R × P Scale	−0.006	0.011	0.591	−0.028	0.016	

Note. IUS-R: Intolerance of Uncertainty Scale Revised; P Scale: Positivity scale. Unstandardized coefficients (B) are displayed for sex which is a categorical predictor.

Pertaining to the second model (T3, April 2020), results are reported in Table 3. The IUS-R emerged as a significant positive predictor of the YSR internalizing problems scale

($t = 5.837$, $p < 0.001$, $\beta = 0.45$, Adjusted $R^2 = 0.202$, $f^2 = 0.28$). The P Scale score then emerged as a significant negative predictor, over and above the effects of the IUS-R ($t = -3.976$, $p < 0.001$, $\beta = -0.29$, Adjusted $R^2 = 0.282$, $f^2 = 0.092$). Finally, and differently from the first model, the interaction between the IUS-R and P Scale emerged to significantly predict the YSR internalizing problems scale ($t = -3.52$, $p < 0.001$, $\beta = -0.02$, Adjusted $R^2 = 0.340$, $f^2 = 0.06$). No significant effect of sex or age emerged for this model.

Table 3. Results of hierarchical linear regression model examining the conditional and interactive effects of the IUS-R and P scale on the YSR internalizing problems scale at T3 ($N = 136$).

	β	SE	p	95% CI Lower	95% CI Upper	ΔR^2
Model 1			<0.001			
Age	−0.002	0.643	0.975	−1.293	1.252	
Sex	2.357	1.484	0.115	−0.578	5.291	
IUS-R	0.449	0.067	<0.001	0.258	0.523	
Model 2			<0.001			0.084
Age	−0.012	0.61	0.874	−1.304	1.110	
Sex	2.082	1.409	0.142	−0.705	4.868	
IUS-R	0.450	0.063	<0.001	0.266	0.517	
P Scale	−0.290	0.102	<0.001	−0.606	−0.203	
Model 3			<0.001			0.06
Age	−0.169	0.586	0.774	−1.327	0.99	
Sex	2.576	1.358	0.06	−0.111	5.263	
IUS-R	0.347	0.062	<0.001	0.225	0.47	
P Scale	−0.501	0.101	<0.001	−0.701	−0.3	
IUS-R × P Scale	−0.024	0.007	<0.001	−0.038	−0.011	

Note. IUS-R: Intolerance of Uncertainty scale Revised; P Scale: Positivity scale. Unstandardized coefficients (B) are displayed for sex which is a categorical predictor.

Figure 2 illustrates the interaction at T3 by depicting the regression lines of the relation between the IUS-R and the internalizing problems scale of the YSR, at high, medium, and low (+1 SD, mean, −1 SD) scores of the P Scale. Decreases in the slope of the regression line with increasing P Scale scores show that the relation between IUS-R and internalizing symptoms becomes weaker with higher scores on the P Scale.

The JN technique showed that the conditional effect of the IUS-R on the YSR internalizing problems scale reached significance at a P Scale score of 32.47 (with P Scale scores in our sample ranging between 0 and 38) ($B = 0.17$, $SE = 0.09$, $t = 1.97$, $p = 0.05$, 95% CIs [0.00, 0.34]), at the 90th percentile of the distribution in our sample. Expressly, the relation between IUS-R and internalizing problems was significant at P Scale scores below this threshold and non-significant at P Scale scores above this threshold.

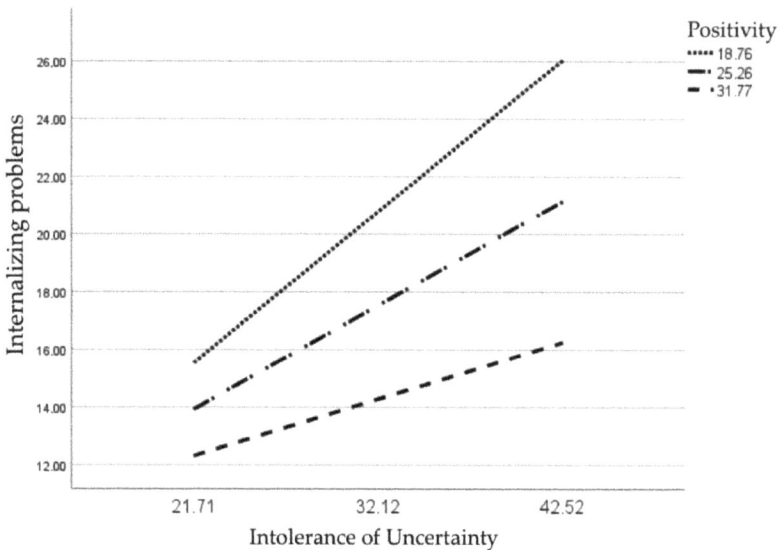

Figure 2. Regression lines of the relation between the IUS-R and the YSR internalizing problems scale scores at high (+1 SD = 18.76), medium (M = 25.26), and low scores (−1 SD = 18.76) on the P Scale.

4. Discussion

The COVID-19 pandemic has exposed youth to a radical change in environment, involving social isolation and pervasive uncertainty [4]. This picture is further worsened by the fact that adolescence is per se characterized by elevated uncertainty [27] and a heightened vulnerability to psychopathology [14]. However, no research has examined IU and psychopathology in Italian adolescents during the pandemic yet; hence the need for works investigating this topic. In particular, in such a context, it is of the utmost importance that studies focus on risk and protective factors since progress in this line of research might provide healthcare professionals with relevant information in their effort to support young people in these uncertain times, while also contributing to the knowledge surrounding resilience in face of majorly stressful environmental contingencies. In this regard, two well-known risk and protective factors of internalizing outcomes are IU and Positivity.

Bearing all these in mind, the present study aimed to investigate what changes, if any, might have co-occurred with the first COVID-19 lockdown in the psychological well-being and psychopathological symptoms of a group of nonclinical Italian adolescents. Moreover, we sought to explore the unique expression of stable dispositions by investigating the moderating role of a key protective trait (i.e., Positivity) in the relationship between IU and internalizing symptoms before and during the COVID-19 pandemic. Table 4 summarizes which initial hypotheses were confirmed and which were not.

Table 4. Hypotheses confirmation or rejection.

Hypotheses	Expected Statistical Significance	Expected Sign	Obtained Sign	Supported/Not Supported
H1a	Not significant			Supported
H1b	Not significant			Supported
H1c	Not significant			Supported
H1d	Not significant			Supported
H1e	Not significant			Supported
H2 at T1	Significant	+	+	Supported
H3 at T1	Significant	−	−	Supported
H4 at T1	Significant	+	+	Supported
H5 at T1	Significant	+		Not supported
H2 at T3	Significant	+	+	Supported
H3 at T3	Significant	−	−	Supported
H4 at T3	Significant	+		Not Supported
H5 at T3	Significant	+		Not supported

With specific regard to the first objective, no significant changes over time emerged for internalizing, externalizing, and attention problems, generalized anxiety, social anxiety, and psychological well-being. These results seem to describe substantial stability in the mental health of our adolescent sample, in line with our hypotheses (H1a–H1e) and the most relevant literature on these measures during early pandemic months [15,55]. It appears that our group of adolescents showed a fairly good adjustment to the pandemic situation, at least in its first phase. It seems safe to reason that a decreased exposure to an in-person school environment might have led to a reduction in several peer stressors and victimization (for those who experienced it), and academic performance triggers [72,73], which would normally cause distress, anxiety, and depression [74]. The shift to a rather "safe" environment such as the domestic one might not have weighted as much on our sample's psychological well-being, producing relative stability. Moreover, no significant differences emerged across time points for school and separation anxiety. Presumably, in the early pandemic phase, adolescents still had not come to realize the extent and real significance of this consequential event, and this may have led them to experience it as a break from normal responsibilities. Indeed, it seems fitting to observe that the three measurements are relatively close in time (T1 and T3 are six months apart) and at T3 only two months had passed since the pandemic outbreak. Therefore, it is possible that an early measurement was not able to fully reflect the psychological footprint of the pandemic on Italian adolescents [15–17]. Observed under this light, our results would align with the somewhat contradictory evidence [15–17], described in the introduction, pointing to a preserved mental health of adolescents during the early months of the pandemic. However, further longitudinal studies are needed to shed light on the long-term consequences of the COVID-19 pandemic on the psychological well-being of youth.

Pertaining to our second aim, we explored the expression of two trait-like dispositions (i.e., IU and Positivity) in two radically different environmental contingencies (i.e., pre-pandemic and during the first national lockdown). In particular, we tested if Positivity had a moderating effect on the relationship between IU and internalizing symptoms and whether the role of Positivity may have changed in the two time points. Findings showed that Positivity significantly moderated the relationship between IU and internalizing problems during the COVID-19 lockdown only, with a small to medium effect size; specifically, the higher an individual's level of dispositional Positivity, the weaker the relation between IU and internalizing symptoms. These results may suggest that IU is less likely to promote anxiety and depressive symptoms, during a stressful situation, in adolescents with higher levels of Positivity. We speculate that this moderation did not emerge in the pre-pandemic measurement because Positivity might have a resilience-specific nature, waxing in stressful times, but waning in "normal" ones. It is also relevant to note that IU has also been recently conceptualized as a construct that is potentially influenced by situational demands, leading authors to describe it as a trans-situational factor [52,75].

At what levels of Positivity, however, do the protective effects become evident? Probing the interaction between IU and Positivity through the JN technique, we found that the significance of the relation between IU and internalizing problems turned at a Positivity score of 32.47, which within our sample was located at the 90th percentile of the distribution. This value describes how IU exerts its known negative effects on most of our participants and that these effects become entirely offset at relatively high levels of Positivity. As can be seen in Figure 1, these results also tell us that Positivity consistently contributes to the reduction of the negative effect of IU, linearly, across the entire range of values. Summing up, high levels of Positivity fully counteract IU's negative effect on anxiety and depression, but lower levels linearly contribute to attenuating them, with a small to moderate effect size.

This result is particularly interesting when examined in light of existing literature highlighting the markedly stable nature of these two cognitive components [27,44]. However, it aligns with those studies showing that both Positivity and IU trait expressions are influenced by situational demands [41,42,76]. The literature on Positivity posits that this disposition might represent an influential genetic endowment that can also be subject to modification under the influence of different environmental factors, which account for our position within our personal range of variation at any particular time [39]. Accordingly, it may be that Positivity is a 'silent' trait, which increases in weight under uncertain environmental conditions, thus protecting adolescents with high IU levels from developing internalizing symptoms. The striking stability in our psychopathology scores might be read in this light, observing how Positivity, by displaying its malleability, could have protected our adolescent sample from developing a wide range of symptoms. This finding seems to further support the key role played by Positivity in fostering resilience in stressful times [40,45,48,49]. One might speculate that Positivity covaried with IU at T3 because these two cognitive components become tied in the face of uncertain and stressful situations. To some extent Positivity's weight on IU increased at T3. However, we are not able to dissect this result to determine whether it is specific to the uncertainty component or if it developed a non-specific counteracting effect on other transdiagnostic risk factors. Finally, our results contribute to the growing body of research that signals IU as a risk factor for internalizing symptomatology in adolescence [14].

Concerning the selected control variables (i.e., sex and age) it is worth noting that sex showed a significant predictive effect on internalizing symptoms at T1 only. This result seems at odds with the existing literature [56,57] and suggests a possible transitory interruption in girls' heightened vulnerability to internalizing symptomatology during the COVID-19 lockdown. As regards the age variable, no effect emerged in either model; this finding is in contrast with our hypothesis (H5) and with a study [58] finding increases in any anxiety and depressive disorder from childhood to adolescence. Generally speaking, these results should be read in light of the specific pandemic phase and its peculiarities, which may have (temporarily) modified some trends in adolescent psychopathology.

Notwithstanding the novel findings that emerged from the present study, some limitations need to be mentioned. Our sample size was reduced in number and limited to only one Italian region which hinders the generalizability of our results. Moreover, the sample is not exhaustive of the adolescent population since we did not benefit from data from early adolescents. Since a clinical sample is missing, we could not examine the exploratory moderation model on individuals suffering from clinical levels of internalizing symptomatology. Future studies should capitalize on these preliminary results to further examine the potential of Positivity in sustaining mental health in at-risk or clinical adolescent samples. Furthermore, an important shortcoming comes from the lack of COVID-19 and lockdown-related control questions addressing key elements such as presence of illness in the family, state of isolation (i.e., quarantine vs. non-quarantined), possible deaths or loss of livelihood in the family, all factors that might have somewhat affected the psychopathological domains addressed in the present study. While the lack of such information does not impact our conclusions, it might have enriched them.

Future research could build upon these initial findings to explore the context-dependent expression of Positivity and IU, both independently and concertedly, in specific transitional phases of adolescence and young adulthood, such as transitions to high school or college [28]. Moreover, the role of Positivity in the relation between IU and anxiety and depressive symptoms could also be explored in the adult population, serving a twofold aim: exploring protective factors to symptomatology during stressful times (i.e., not merely pandemics) and whether our findings are phase-specific to adolescence or can be extended to adulthood.

The present results constitute a novel contribution in that they provide same sample data on early mental health response with baseline pre-pandemic measurements on adolescent mental health during the pandemic. Moreover, to our knowledge, this is the first study to provide data on Positivity in a sample aged 14–18 and to detect a situational effect on Positivity or IU. Such an effort, while explorative in nature, might add to current knowledge on patterns of resilience for these two key constructs, observed in the light of environmentally driven changes, as called for by some authors [39,52]. Additionally, this result appears to tie in with the positive psychology framework, which encourages a shift in focus to how positive and negative factors act concertedly, as opposed to solely on negative factors [31]. Crucially, while these factors were examined under the light of a pandemic outbreak, our results can and should be extended to stressful and uncertain contingencies in general, especially considering the wide range of challenges that adolescents face daily [77].

5. Conclusions

In conclusion, this study adds to the extant literature on early mental health response to the COVID-19 pandemic, a large-scale, highly impactful environmental stressor, indicating that our adolescent sample fared well at first. Such a result, along with the literature that supported our hypotheses [15,55] conveys the impression that the initial phase of this pandemic misguided us into observing preserved adolescent psychological functioning. On the contrary, literature addressing later results [78] showed a progressive impairment in adolescent mental health co-occurring with the progression of the COVID-19 pandemic, suggesting that individual protective factors such as Positivity might support psychological well-being, albeit not indefinitely. Additionally, it provides tentative evidence on how two key cognitive contributors to internalizing symptomatology (i.e., Positivity and IU) may act jointly in face of a significant stressor, although further investigations are warranted. Altogether, these considerations support extant literature [79,80] in calling for raised attention towards adolescents' vulnerable mental health, especially in acute times of uncertainty but also considering the long-term effects of the COVID-19 pandemic. In particular, the observed malleability of Positivity expression hints at the clinical potential of this cognitive construct. As already mentioned, adolescents are under a heightened vulnerability to internalizing problems [14], and uncertainty and IU are elevated in this crucially developmental phase [27]; consequently, interventions aimed at prevention and treatment of such problems might benefit from a focus on positive orientation, which has repeatedly proved critical in supporting resilience, especially during uncertain times.

Author Contributions: Conceptualization, G.B.; methodology, M.L. and G.B.; formal analysis, A.M.; investigation, G.C. and G.B.; data curation, A.M. and S.I.; writing—original draft preparation, A.M.; writing—review and editing, S.I.; supervision, M.L. and G.B.; project administration, G.B. All authors have read and agreed to the published version of the manuscript.

Funding: This research received no external funding.

Institutional Review Board Statement: The study was conducted in accordance with the Declaration of Helsinki, and approved by the Ethics Committee of the University of Padua (protocol code 2711, date of approval 4 July 2018).

Informed Consent Statement: Informed consent was obtained from all subjects involved in the study.

Data Availability Statement: The data presented in this study are available on reasonable request from the corresponding author (S.I.). The data are not publicly available because they report private information about participants.

Acknowledgments: This work was carried out within the scope of the project "use-inspired basic research", for which the Department of General Psychology of the University of Padova has been recognized as "Dipartimento di eccellenza" by the Ministry of University and Research.

Conflicts of Interest: The authors declare no conflict of interest.

Appendix A

Table A1. Zero-order correlations for total scores at two time points (T1 and T3).

Time	Variable	1	2	3	4	5	6
Time 1	1. IUS-R	-					
	2. P Scale	−0.199 *	-				
	3. YSR Int.	0.519 ***	−0.479 ***	-			
Time 3	4. IUS-R	0.565 ***	−0.140	0.293 ***	-		
	5. P Scale	−0.142	0.371 ***	−0.326 ***	0.002	-	
	6. YSR Int.	0.408 ***	−0.410 ***	0.603 ***	0.453 ***	−0.295 ***	-

Note. IUS-R = Intolerance of Uncertainty Scale—Revised total score; P Scale = Positivity Scale total score; YSR Int. = Youth Self Report Internalizing problems scale score. * $p < 0.05$; *** $p < 0.001$.

References

1. Delmastro, M.; Zamariola, G. Depressive Symptoms in Response to COVID-19 and Lockdown: A Cross-Sectional Study on the Italian Population. *Sci. Rep.* **2020**, *10*, 22457. [CrossRef] [PubMed]
2. WHO. Headquarters (HQ) Mental Health and COVID-19: Early Evidence of the Pandemic's Impact: Scientific Brief, 2 March 2022. Available online: https://www.who.int/publications-detail-redirect/WHO-2019-nCoV-Sci_Brief-Mental_health-2022.1 (accessed on 24 August 2022).
3. Santomauro, D.F.; Herrera, A.M.M.; Shadid, J.; Zheng, P.; Ashbaugh, C.; Pigott, D.M.; Abbafati, C.; Adolph, C.; Amlag, J.O.; Aravkin, A.Y.; et al. Global Prevalence and Burden of Depressive and Anxiety Disorders in 204 Countries and Territories in 2020 Due to the COVID-19 Pandemic. *Lancet* **2021**, *398*, 1700–1712. [CrossRef]
4. COVID Impact On Young People With Mental Health Needs. Available online: https://www.youngminds.org.uk/about-us/reports-and-impact/coronavirus-impact-on-young-people-with-mental-health-needs/ (accessed on 1 August 2022).
5. Marengo, D.; Angelo Fabris, M.; Longobardi, C.; Settanni, M. Smartphone and Social Media Use Contributed to Individual Tendencies towards Social Media Addiction in Italian Adolescents during the COVID-19 Pandemic. *Addict. Behav.* **2022**, *126*, 107204. [CrossRef]
6. UNICEF Innocenti Research Centre. *Life in Lockdown: Child and Adolescent Mental Health and Well-Being in the Time of COVID-19*; Innocenti Research Reports; United Nations: New York, NY, USA, 2021; ISBN 978-92-1-001075-7.
7. Colì, E.; Norcia, M.; Bruzzone, A. What Do Italians Think About Coronavirus? An Exploratory Study on Social Representations. *Pap. Soc. Represent.* **2020**, *29*, 1–29.
8. Nearchou, F.; Flinn, C.; Niland, R.; Subramaniam, S.S.; Hennessy, E. Exploring the Impact of COVID-19 on Mental Health Outcomes in Children and Adolescents: A Systematic Review. *Int. J. Environ. Res. Public. Health* **2020**, *17*, 8479. [CrossRef]
9. Thorisdottir, I.E.; Asgeirsdottir, B.B.; Kristjansson, A.L.; Valdimarsdottir, H.B.; Tolgyes, E.M.J.; Sigfusson, J.; Allegrante, J.P.; Sigfusdottir, I.D.; Halldorsdottir, T. Depressive Symptoms, Mental Wellbeing, and Substance Use among Adolescents before and during the COVID-19 Pandemic in Iceland: A Longitudinal, Population-Based Study. *Lancet Psychiatry* **2021**, *8*, 663–672. [CrossRef]
10. Fioretti, C.; Palladino, B.E.; Nocentini, A.; Menesini, E. Positive and Negative Experiences of Living in COVID-19 Pandemic: Analysis of Italian Adolescents' Narratives. *Front. Psychol.* **2020**, *11*, 599531. [CrossRef]
11. Havighurst, R.J. *Developmental Tasks and Education*; University of Chicago Press: Chicago, IL, USA, 1948.
12. Berger, E.; Jamshidi, N.; Reupert, A.; Jobson, L.; Miko, A. Review: The Mental Health Implications for Children and Adolescents Impacted by Infectious Outbreaks-a Systematic Review. *Child Adolesc. Ment. Health* **2021**, *26*, 157–166. [CrossRef]
13. Kazi, F.; Mushtaq, A. Adolescents Navigating the COVID-19 Pandemic. *Lancet Child Adolesc. Health* **2021**, *5*, 692–693. [CrossRef]
14. Bottesi, G. Vulnerabilità Psicopatologica in Adolescenza: Intolleranza All'incertezza Come Fattore Di Rischio Transdiagnostico. *Psicol. Clin. Dello Sviluppo* **2022**, *1*, 1–26. [CrossRef]
15. Robinson, E.; Sutin, A.R.; Daly, M.; Jones, A. A Systematic Review and Meta-Analysis of Longitudinal Cohort Studies Comparing Mental Health before versus during the COVID-19 Pandemic in 2020. *J. Affect. Disord.* **2022**, *296*, 567. [CrossRef] [PubMed]
16. Racine, N.; McArthur, B.A.; Cooke, J.E.; Eirich, R.; Zhu, J.; Madigan, S. Global Prevalence of Depressive and Anxiety Symptoms in Children and Adolescents During COVID-19: A Meta-Analysis. *JAMA Pediatr.* **2021**, *175*, 1142–1150. [CrossRef]

17. Ma, L.; Mazidi, M.; Li, K.; Li, Y.; Chen, S.; Kirwan, R.; Zhou, H.; Yan, N.; Rahman, A.; Wang, W.; et al. Prevalence of Mental Health Problems among Children and Adolescents during the COVID-19 Pandemic: A Systematic Review and Meta-Analysis. *J. Affect. Disord.* **2021**, *293*, 78–89. [CrossRef]
18. Solmi, M.; Estradé, A.; Thompson, T.; Agorastos, A.; Radua, J.; Cortese, S.; Dragioti, E.; Leisch, F.; Vancampfort, D.; Thygesen, L.C.; et al. Physical and Mental Health Impact of COVID-19 on Children, Adolescents, and Their Families: The Collaborative Outcomes Study on Health and Functioning during Infection Times-Children and Adolescents (COH-FIT-C&A). *J. Affect. Disord.* **2022**, *299*, 367–376. [CrossRef] [PubMed]
19. Zuffianò, A.; López-Pérez, B.; Cirimele, F.; Kvapilová, J.; Caprara, G.V. The Positivity Scale: Concurrent and Factorial Validity Across Late Childhood and Early Adolescence. *Front. Psychol.* **2019**, *10*, 831. [CrossRef] [PubMed]
20. Poh, R.Y.N.; Zhuang, S.; Ong, X.L.; Hong, R.Y. Evaluating Structural Models of Cognitive Vulnerabilities: Transdiagnostic and Specific Pathways to Internalizing Symptoms. *Assessment* **2021**, *28*, 1635–1655. [CrossRef] [PubMed]
21. Hong, R.Y.; Cheung, M.W.-L. The Structure of Cognitive Vulnerabilities to Depression and Anxiety: Evidence for a Common Core Etiologic Process Based on a Meta-Analytic Review. *Clin. Psychol. Sci.* **2015**, *3*, 892–912. [CrossRef]
22. Kuang, K.; Wilson, S.R. A Meta-Analysis of Uncertainty and Information Management in Illness Contexts. *J. Commun.* **2017**, *67*, 378–401. [CrossRef]
23. Carleton, R.N. Into the Unknown: A Review and Synthesis of Contemporary Models Involving Uncertainty. *J. Anxiety Disord.* **2016**, *39*, 30–43. [CrossRef]
24. Freeston, M.H.; Rhéaume, J.; Letarte, H.; Dugas, M.J.; Ladouceur, R. Why Do People Worry? *Personal. Individ. Differ.* **1994**, *17*, 791–802. [CrossRef]
25. Carleton, R.N.; Thibodeau, M.; Osborne, J.; Taylor, S.; Asmundson, G. Revisiting the Fundamental Fears: Towards Establishing Construct Independence. *Personal. Individ. Differ.* **2014**, *63*, 94–99. [CrossRef]
26. Gentes, E.L.; Ruscio, A.M. A Meta-Analysis of the Relation of Intolerance of Uncertainty to Symptoms of Generalized Anxiety Disorder, Major Depressive Disorder, and Obsessive–Compulsive Disorder. *Clin. Psychol. Rev.* **2011**, *31*, 923–933. [CrossRef] [PubMed]
27. Bottesi, G.; Iannattone, S.; Carraro, E.; Lauriola, M. The Assessment of Intolerance of Uncertainty in Youth: An Examination of the Intolerance of Uncertainty Scale-Revised in Italian Nonclinical Boys and Girls. *Res. Child Adolesc. Psychopathol.* **2022**. [CrossRef] [PubMed]
28. Dugas, M.J.; Laugesen, N.; Bukowski, W.M. Intolerance of Uncertainty, Fear of Anxiety, and Adolescent Worry. *J. Abnorm. Child Psychol.* **2012**, *40*, 863–870. [CrossRef]
29. World Health Organization. *World Mental Health Report: Transforming Mental Health for All*; World Health Organization: New York, NY, USA, 2022.
30. Taylor, S. *The Psychology of Pandemics: Preparing for the Next Global Outbreak of Infectious Disease*; Cambridge Scholars Publishing: Newcastle upon Tyne, UK, 2019; ISBN 978-1-5275-3959-4.
31. Bakioğlu, F.; Korkmaz, O.; Ercan, H. Fear of COVID-19 and Positivity: Mediating Role of Intolerance of Uncertainty, Depression, Anxiety, and Stress. *Int. J. Ment. Health Addict.* **2021**, *19*, 2369–2382. [CrossRef]
32. Korte, C.; Friedberg, R.D.; Wilgenbusch, T.; Paternostro, J.K.; Brown, K.; Kakolu, A.; Tiller-Ormord, J.; Baweja, R.; Cassar, M.; Barnowski, A.; et al. Intolerance of Uncertainty and Health-Related Anxiety in Youth amid the COVID-19 Pandemic: Understanding and Weathering the Continuing Storm. *J. Clin. Psychol. Med. Settings* **2022**, *29*, 645–653. [CrossRef]
33. World Health Organization. *The World Health Report: 2004: Changing History*; World Health Organization: New York, NY, USA, 2004.
34. Caprara, G.V.; Steca, P.; Alessandri, G.; Abela, J.R.; McWhinnie, C.M. Positive Orientation: Explorations on What Is Common to Life Satisfaction, Self-Esteem, and Optimism. *Epidemiol. Psichiatr. Soc.* **2010**, *19*, 63–71. [CrossRef]
35. Keyes, C.L.M. Promoting and Protecting Mental Health as Flourishing: A Complementary Strategy for Improving National Mental Health. *Am. Psychol.* **2007**, *62*, 95–108. [CrossRef]
36. Baumeister, R.F. *Self-Esteem: The Puzzle of Low Self-Regard*; Springer Science & Business Media: Berlin, Germany, 2013; ISBN 978-1-4684-8956-9.
37. Diener, E.; Emmons, R.A.; Larsen, R.J.; Griffin, S. The Satisfaction With Life Scale. *J. Pers. Assess.* **1985**, *49*, 71–75. [CrossRef]
38. Scheier, M.F.; Carver, C.S. On the Power of Positive Thinking: The Benefits of Being Optimistic. *Curr. Dir. Psychol. Sci.* **1993**, *2*, 26–30. [CrossRef]
39. Caprara, G.V.; Fagnani, C.; Alessandri, G.; Steca, P.; Gigantesco, A.; Cavalli Sforza, L.L.; Sforza, L.L.C.; Stazi, M.A. Human Optimal Functioning: The Genetics of Positive Orientation towards Self, Life, and the Future. *Behav. Genet.* **2009**, *39*, 277–284. [CrossRef] [PubMed]
40. Caprara, G.V.; Eisenberg, N.; Alessandri, G. Positivity: The Dispositional Basis of Happiness. *J. Happiness Stud.* **2017**, *18*, 353–371. [CrossRef]
41. Caprara, G.V.; Alessandri, G.; Caprara, M.G. A Response to Commentaries on Positivity. *Asian J. Soc. Psychol.* **2019**, *22*, 146–150. [CrossRef]
42. Fagnani, C.; Medda, E.; Stazi, M.A.; Caprara, G.V.; Alessandri, G. Investigation of Age and Gender Effects on Positive Orientation in Italian Twins. *Int. J. Psychol.* **2014**, *49*, 453–461. [CrossRef]

43. Alessandri, G.; Zuffianò, A.; Fabes, R.; Vecchione, M.; Martin, C. Linking Positive Affect and Positive Self-Beliefs in Daily Life. *J. Happiness Stud.* **2014**, *15*, 1479–1493. [CrossRef]
44. Alessandri, G.; Caprara, G.V.; Tisak, J. A Unified Latent Curve, Latent State-Trait Analysis of the Developmental Trajectories and Correlates of Positive Orientation. *Multivar. Behav. Res.* **2012**, *47*, 341–368. [CrossRef] [PubMed]
45. Caprara, M.; Di Giunta, L.; Caprara, G.V. Association of Positivity with Health Problems in Old Age: Preliminary Findings from Spanish Middle Class Seniors. *J. Happiness Stud.* **2017**, *18*, 1339–1358. [CrossRef]
46. Caprara, G.V.; Alessandri, G.; Colaiaco, F.; Zuffianò, A. Dispositional Bases of Self-Serving Positive Evaluations. *Personal. Individ. Differ.* **2013**, *55*, 864–867. [CrossRef]
47. Castellani, V.; Perinelli, E.; Gerbino, M.; Caprara, G.V. Positive Orientation and Interpersonal Styles. *Personal. Individ. Differ.* **2016**, *98*, 229–234. [CrossRef]
48. Milioni, M.; Alessandri, G.; Eisenberg, N.; Caprara, G.V. The Role of Positivity as Predictor of Ego-Resiliency from Adolescence to Young Adulthood. *Personal. Individ. Differ.* **2016**, *101*, 306–311. [CrossRef]
49. Thartori, E.; Pastorelli, C.; Cirimele, F.; Remondi, C.; Gerbino, M.; Basili, E.; Favini, A.; Lunetti, C.; Fiasconaro, I.; Caprara, G.V. Exploring the Protective Function of Positivity and Regulatory Emotional Self-Efficacy in Time of Pandemic COVID-19. *Int. J. Environ. Res. Public. Health* **2021**, *18*, 13171. [CrossRef] [PubMed]
50. Tian, L.; Zhang, D.; Huebner, E.S. Psychometric Properties of the Positivity Scale among Chinese Adults and Early Adolescents. *Front. Psychol.* **2018**, *9*, 197. [CrossRef] [PubMed]
51. Clark, D.A.; Beck, A.T.; Alford, B.A. *Scientific Foundations of Cognitive Theory and Therapy of Depression*; John Wiley & Sons Inc: Hoboken, NJ, USA, 1999; ISBN 978-0-471-18970-1.
52. Freeston, M.; Tiplady, A.; Mawn, L.; Bottesi, G.; Thwaites, S. Towards a Model of Uncertainty Distress in the Context of Coronavirus (COVID-19). *Cogn. Behav. Ther.* **2020**, *13*, e31. [CrossRef]
53. Janssen, L.H.C.; Kullberg, M.-L.J.; Verkuil, B.; van Zwieten, N.; Wever, M.C.M.; van Houtum, L.A.E.M.; Wentholt, W.G.M.; Elzinga, B.M. Does the COVID-19 Pandemic Impact Parents' and Adolescents' Well-Being? An EMA-Study on Daily Affect and Parenting. *PLoS ONE* **2020**, *15*, e0240962. [CrossRef] [PubMed]
54. Carleton, R.N.; Mulvogue, M.K.; Thibodeau, M.A.; McCabe, R.E.; Antony, M.M.; Asmundson, G.J.G. Increasingly Certain about Uncertainty: Intolerance of Uncertainty across Anxiety and Depression. *J. Anxiety Disord.* **2012**, *26*, 468–479. [CrossRef]
55. Penner, F.; Ortiz, J.H.; Sharp, C. Change in Youth Mental Health During the COVID-19 Pandemic in a Majority Hispanic/Latinx US Sample. *J. Am. Acad. Child Adolesc. Psychiatry* **2021**, *60*, 513–523. [CrossRef] [PubMed]
56. Hayward, C.; Sanborn, K. Puberty and the Emergence of Gender Differences in Psychopathology. *J. Adolesc. Health* **2002**, *30*, 49–58. [CrossRef]
57. Zahn-Waxler, C.; Shirtcliff, E.A.; Marceau, K. Disorders of Childhood and Adolescence: Gender and Psychopathology. *Annu. Rev. Clin. Psychol.* **2008**, *4*, 275–303. [CrossRef]
58. Costello, E.J.; Copeland, W.; Angold, A. Trends in Psychopathology across the Adolescent Years: What Changes When Children Become Adolescents, and When Adolescents Become Adults? *J. Child Psychol. Psychiatry* **2011**, *52*, 1015–1025. [CrossRef]
59. Cracco, E.; Goossens, L.; Braet, C. Emotion Regulation across Childhood and Adolescence: Evidence for a Maladaptive Shift in Adolescence. *Eur. Child Adolesc. Psychiatry* **2017**, *26*, 909–921. [CrossRef]
60. Fedeli, U. Mortalità Generale in Veneto, 1 Gennaio–30 Novembre 2020. 14. Available online: https://www.ser-veneto.it/public/Mortalit%C3%A0_agg20201214.pdf (accessed on 14 July 2022).
61. Caprara, G.V.; Alessandri, G.; Eisenberg, N.; Kupfer, A.; Steca, P.; Caprara, M.G.; Yamaguchi, S.; Fukuzawa, A.; Abela, J. The Positivity Scale. *Psychol. Assess.* **2012**, *24*, 701–712. [CrossRef] [PubMed]
62. Bottesi, G.; Noventa, S.; Freeston, M.H.; Ghisi, M. Seeking Certainty about Intolerance of Uncertainty: Addressing Old and New Issues through the Intolerance of Uncertainty Scale-Revised. *PLoS ONE* **2019**, *14*, e0211929. [CrossRef] [PubMed]
63. Frigerio, A.; Vanzin, L.; Pastore, V.; Nobile, M.; Giorda, R.; Marino, C.; Molteni, M.; Rucci, P.; Ammaniti, M.; Lucarelli, L.; et al. The Italian Preadolescent Mental Health Project (PrISMA): Rationale and Methods. *Int. J. Methods Psychiatr. Res.* **2006**, *15*, 22–35. [CrossRef]
64. Achenbach, T.M. *Manual for ASEBA School-Age Forms & Profiles*; University of Vermont, Research Center for Children, Youth & Families: Burlington, VT, USA, 2001.
65. Cianchetti, C.; Fancello, G.S. *SAFA: Scale Psichiatriche Di Autosomministrazione per Fanciulli e Adolescenti: Manuale*; Giunti Psychometrics: Firenze, Italy, 2001.
66. Ryff, C.D.; Keyes, C.L.M. The Structure of Psychological Well-Being Revisited. *J. Pers. Soc. Psychol.* **1995**, *69*, 719–727. [CrossRef] [PubMed]
67. Ruini, C.; Ottolini, F.; Rafanelli, C.; Ryff, C.; Fava, G.A. La Validazione Italiana Delle Psychological Well-Being Scales (PWB). [Italian Validation of Psychological Well-Being Scales (PWB). *Riv. Psichiatr.* **2003**, *38*, 117–130.
68. Sirigatti, S.; Stefanile, C.; Giannetti, E.; Iani, L.; Annamaria, M. Assessment of Factor Structure of Ryff's Psychological Well-Being Scales in Italian Adolescents. *Boll. Psicol. Appl.* **2009**, *56*, 30–50.
69. Viola, M.M.; Musso, P.; Inguglia, C.; Lo Coco, A. Psychological Well-Being and Career Indecision in Emerging Adulthood: The Moderating Role of Hardiness. *Career Dev. Q.* **2016**, *64*, 387–396. [CrossRef]
70. Hayes, A.F. *Introduction to Mediation, Moderation, and Conditional Process Analysis, Third Edition: A Regression-Based Approach (Methodology in the Social Sciences)*, 3rd ed.; The Guilford Press: New York, NY, USA, 2022; ISBN 978-1-4625-4903-0.

71. JASP Team. *JASP*, Version 0.16.3. 2022.
72. Hoekstra, P.J. Suicidality in Children and Adolescents: Lessons to Be Learned from the COVID-19 Crisis. *Eur. Child Adolesc. Psychiatry* **2020**, *29*, 737–738. [CrossRef]
73. Becker, S.P.; Gregory, A.M. Editorial Perspective: Perils and Promise for Child and Adolescent Sleep and Associated Psychopathology during the COVID-19 Pandemic. *J. Child Psychol. Psychiatry* **2020**, *61*, 757–759. [CrossRef] [PubMed]
74. Raffagnato, A.; Iannattone, S.; Tascini, B.; Venchiarutti, M.; Broggio, A.; Zanato, S.; Traverso, A.; Mascoli, C.; Manganiello, A.; Miscioscia, M.; et al. The COVID-19 Pandemic: A Longitudinal Study on the Emotional-Behavioral Sequelae for Children and Adolescents with Neuropsychiatric Disorders and Their Families. *Int. J. Environ. Res. Public. Health* **2021**, *18*, 9880. [CrossRef]
75. Lauriola, M.; Iannattone, S.; Bottesi, G. Intolerance of Uncertainty and Emotional Processing in Adolescence: Separating between-Person Stability and within-Person Change. *Res. Child Adolesc. Psychopathol.* 2022; *submitted*.
76. Caprara, G.V.; Alessandri, G.; Caprara, M. Associations of Positive Orientation with Health and Psychosocial Adaptation: A Review of Findings and Perspectives. *Asian J. Soc. Psychol.* **2019**, *22*, 126–132. [CrossRef]
77. World Health Organization. Regional Office for Europe. *Growing up Unequal: Gender and Socioeconomic Differences in Young People's Health and Well-Being*; World Health Organization. Regional Office for Europe: København, Denmark, 2016; ISBN 978-92-890-5136-1.
78. Wang, S.; Chen, L.; Ran, H.; Che, Y.; Fang, D.; Sun, H.; Peng, J.; Liang, X.; Xiao, Y. Depression and Anxiety among Children and Adolescents Pre and Post COVID-19: A Comparative Meta-Analysis. *Front. Psychiatry* **2022**, *13*, 917552. [CrossRef] [PubMed]
79. Cusinato, M.; Iannattone, S.; Spoto, A.; Poli, M.; Moretti, C.; Gatta, M.; Miscioscia, M. Stress, Resilience, and Well-Being in Italian Children and Their Parents during the COVID-19 Pandemic. *Int. J. Environ. Res. Public. Health* **2020**, *17*, 8297. [CrossRef]
80. Iannattone, S.; Raffagnato, A.; Zanato, S.; Traverso, A.; Tascini, B.; Del Col, L.; Miscioscia, M.; Gatta, M. Children with Psychopathology and Their Parents Facing the COVID-19 Pandemic: A Case-Control Study. *Clin. Neuropsychiatry* **2021**, *18*, 324–333. [CrossRef]

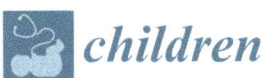

Article

Depressive Anxiety Symptoms in Hospitalized Children with Chronic Illness during the First Italian COVID-19 Lockdown

Cinzia Correale [1,*], Chiara Falamesca [1], Ilaria Tondo [1], Marta Borgi [2], Francesca Cirulli [2], Mauro Truglio [3], Oriana Papa [4], Laura Vagnoli [5], Cinzia Arzilli [5], Cristina Venturino [6], Michele Pellegrini [7], Valentina Manfredi [8], Rossella Sterpone [8], Teresa Grimaldi Capitello [1], Simonetta Gentile [9] and Simona Cappelletti [1]

1. Clinical Psychology Unit, IRCCS Bambino Gesù Children Hospital, 00146 Rome, Italy; chiara.falamesca@opbg.net (C.F.); ilaria.tondo@opbg.net (I.T.); teresa.grimaldi@opbg.net (T.G.C.); simona.cappelletti@opbg.net (S.C.)
2. Center for Behavioral Sciences and Mental Health, Istituto Superiore di Sanità, 00161 Rome, Italy; marta.borgi@iss.it (M.B.); francesca.cirulli@iss.it (F.C.)
3. School of Fundamental Sciences, Massey University, Palmerston North 4442, New Zealand; mauro.truglio@gmail.com
4. Children's Neuropsychiatric Ward, Regional Pediatric Hospital "G. Salesi", 60123 Ancona, Italy; oriana.papa@ospedaliriuniti.marche.it
5. Pediatric Psychology, Meyer Children's Hospital, 50139 Florence, Italy; laura.vagnoli@meyer.it (L.V.); cinzia.arzilli@meyer.it (C.A.)
6. Psychology Unit, IRCCS Istituto Giannina Gaslini, 16147 Genoa, Italy; cristinaventurino@gaslini.org
7. Azienda Ospedaliera Universitaria Policlinico—Giovanni XXIII, 70124 Bari, Italy; michele.pellegrini@policlinico.ba.it
8. Psychology Unit, A.O. S.S. Antonio Biagio and C. Arrigo Hospital, 15121 Alessandria, Italy; valentina.manfredi@ospedale.al.it (V.M.); rsterpone@ospedale.al.it (R.S.)
9. Department of Humanities, LUMSA University, 00193 Rome, Italy; s.gentile6@lumsa.it
* Correspondence: cinzia.correale@opbg.net

Abstract: COVID-19 is continuing to spread around the world, having a direct impact on people's daily lives and health. Although the knowledge of the impact of the COVID-19 pandemic on mental health in the general population is now well established, there is less information on its effect on specific and vulnerable populations, such as children with chronic illness (CI). We conducted a multi-centered cross-sectional study among pediatric patients in six public children's hospitals in Italy during the first lockdown, with the aim of assessing the proportion of children with CI presenting anxiety and depressive symptoms, and the clinical and demographic characteristics affecting such symptomatology. We included children with at least one chronic condition, with no cognitive delay, aged between 11 and 18 years. Brief standardized questionnaires were administered during medical scheduled visits to screen anxiety and depressive symptoms. We found a very high proportion of children showing mild to severe depressive and anxiety symptomatology (approximately 68% and 63%, respectively). Our results highlight the need of ensuring tailored psychological interventions to protect children with CI from the effect of the pandemic (and related restrictive measures such as quarantine and social distancing), with the final aim of promoting mental health and psychological well-being in this vulnerable population.

Keywords: COVID-19; lockdown; mood disorders; chronic illness; anxiety; depression; pandemic; mental health; childhood

1. Introduction

Although more than two years have passed since the first case, the COVID-19 pandemic is still ongoing across most of the world's populations, having a direct impact on people's lives and health [1]. Although the knowledge of the effects of the COVID-19 pandemic on mental health in the general population is now well established, less is known about its impact on specific and vulnerable populations. This information is particularly important to further enhance the potential to prepare for future epidemics and pandemics, as well as providing targeted intervention and support measures for particularly affected groups, such as children with chronic illness [2].

Chronic illness (CI) in childhood is a heterogeneous category encompassing diverse diseases with varying degrees of impact on children and their families [3,4]. Prevalence rates of CI in children vary greatly, ranging from 3.5% to 35.3% [5]. Rates of childhood CI have steadily increased from 1.8% in 1960 to 7% in 2004, mostly as a result of advances in healthcare, which have allowed children to live longer [6], as well as of changes in diagnostic processes and management. The diagnosis of CI is often associated with multi-morbidity (e.g., IBD and psoriatic arthritis) and can have a life-long impact on children's well-being and quality of life, leading to a greater risk of developing psychological and mental problems, especially mood disorders [7–9].

As a result of the COVID-19 pandemic, a substantial increase in the prevalence and burden of major depressive and anxiety disorders has been observed in the general population [10–12]. Social restrictions, lockdowns, school and business closures, loss of income, and the shifting priorities of governments in their attempts to control COVID-19 outbreaks all have negatively affected people's mental health. Emerging evidence on the impact of the coronavirus (COVID-19) pandemic shows that young people are among the groups who are disproportionately affected by the current pandemic, particularly in terms of mental well-being, education, training, and employment. As a result, higher rates of anxiety and depression have been observed, as shown by a meta-analysis on the global prevalence of depressive and anxiety symptoms in children and adolescents during COVID-19 [13]. The spread of the disease and social distancing measures have even more strongly impacted vulnerable target groups with pre-existing mental health conditions or those already facing social integration barriers and daily routine disruption, such as children with CI.

Moreover, during the COVID-19 pandemic, this population had to face the interruption—or delay—of medical assistance, hospital treatment, and diagnostic procedures. In Italy, one of the countries most affected by COVID-19, Lazzerini and colleagues [14] reported 12 pediatric cases of delayed access to hospital care during the week of 23–27 March 2020 across five hospitals. Of these cases, half were admitted to an Intensive Care Unit and four died of medical diseases that, if treated in time, could have had a better outcome. All patients were affected by a CI and parents reported delaying access to care because of concerns about being exposed to COVID-19 infection (fear of contagion). Considering that a family with a child with CI commonly suffers a significant burden of care associated with financial and social problems, the COVID-19 pandemic has exacerbated the gap between the family's needs and the healthcare provided. As an example, Zhang and colleagues [15] conducted research among a group of parents of children with Chronic Kidney Disease (CKD) in China, confirming that 62.3% of parents were worried that the CKD might relapse or be aggravated during the pandemic since they could not regularly see a doctor.

Notwithstanding the very first recommendations promoted by several scientific and academic committees to address particular attention to vulnerable groups [16], to date, we have still little information on how the COVID-pandemic has affected the mental health of children with CI.

We conducted a multi-centered cross-sectional study among pediatric patients in six public children's hospitals in Italy, with the aim of exploring the manifestations of anxiety and depression symptomatology among children with CI in the very first phase of the Italian lockdown.

2. Materials and Methods

We conducted a multi-centered cross-sectional study among pediatric patients in six public children's hospitals in Italy (Table 1). We collected data from 3 March 2020 to 17 May 2021, performing face-to-face interviews during scheduled medical examinations (day hospital, hospitalization, and follow-up), medical follow-up teleconsultation, or via online survey forms. Upon completion of the evaluation interviews, the questionnaires were delivered and scored by a qualified clinical psychologist of the Clinical Psychology Unit (CPU). The clinical psychologist then recorded the results in the appropriate CRF and entered the values into the database, following the appropriate de-identification strategy. The response rate for this study was roughly 100%, since the delivery of the questionnaires took place before or during the interview with the clinical psychologist, who made sure, before the resignation, that the patient had completed the whole questionnaire. This was also true in the few instances where questionnaires were delivered through Google modules. If the questionnaire was not delivered by the patient, it was completed by the clinical psychologist via a telephone interview.

Table 1. Participants' sample size: patients per center (n = 334).

Pediatric Center	Patients (n)
IRCCS O.P. Bambino Gesù	242
IRCCS Istituto Giannina Gaslini	5
O.P. Giovanni XXIII	17
A.O.U. Meyer	35
A.O.U. Ospedali Riuniti di Ancona	28
A.O. SS. Antonio e Biagio e C. Arrigo	7

IRCCS: Istituto di Ricovero e Cura a Carattere Scientifico; O.P.: Ospedale Pediatrico; A.O.U.: Azienza Ospedaliera Universitaria; A.O.: Azienda Ospedaliera.

2.1. Participants

Starting from the more conservative hypothesis of a prevalence of 50%, we calculated that a sample of at least 380 individuals would allow us to estimate the prevalence of psychological discomfort with a margin of error of 10% and a confidence level of 5% (95% confidence interval). Then, we were able to recruit a total sample of 334 children (60% F) aged between 11 and 18 years (mean 14.44; SD 1.85). The inclusion criterion was children with at least one chronic condition, while the exclusion criterion was children with cognitive delay (IQ $\leq$ 85). Participants were recruited through the Clinical Psychology Units of the children's hospitals participating in the project, and the CPU's personnel carried out assessments during routine or scheduled examinations. Each participant spent no more than 10 min approximately in completing both questionnaires. Table 2 describes the clinical characteristics of the study sample.

Table 2. Clinical characteristics (CI diagnosis) of the study sample (n = 334).

CI Diagnosis		n
Epilepsy		53
	Generalized	10
	Focal	34
	Others	9
Heart Disease		14
	Fontan	6
	Cardiomyopathy Hypertrophic	1
	Interventricular Defect	3
	Defect Transposition of Large Vessels	1
	Congenital Cardiopathy	2
	Third-Degree Ventricular Atrium Block	1
AIDS		16
Cystic Fibrosis		22
Gastrointestinal Diseases		20
	Chron disease	10

Table 2. *Cont.*

CI Diagnosis		n
	Ulcerative Colitis	7
	Pancolitis	2
	Hirschsprung disease	1
Onco-Hematological Diseases		9
	Acute Lymphoblastic Leukemia	3
	Histiocytosis	1
	Hypothalamic Hamartoma	1
	Osteosarcoma	2
	Desmoplastic Small Round Cell Tumor	1
	Parietal Cavernoma	1
Migraines		151
Diabetes		19
Asthma		4
Scoliosis		4
Arthritis		2
Kidney Disease		7
	Chronic Kidney Failure	2
	Renal Dysplasia	1
	Renal Agenesis	1
	Nephrophysis	1
	Hemolytic Uremic Syndrome	1
	Glomerulonephritis Membranoproliferatin	1
Other Rare Diseases		13
	Duchenne Syndrome	1
	GLUT1 Deficiency Syndrome	1
	Schizotypic Disorder	1
	Primitive Sclerosing Cholangitis	1
	Atopic Dermatitis	1
	Coeliac Disease	1
	Schimke Immuno-Osseous Dysplasia	1
	Lupus	1
	Primary Hyperoxaluria Type I	1
	Thrombocytopenia	1
	Dravet Syndrome	1
	Janz Syndrome	1
	Optical Neuromyelitis	1

AIDS: Acquired Immune Deficiency Syndrome.

2.2. Measures

In order to assess anxious–depressive symptoms, we administered the Generalized Anxiety Disorder scale (GAD-7) [17] and the Patient Health Questionnaire (PHQ-9) [18–21]. The Generalized Anxiety Disorder (GAD-7) scale measures seven symptoms. Participants are asked how often they have experienced each symptom in the past two weeks. The response options are "not at all," "several days," "more than half the days," and "nearly every day," scored as 0, 1, 2, and 3, respectively. The thresholds for symptom severity are: 5–9 mild, 10–14 moderate, and 15–21 severe. This tool has been used in a variety of studies to assess anxiety symptoms in a wide range of chronic conditions [22,23]. The PHQ-9 is a simple, very effective self-assessment test for depressive symptomatology. Participants are asked to indicate the presence of nine issues, including depression and interest decline, in the last 2 weeks on a 4-point scale ranging from "nearly every day" (3 points) to "not at all" (0 points). The thresholds for symptom severity are: 5–9 mild, 10–14 moderate, 15–19 moderately severe, and 20–27 severe. The PHQ-9 has good internal consistency, with a Cronbach's alpha coefficient between 0.80 and 0.90. Both the PHQ-9 and GAD-7 measures are suitable for use with persons 11 years of age and older.

2.3. Data Analysis

All the statistical analyses were performed using JASP, R [24,25], and custom Python scripts. The analysis was organized into two stages. For the first one, our sample was divided into subgroups according to various parameters (clinical, i.e., disease-specific groups, and demographic) and Wilcoxon's signed-rank one-sample test was used to assess whether PHQ-9 and GAD-7 scores were substantially different from the threshold score of 5 for any symptomatology. For the second stage, we carried out comparisons between said subgroups, using Mann–Whitney's U test and Kruskal–Wallis with Dunn's post-hoc test with Bonferroni–Holm correction. The only exception was the "continuity of care during COVID-19's first lockdown" variable, where we used Welch's t-test as the dataset was unbalanced. All the correlations were calculated using Spearman's Rho. The significance threshold for all tests was set at $p < 0.05$.

3. Results

Table 3 shows the proportions of patients with different levels of depressive and anxiety symptoms. Mild and moderate depressive and anxiety symptoms were most common. The rate of mild depression was 36.23%, while that of moderate depression was 23.65%; meanwhile, the rate of mild anxiety was 33.53%, and that of moderate anxiety was 19.76%. The proportion of all of the participating patients with mild-to-severe depressive symptoms was 67.96%, and the proportion of all of the patients with mild-to-severe anxiety was 62.87%. The prevalence of comorbid depressive and anxiety symptoms was 53.89% among all the participants.

Table 3. The rates of different severities of depressive and anxiety symptoms (n = 334).

Variables	Depressive Symptoms (PHQ-9)		Anxiety Symptoms (GAD-7)		Comorbid Depression and Anxiety Symptoms	
	n	%	n	%	n	%
None	106	31.74	123	36.83	-	-
Mild	121	36.23	112	33.53	-	-
Moderate	79	23.65	66	19.76	-	-
Severe	27	8.08	32	9.58	-	-
Total symptoms	227	67.96	210	62.87	180	53.89

Table 4 shows that, according to the Wilcoxon one-sample test, patients diagnosed with migraines, diabetes, and gastrointestinal diseases had statistically significant rates of anxious symptomatology compared to the mild-to-severe threshold of 5, while only migraines and diabetes showed statistically significantly higher rates of depressive symptomatology than the mild-to-severe threshold of 5.

The overall sample of children with CI showed strong statistically significant anxiety and depressive scores and symptomatology (p-value < 0.001) (Table 5). Females exhibited a significantly higher mean score for anxious and depressive symptoms (p-value < 0.001) while males did not. Both patients receiving and not receiving pharmacological treatment showed statistically significant scores for depressive and anxiety symptomatology. Similarly, all patients following and not following non-pharmacological therapies (i.e., psychotherapy, speech therapy, etc.) showed very high scores for mood symptoms (p-value < 0.001). Among patients receiving continuity of care during the COVID-19 lockdown and suspension of deferrable medical examinations, both groups showed significantly elevated rates of mood disorders, even if those who had had the opportunity to see a doctor showed less statistically significant scores of mood impairment (p-value < 0.01) than those who suspended visits (p-value < 0.001). In terms of years of illness, again, the overall group showed statistically significant scores of mood impairment, even if the group of patients with $\geq$5 years of illness showed the lower statistical significance score for depression (*p*-value < 0.05). Finally, children diagnosed with CI at school had statistically significant depression and anxiety symptomatology scores, whereas those diagnosed in preschool showed average rates below the clinical cut-off.

Table 4. Description of disease distributions, with significance determined by Wilcoxon's signed-rank one-sample test.

Diagnosis	n	%	Anxiety Symptoms (GAD-7) M	SD	Depressive Symptoms (PHQ-9) M	SD
Migraines	151	45.21	**7.81 *****	4.90	**8.57 *****	4.62
Diabetes	19	5.69	**9.21 ** **	5.45	**9.89 ** **	5.92
Gastrointestinal Diseases	20	5.99	**7.45 ***	4.19	6.55	5.29
Epilepsy	53	15.87	6.94	5.25	6.23	4.97
Cystic Fibrosis	22	6.59	4.73	3.53	5.68	3.56
AIDS	16	4.79	4.87	3.04	6.80	5.36
Heart Diseases	14	4.19	4.71	4.18	5.07	4.57
Onco-Hemat. Diseases	9	2.69	6.78	3.53	6.56	2.74
Kidney Disease	7	2.09	8.29	6.16	5.57	4.12
Asthma	4	1.20	5.00	3.65	8.25	4.03
Scoliosis	4	1.20	3.75	2.75	3.25	1.50
Arthritis	2	0.60	2.50	2.12	3.50	3.54
Other Rare Diseases	13	3.89	7.85	4.41	8.23	7.05

*: *p*-value < 0.05; **: *p*-value < 0.01; ***: *p*-value < 0.001. Statistically significant results are marked in bold.

Table 5. Description of clinical and demographical distributions, with significance determined by Wilcoxon's signed-rank one-sample test.

Variables		n	%	Anxiety Symptoms (GAD-7) M	SD	Max Tot Score	Depressive Symptoms (PHQ-9) M	SD	Max Tot Score
Overall		334	100	**7.132 *****	4.83		**7.505 *****	4.94	
Sex	Male	133	39.82	5.64	4.03	18 *	5.70	4.12	23 *
	Female	201	60.18	**8.11 *****	5.06	21 *	**8.69 *****	5.08	26 *
Pharmacological therapy	Yes	186	55.69	**7.05 *****	4.88	21 *	**7.20 *****	5.04	26 *
	No	148	44.31	**7.24 *****	4.78	19 *	**7.92 *****	4.80	22 *
Other (non-pharmacological) therapies	Yes	84	25.15	**7.60 *****	4.73 *	18 *	**8.13 *****	5.06	22 *
	No	240	71.86	**7.02 *****	4.89	21 *	**7.31 *****	4.85	26 *
Continuity of care during COVID-19 first lockdown	Yes	35	10.48	**7.51 ** **	4.72	17 *	**8.03 ** **	5.28	24 *
	No	293	87.72	**7.11 *****	4.86	21 *	**7.43 *****	4.61	26 *
Years of illness	≤1	48	14.37	**8.15 *****	4.80	17 *	**8.78 *****	5.75	24 *
	1 < 5	134	40.12	**6.85 *****	4.91	21 *	**7.70 *****	4.89	26 *
	≥5	111	33.23	**6.82 *****	4.64	18 *	**6.50 ***	4.64	19 *
Age at diagnosis	Preschool	65	19.46	6.14	4.41	18 *	6.22	4.35	19 *
	School	227	67.96	**7.29 *****	4.89	21 *	**7.77 *****	5.14	26 *

*: *p*-value < 0.05; **: *p*-value < 0.01; ***: *p*-value < 0.001. Statistically significant results are marked in bold.

Next, we found that, as years of illness increase, there is a downward trend in anxiety and depression scores, even if it is not statistically significant (anticorrelation −0.140). Moreover, depressive–anxious scores do not depend on the patient's age.

Next, we were interested in investigating whether some variables had an impact on depressive–anxious symptoms.

Figures 1 and 2 present the relationship between anxiety and depression scores and single diagnosis of CI. The Kruskal–Wallis test found no significant difference in scores between diagnoses, so we could conclude that there was no precise diagnosis that influenced mood scores (data omitted).

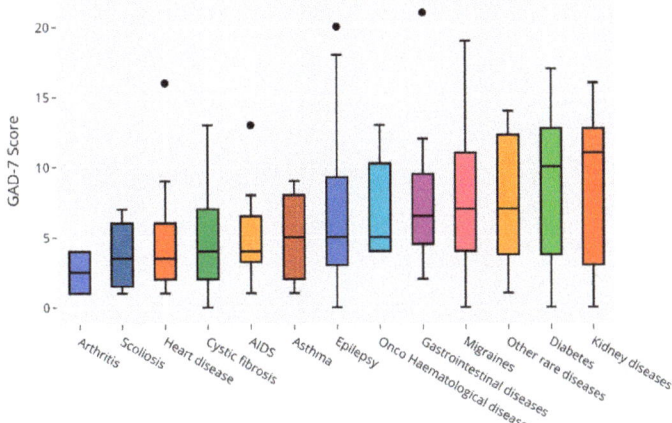

Figure 1. Relationship between anxiety scores and single diagnosis of CI.

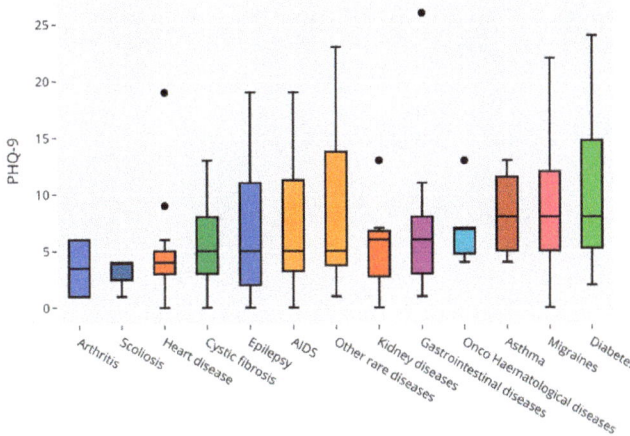

Figure 2. Relationship between depression scores and single diagnosis of CI.

Then, we proceeded to investigate whether there was a statistically significant difference in mood scores between sub-groups (Table 6), using Mann–Whitney's and Kruskal–Wallis' tests. We were interested in investigating the effect of children's demographic and clinical characteristics, such as age at diagnosis (preschool vs. school age), being under pharmacological therapy (yes or not), being under non-pharmacological treatment (speech therapy, psychotherapy, etc., or not), having continuity of care while in lockdown or restriction period, and sex, on depressive and anxiety symptoms. No differences between groups were found, except for age at diagnosis and sex. More specifically, children who received the diagnosis of CI during school age and girls had statistically significantly higher scores of depressive symptoms than children who were diagnosed during preschool and boys.

Lastly, we found that anxiety and depression scores were strongly correlated (rh0 = 0.671, $p < 0.001$)

Table 6. Differences in mood scores between clinical and demographical sub-groups.

	W	df	p
Age at diagnosis (preschool vs. school) [†]			
Tot score GAD-7	5432.000		0.073
Tot score PHQ-9	5553.000		0.039 *
Pharmacological therapy (Y/N) [†]			
Tot score GAD-7	11094.000		0.217
Tot score PHQ-9	11592.500		0.051
Other (non-pharmacological) therapies (Y/N) [†]			
Tot score GAD-7	6387.500		0.183
Tot score PHQ-9	6307.000		0.142
Continuity of care during COVID-19 first lockdown (Y/N) [‡]			
Tot score GAD-7	−0.553	39.746	0.584
Tot score PHQ-9	−0.657	38.774	0.515
Sex (m/f) [†]			
Tot score GAD-7	13,017.500		**<0.001 ***
Tot score PHQ-9	13,522.000		**<0.001 ***

*: p-value < 0.05; ***: p-value < 0.001. Note. [†]: Mann–Whitney U-test; [‡]: Welch's t-test. Statistically significant results are marked in bold.

4. Discussion

The aim of the present study was to assess the proportion of children with CI presenting anxiety and depressive symptoms, and the clinical and demographic characteristics affecting such symptomatology.

Depressive and anxiety symptomatology was assessed using standardized questionnaires largely used in populations with chronic conditions [26]. Our study population represents various regions in Italy, although the majority resided in the central area of the country and were affected by a wide variety of chronic conditions. The majority of the participants were adolescents or pre-adolescents (mean age 14.44, range 11–18) and female (201F; 133M).

We found a very high proportion of children showing mild to severe depressive and anxiety symptomatology (approximately 68% and 63%, respectively). No differences were found among children affected by different CI, although the lack of significance may be due to the small sample size. Future studies with larger sample sizes should investigate whether children with specific conditions are more at risk of mental health issues.

Concerning the pharmacological and other (non-pharmacological) therapies, again, very high scores of anxiety and depression symptomatology were found in those receiving or not receiving the treatment, but no statistical differences were found between groups. Regarding the impact of the duration of the chronic condition (years of illness), our analysis showed an inverse downward trend—the longer the years of the disease, the lower the levels of anxiety and depression—even if this result did not reach statistical significance. This finding is consistent with previous literature, presuming a process of long-term adaptation to the disease [27].

Regarding the sex, girls in our sample showed significantly higher scores of symptoms, both anxiety and depression, than boys. This has been already documented in the general population [28], but is in contrast with previous findings in some chronic conditions [29–31]. Further research should better understand the factors involved in differentiating the symptomatology between males and females, related also to the agreement between self-report measures and proxy reports.

Lastly, we found high levels of mood disorders only in children who had been diagnosed with CI at school age, a result confirmed by a statistically significant correlation between the age at diagnosis and depression scores. These results could be due to the processes of adaptation to the illness, which can be enhanced also by early detection and diagnosis of the disease, where possible. In addition, timely detection and communication of diagnosis can be used to promote early coping strategies in patients with chronic illness, and to buffer some disease-related outcomes, such as behavioral problems [32].

4.1. Depression and Anxiety Manifestations and Proportions

Mental disorders are increasingly identified as the main cause of the burden of illness in the general population [33]. According to the Global Burden of Diseases, Injuries, and Risk Factors Study 2019 (GBD), between 1990 and 2019, mental health disorders increased by 48.1% worldwide, with the two most common conditions represented by depressive and anxiety disorders [1]. A recent review conducted by LaGrant and colleagues (2020) found that, among children with epilepsy and other chronic conditions living in the United States during the pre-pandemic period, 25% of children aged 5–17 with epilepsy and 22.1% of children with other conditions had depression and/or anxiety symptoms [31].

The authors of this study note that many previous studies have estimated the prevalence of depression and anxiety in children suffering from chronic illness [34–36]: in the case of epilepsy, estimates vary widely between studies—rates of depression range from 8 to 33%, while rates of anxiety range from 5 to 48.5%. Regarding comorbidity, 11.5% of all children with epilepsy had both depression and anxiety. For other chronic conditions, such as asthma, migraines, and allergies, reported overall rates of depression range from 2.8% to 7%, while rates of anxiety range from 7.5% to 15.8%. Comorbidity among these conditions ranges from 6.2% to 20.4%. When compared to these data, we found far greater proportions among our sample: depressive symptoms at 67.96% and anxiety symptoms at 62.87%, with a prevalence of comorbidity of 53.89%.

According to these results and considerations, the COVID-19 pandemic appears to have exacerbated the psychological burden on this population, but it is not limited to this group. Indeed, a recent systematic review conducted by Ma and colleagues (2021) [37] found a pooled prevalence of depression among children of 29% (ranging from 10% to 71%) and a pooled prevalence of anxiety of 26% (ranging from 7% to 55%) during the COVID-19 pandemic.

However, further investigations are needed to obtain a clearer picture of children with chronic illness worldwide. It is important to note that during the COVID-19 pandemic, school closures were one of the first containment measures implemented by governments around the world. School is an important social and support resource for children with chronic conditions, which provides rehabilitation interventions, special learning programs, coping routines, and socialization among peers. As stated by Lee [13], social restrictions exposed high-risk populations, such as pediatric CI patients, to the onset or relapse of anxious–depressive symptoms.

Even though our study has some limitations, such as a more representative sample from Central Italy and fewer from other regions, these preliminary data show alarming percentages of depressive and anxiety symptoms, calling for an urgent effort to implement tailored prevention and public treatment programs addressing the needs of this vulnerable group of patients.

4.2. Continuity of Care

Of the overall sample of 334 children, only 35 of them (10,48%) received continuity of care, while 293 children (89,52%) did not. In both groups, we found very high levels of depressive and anxiety symptoms, which are consistent with previous findings showing children with CI as an "at-risk" group for mood impairment [38]. Even if no statistical significance was reached, lower levels of mood symptomatology were found in the group of patients receiving continuity of care during the early phase of the COVID-19 pandemic in Italy, suggesting the role that continuity of care may play as a protective factor for the emergence of mental disorders.

The COVID-19 pandemic caused the disruption of medical essential services and delayed care-seeking due to fear of contracting the virus [14]. Guaranteeing continuity of care is a critical factor, not only to provide stable monitoring and managing of their chronic condition, to prevent relapses, and to ensure medical prescriptions, but also to promote mental health and ensure resilience in this population. Resilience implies having skills that can help a person facing (and coping with) stressful/threatening events. The presence of risk and protective factors have a strong impact in the promotion of positive outcomes, as well as in the reduction of the negative ones [39].

The "state of emergency" caused by the COVID-19 pandemic focused on hospital care to prevent the health system from being over-burdened, overlooking the importance of primary care in guaranteeing continuity of care. This contributed to a rupture and loss of references and services, essential to promote the sense of safety and protection that the chronic patient and his/her family can benefit from. Ensuring continuity of care during critical times, especially for those in vulnerable categories such as children with CI, should be prioritized also as an inherent path to promote resilience and mental health. As Prof. Prince and colleagues (2007) stated in their famous article published in the prestigious journal "The Lancet", "There is no health without mental health" [40].

5. Conclusions

Our analysis showed a very high proportion of anxious–depressive symptomatology in a sample of children and adolescents with CI during the first COVID-19 lockdown in Italy. As the pandemic is still ongoing, continuity of care must be ensured and tailored psychological assistance should be enhanced in order to promote and manage their mental health. Further longitudinal and larger studies are still needed to obtain deeper knowledge of the phenomenon and related risk/protective factors.

Author Contributions: Conceptualization, C.C., S.G. and S.C.; methodology, C.C. and M.T.; formal analysis, C.C., C.F. and M.T.; investigation, I.T., O.P., L.V., C.A., C.V., M.P., V.M., R.S. and C.C.; data curation, C.C., C.F. and S.C.; writing—original draft preparation, C.C. and C.F.; writing—review and editing, C.C., C.F., I.T., S.C., M.B. and F.C.; supervision, S.C., T.G.C. and S.G.; project administration, C.C. and S.C. All authors have read and agreed to the published version of the manuscript.

Funding: This work was supported by the Italian Ministry of Health with "Current Research" funds.

Institutional Review Board Statement: Our study was approved by the Ethics Committee Board of the Bambino Gesù Children Hospital (protocol code 2162_OPBG_2020, date of approval 6 July 2020). When necessary, partner centers sought and obtained approval from their local Ethics Committee.

Informed Consent Statement: Informed consent was obtained from all subjects involved in the study.

Data Availability Statement: The data presented in this study are available on request from the corresponding author. The data are not publicly available due to privacy and ethical reasons.

Acknowledgments: The authors thank Martina Checchi Proietti (Bambino Gesù Children Hospital), Grazia Foschino Barbaro (Azienda Ospedaliera Universitaria Policlinico—Giovanni XXII) and Pasquale Capuozzo (IRCCS Istituto Giannina Gaslini) for their valuable contributions to the data collection.

Conflicts of Interest: The authors declare no conflict of interest.

References

1. GBD 2019 Mental Disorders Collaborators. Global, regional, and national burden of 12 mental disorders in 204 countries and territories, 1990–2019: A systematic analysis for the Global Burden of Disease Study 2019. *Lancet Psychiatry* **2022**, *9*, 137–150. [CrossRef]
2. Fridell, A.; Norrman, H.N.; Girke, L.; Bölte, S. Effects of the Early Phase of COVID-19 on the Autistic Community in Sweden: A Qualitative Multi-Informant Study Linking to ICF. *Int. J. Environ. Res. Public Health* **2022**, *19*, 1268. [CrossRef]

3. Newacheck, P.W.; Taylor, W.R. Childhood chronic illness: Prevalence, severity, and impact. *Am. J. Public Health* **1992**, *82*, 364–371. [CrossRef] [PubMed]
4. Martinez, W.; Carter, J.S.; Legato, L.J. Social competence in children with chronic illness: A meta-analytic review. *J. Pediatr. Psychol.* **2011**, *36*, 878–890. [CrossRef] [PubMed]
5. Van der Lee, J.H.; Mokkink, L.B.; Grootenhuis, M.A.; Heymans, H.S.; Offringa, M. Definitions and measurement of chronic health conditions in childhood: A systematic review. *JAMA* **2007**, *297*, 2741. [CrossRef] [PubMed]
6. Van Cleave, J.; Gortmaker, S.L.; Perrin, J.M. Dynamics of obesity and chronic health conditions among children and youth. *JAMA* **2010**, *303*, 623–630. [CrossRef] [PubMed]
7. Serlachius, A.; Badawy, S.M.; Thabrew, H. Psychosocial challenges and opportunities for youth with chronic health conditions during the COVID-19 pandemic. *JMIR Pediatr Parent.* **2020**, *3*, e23057. [CrossRef]
8. Cobham, V.E.; Hickling, A.; Kimball, H.; Thomas, H.J.; Scott, J.G.; Middeldorp, C.M. Systematic review: Anxiety in children and adolescents with chronic medical conditions. *J. Am. Acad. Child Adolesc. Psychiatry* **2020**, *59*, 595–618. [CrossRef]
9. Curtis, C.E.; Luby, J.L. Depression and social functioning in preschool children with chronic medical conditions. *J. Pediatr.* **2008**, *153*, 408–413. [CrossRef]
10. Santomauro, D.F.; Herrera AM, M.; Shadid, J.; Zheng, P.; Ashbaugh, C.; Pigott, D.M.; Ferrari, A.J. Global prevalence and burden of depressive and anxiety disorders in 204 countries and territories in 2020 due to the COVID-19 pandemic. *Lancet* **2021**, *398*, 1700–1712. [CrossRef]
11. World Health Organization. *Mental Health and COVID-19: Early Evidence of the Pandemic's Impact: Scientific Brief*; World Health Organization: Geneva, Switzerland, 2022.
12. Racine, N.; McArthur, B.A.; Cooke, J.E.; Eirich, R.; Zhu, J.; Madigan, S. Global prevalence of depressive and anxiety symptoms in children and adolescents during COVID-19: A meta-analysis. *JAMA Pediatrics* **2021**, *175*, 1142–1150. [CrossRef] [PubMed]
13. Lee, J. Effetti sulla salute mentale della chiusura delle scuole durante il COVID-19. *Lancet Child Adolesc. Health* **2020**, *4*, 421. [CrossRef]
14. Lazzerini, M.; Barbi, E.; Apicella, A.; Marchetti, F.; Cardinale, F.; Trobia, G. Delayed access or provision of care in Italy resulting from fear of COVID-19. *Lancet Child Adolesc Health* **2020**, *4*, e10–e11. [CrossRef]
15. Zhang, G.; Yang, H.; Zhang, A.; Shen, Q.; Wang, L.; Li, Z.; Zhao, B. The Impact of the COVID-19 Outbreak on the Medical Treatment of Chinese Children with Chronic Kidney Disease (CKD): A Multicenter Cross-section Study in the Context of a Public Health Emergency of International Concern. *medRxiv* **2020**. [CrossRef]
16. Holmes, E.A.; O'Connor, R.C.; Perry, V.H.; Tracey, I.; Wessely, S.; Arseneault, L.; Ford, T. Multidisciplinary research priorities for the COVID-19 pandemic: A call for action for mental health science. *Lancet Psychiatry* **2020**, *7*, 547–560. [CrossRef]
17. Spitzer, R.L.; Kroenke, K.; Williams, J.B.; Löwe, B. A brief measure for assessing generalized anxiety disorder: The GAD-7. *Arch. Intern. Med.* **2006**, *166*, 1092–1097. [CrossRef] [PubMed]
18. Spitzer, R.L.; Kroenke, K.; Williams, J.B. Patient Health Questionnaire Primary Care Study Group, & Patient Health Questionnaire Primary Care Study Group. Validation and utility of a self-report version of PRIME-MD: The PHQ primary care study. *JAMA* **1999**, *282*, 1737–1744.
19. Kroenke, K.; Spitzer, R.L.; Williams, J.B. The PHQ-9: Validity of a brief depression severity measure. *J. Gen. Intern. Med.* **2001**, *16*, 606–613. [CrossRef] [PubMed]
20. Wittkampf, K.A.; Naeije, L.; Schene, A.H.; Huyser, J.; van Weert, H.C. Diagnostic accuracy of the mood module of the Patient Health Questionnaire: A systematic review. *Gen. Hosp. Psychiatry* **2007**, *29*, 388–395. [CrossRef] [PubMed]
21. Levis, B.; Benedetti, A.; Thombs, B.D. Accuracy of Patient Health Questionnaire-9 (PHQ-9) for screening to detect major depression: Individual participant data meta-analysis. *BMJ* **2019**, *365*, 1476. [CrossRef]
22. Alharbi, R.; Alsuhaibani, K.; Almarshad, A.; Alyahya, A. Depression and anxiety among high school student at Qassim Region. *Fam. Med. Prim. Care Rev.* **2019**, *8*, 504. [CrossRef] [PubMed]
23. Tiirikainen, K.; Haravuori, H.; Ranta, K.; Kaltiala-Heino, R.; Marttunen, M. Psychometric properties of the 7-item Generalized Anxiety Disorder Scale (GAD-7) in a large representative sample of Finnish adolescents. *Psychiatry Res.* **2019**, *272*, 30–35. [CrossRef] [PubMed]
24. JASP Team. *JASP v. 0.16.1*; JASP: Amsterdam, The Netherlands, 2022.
25. Core Team. *R: A Language and Environment for Statistical Computing*; R Foundation for Statistical Computing, R: Vienna, Austria, 2021.
26. Quittner, A.L.; Abbott, J.; Georgiopoulos, A.M.; Goldbeck, L.; Smith, B.; Hempstead, S.E.; Elborn, S. International committee on mental health in cystic fibrosis: Cystic fibrosis foundation and European cystic fibrosis society consensus statements for screening and treating depression and anxiety. *Thorax* **2016**, *71*, 26–34. [CrossRef] [PubMed]
27. Mussatto, K. Adaptation of the child and family to life with a chronic illness. *Cardiol. Young* **2006**, *16*, 110–116. [CrossRef] [PubMed]
28. Merikangas, K.R.; He, J.P.; Burstein, M.; Swanson, S.A.; Avenevoli, S.; Cui, L.; Benjet, C.; Georgiades, K.; Swendsen, J. Lifetime prevalence of mental disorders in U.S. adolescents: Results from the National Comorbidity Survey Replication–Adolescent Supplement (NCS-A). *J. Am. Acad. Child. Adolesc. Psychiatry* **2010**, *49*, 980–989. [CrossRef]
29. Ekinci, O.; Titus, J.B.; Rodopman, A.A.; Berkem, M.; Trevathan, E. Depression and anxiety in children and adolescents with epilepsy: Prevalence, risk factors, and treatment. *Epilepsy Behav.* **2009**, *14*, 8–18. [CrossRef]
30. Reilly, C.; Agnew, R.; Neville, B.G. Depression and anxiety in childhood epilepsy: A review. *Seizure* **2011**, *20*, 589–597. [CrossRef]

31. LaGrant, B.; Marquis, B.O.; Berg, A.T.; Grinspan, Z.M. Depression and anxiety in children with epilepsy and other chronic health conditions: National estimates of prevalence and risk factors. *Epilepsy Behav.* **2020**, *103*, 106828. [CrossRef]
32. Schmidt, S.; Petersen, C.; Bullinger, M. Coping with chronic disease from the perspective of children and adolescents–a conceptual framework and its implications for participation. *Child Care Health Dev.* **2003**, *29*, 63–75. [CrossRef]
33. Patel, V.; Saxena, S.; Lund, C.; Thornicroft, G.; Baingana, F.; Bolton, P.; Chisholm, D.; Collins, P.Y.; Cooper, J.L.; Eaton, J.; et al. The Lancet Commission on global mental health and sustainable development. *Lancet* **2018**, *392*, 1553–1598. [CrossRef]
34. Russ, S.A.; Larson, K.; Halfon, N. A national profile of childhood epilepsy and seizure disorder. *Pediatrics* **2012**, *129*, 256–264. [CrossRef] [PubMed]
35. Berg, A.T.; Caplan, R.; Hesdorffer, D.C. Psychiatric and neurodevelopmental disorders in childhood-onset epilepsy. *Epilepsy Behav.* **2011**, *20*, 550–555. [CrossRef] [PubMed]
36. Clarke, D.M.; Currie, K.C. Depression, anxiety and their relationship with chronic diseases: A review of the epidemiology, risk and treatment evidence. *Med. J. Aust.* **2009**, *190*, S54–S60. [CrossRef]
37. Ma, L.; Mazidi, M.; Li, K.; Li, Y.; Chen, S.; Kirwan, R.; Wang, Y. Prevalence of mental health problems among children and adolescents during the COVID-19 pandemic: A systematic review and meta-analysis. *J. Affect. Disord.* **2021**, *293*, 78–89. [CrossRef]
38. Combs-Orme, T.; Heflinger, C.A.; Simpkins, C.G. Comorbidity of mental health problems and chronic health conditions in children. *J. Emot. Behav. Disord.* **2002**, *10*, 116–125. [CrossRef]
39. Zolkoski, S.M.; Bullock, L.M. Resilience in children and youth: A review. *Child. Youth Serv. Rev.* **2012**, *34*, 2295–2303. [CrossRef]
40. Prince, M.; Patel, V.; Saxena, S.; Maj, M.; Maselko, J.; Phillips, M.R.; Rahman, A. No health without mental health. *Lancet* **2007**, *370*, 859–877. [CrossRef]

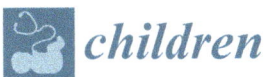

Article

A Comprehensive Analysis of the Relationship between Play Performance and Psychosocial Problems in School-Aged Children

Raúl Vigil-Dopico [1,†], Laura Delgado-Lobete [1,*,†], Rebeca Montes-Montes [2] and José Antonio Prieto-Saborit [1]

1 Faculty Padre Ossó, University of Oviedo, 33008 Oviedo, Spain; raulvigil00@gmail.com (R.V.-D.); josea@facultadpadreosso.es (J.A.P.-S.)
2 Talionis Research Group, Centre for Information and Communications Technology Research (CITIC), Universidade da Coruña, 15008 A Coruña, Spain; rebeca.montes.montes@gmail.com
* Correspondence: lauradelgado@facultadpadreosso.es
† These authors contributed equally to this work.

Abstract: During childhood, play contributes to the physical, emotional, cognitive and social development of infants and children and may enhance future mental health. The aim of this study was to examine the relationship between play performance factors and psychosocial problems in school-aged children. A total of 142 typical Spanish children aged 5 to 9 years were included. Play performance was measured with the My Child's Play questionnaire, while the Strengths and Difficulties Questionnaire was used to evaluate internalizing and externalizing problems. The findings showed that personal, environmental and activity factors of play performance were associated with psychosocial problems and prosocial behavior in children. Moreover, children with high psychosocial difficulties reported significantly poorer play performance. As executive functioning during play was the factor that was most strongly associated with internalizing and externalizing psychosocial difficulties, it is possible that executive functions have a decisive role on both social cognition and self-regulation during play performance.

Keywords: psychosocial difficulties; daily performance; play performance; activities of daily living; occupational therapy; participation; school-aged; typically developing

1. Introduction

Play is described as an intrinsically motivated, internally controlled and freely chosen activity that may involve exploration, fantasy, humor or risk taking [1–3]. Play performance encompasses a broad range of aspects that should be evaluated, including executive functioning, environment and material opportunities and uses, preferences and choices, and parent and peer relationships [4]. Therefore, it is necessary to consider the personal, environmental and activity-related aspects of play. Due to its multidimensional nature, play perception and conceptualization highly depend on sociocultural factors, which makes it a complex construct to assess [5].

The importance of play has been internationally highlighted and recognized, and it is a fundamental right of all children that should be ensured by the public health system [6]. As a main occupation during childhood, play greatly contributes to the physical, emotional, cognitive and social development of infants and children. Play activities allows children to develop the motor, processing, cognitive and social skills needed to participate in their daily present and future contexts [7–10]. Play activities provide a safe and controlled scenario for children to explore, express and learn to regulate their emotional and behavioral responses through interaction with caregivers and peers [11]. Moreover, promoting play and playfulness has proven to be a useful intervention strategy to help children to cope with severe mental health outcomes of trauma or acute medical procedures [12,13], and to enhance social and adaptive skills in children with intellectual, neurodevelopmental and learning disorders [14,15].

Play development and performance during middle childhood is of special relevance as children gain more independence and autonomy and social aspects and personal preferences become more important. Children between 5 and 9 years engage in more structured and organized play activities that usually involve higher psychosocial demands such as following rules or cooperating with peers. In addition, in middle childhood children become interested in achievement through play and form close friendships as they appreciate the social recognition that comes with successful performance of shared play projects [1,4,16]. Social skills and peer rejection are aspects of concern in middle childhood. Therefore, one of the most investigated benefits of play on childhood development is the influence of peer play ability on childhood mental health and psychosocial skills. Based on accumulative experimental and exploratory research [17–20], Zhao and Gibson [21] proposed a theoretical explanation of the relationship between peer play competence and mental health outcomes during early and middle childhood through social cognition and self-regulatory skills. According to this model, early peer play competence promotes socio-cognitive and self-regulation skills that will facilitate engagement in high-quality peer relational networks, which in turn contributes to a lower risk for later psychosocial issues such as anxiety and depression.

In fact, mental health in children and adolescents has become a public health issue of great importance. It is estimated that up to one in five children presents with mental health problems, and, more specifically, with internalizing and externalizing psychosocial problems such as anxiety, hyperactivity, depression or behavioural problems [22]. Although the relationship between social factors of play and psychosocial problems in children have been demonstrated, there are other play-related factors that may underly this link and that could contribute to further understanding it such as the environmental and executive functioning [23].

Overall, previous research has investigated the potential links between the social aspects of play and mental health outcomes in childhood and adolescence [21]. However, a comprehensively analysis of the relationship between the broad range of play performance aspects and psychosocial problems in typically developing children is lacking. It is yet unknown if the executive function, social and environmental aspects of play are equally associated with both externalizing and internalizing symptoms, as it could have important practical implications to developmental and health promotion programs. Moreover, children with psychosocial problems may display specific difficulties to engage in play activities, which would further limit their daily functioning. In addition, it is important to specifically examine this relationship in different cultural contexts, as children perform and participate in their daily occupations differently according to country and cultural setting [24].

Thus, the main aim of this study was to examine comprehensively the relationships between play performance factors and psychosocial problems in typically developing children.

2. Materials and Methods

2.1. Design, Ethical Considerations and Procedure

We conducted a cross-sectional study involving nine public elementary schools in Asturias (Spain). The study was approved by the Research Ethics Committee of the Principality of Asturias (code 2022.028) and was carried out in accordance to the Declaration of Helsinki. Parental consent was obtained from all the parents of the children enrolled in the study and from the schools' boards.

To increase the representativity of the sample, rural and urban schools were invited to participate in the study. This region of Spain has a high percentage of people living in rural or semirural areas (4.0 and 14.9%, respectively) [25]; thus, two of the nine participating schools were gathered rural schools. As this kind of school is difficult to access, they were nonrandomly selected according to availability criteria. The remaining seven schools were located in urban settings and were randomly selected. All families of the students enrolled in the first four grades of elementary education of the participating schools received an online questionnaire between February and March 2022 that included the information form and informed consent, the Spanish versions of the My Child's Play scale (MCP) and the Strengths and Difficulties Questionnaire (SDQ), and a socio-demographic questionnaire to gather information regarding child's age, sex, clinical diagnosis of any neurodevelopmental or learning disorders, mother and father educational level, family structure, prematurity and presence of and age difference between siblings. Additionally, family socio-economic status (SES) was assessed using the family net income per month, which was calculated using the Spanish Public Income Indicator of Multiple Effects (IPREM) [26].

2.2. Sample Size and Participants

According to previous research, it was expected to find a medium-to-large correlation between play-related factors and psychosocial problems in children [19–21]. Thus, a minimum sample size of 138 children was used to measure a correlation of $r \geq 0.3$ [27] with sufficient confidence and power ($\alpha = 0.05$; power $(1 - \beta) = 0.95$). The child inclusion criteria were (a) aged between 5 and 9 years old; (b) no clinical diagnosis of intellectual, neurodevelopmental or learning disorder, and; (c) enrolled in a mainstream school in the 2021–2022 academic year. To ensure the eligibility criteria of the participants, the socio-demographic questionnaires were revised prior to data analysis, and those children who did not meet the criteria were excluded beforehand. A total of 168 parents returned the questionnaires, of which 12 children were excluded due to being younger than 5 years ($n = 2$) or older than 9 years ($n = 10$). In addition, 14 more children were discarded due to a parental report of diagnosed intellectual, neurodevelopmental or learning disorder. The final sample comprised 142 typically developing children: 58.5% girls; mean age (DT) 7.6 y (1.1 y; see Table 1). Participants had a mean of 0.9 siblings (SD = 0.6), and the reported age difference between participants and their siblings was 5.1 years (SD = 4.5).

Table 1. Sociodemographic data of the participants ($n = 142$).

Sociodemographic Characteristics	N (%)
Sex	
• Boys	59 (41.5)
• Girls	83 (58.5)
Questionnaire filled by	
• Mother	131 (92.3)
• Father	10 (7.0)
• Other (legal guardian)	1 (0.7)
Siblings	
• Only child	37 (26.1)
• Has siblings	105 (73.9)
Family structure (including the child)	
• Two members	5 (3.5)
• Three members	35 (24.7)
• Four members	86 (60.6)
• Five members	16 (11.3)
Prematurity	
• Preterm (<37 weeks of pregnancy)	12 (8.5)
• Term (≥37 weeks of pregnancy)	130 (91.5)
Father educational level	
• Incomplete first level studies	3 (2.1)
• First level studies	22 (15.5)
• Second level studies	85 (59.9)
• University studies	32 (22.5)
Mother educational level	
• Incomplete first level studies	1 (0.7)
• First level studies	6 (4.2)
• Second level studies	57 (40.1)
• University studies	78 (54.9)

Table 1. *Cont.*

Sociodemographic Characteristics	N (%)
Family SES (IPREM) [1]	
• <2.5 IPREM	25 (17.6)
• 2.5–5.5 IPREM	78 (54.9)
• 5.5–7.5 IPREM	31 (21.8)
• >7.5 IPREM	8 (5.6)

[1] <2.5 IPREM ≤ 1412 euro per month; 2.5–5.5 IPREM = 1412–3107 euro per month; 5.5–7.5 IPREM = 3108–4237 euro per month; >7.5 IPREM ≥ 4237 euro per month.

2.3. Outcome Variables and Measures

2.3.1. Play

Play performance was measured with the Spanish version of the MCP, a parent questionnaire designed to evaluate different aspects of play performance in children aged 4 to 9 [28]. The Spanish version of the MCP comprises 40 items that assess four factors: (1) play preferences and interpersonal relationships; (2) executive functions: flexibility and executive attention; (3) play characteristics, and; (4) environmental context). Each item is rated on a 5-point Likert scale, where higher scores reflect better play performance. In addition, a cut-off score of <142 on the MCP scale was indicative of atypical play associated with the presence of neurodevelopmental disorders (NDD-play) [29].

The MCP has acceptable internal consistency, construct validity and discriminant validity for Spanish children with and without neurodevelopmental conditions (internal consistency: Cronbach's alpha = 0.695; construct validity: root mean square error of approximation = 0.023 (95% CI = 0.010–0.050), comparative fit index = 0.991, non-normed fit index = 0.990, root mean square of residuals = 0.048; discriminant validity: area under the curve = 0.876 (95% CI = 0.840–0.912)) [29].

2.3.2. Psychosocial Difficulties

The Spanish version of the SDQ was used to measure the emotional, behavioral and social problems of the children [30–32]. It is a parent questionnaire that comprises 25 items divided into two externalizing factors: emotional symptoms and peer problems, and two externalizing factors: conduct problems and hyperactivity symptoms along with a fifth prosocial behavior factor. Each item is rated on a 3-point Likert scale, where higher scores are indicative of more psychosocial problems and less prosocial behavior. The scores of the first four factors are summed to obtain a total score of psychosocial problems. Children who score > 90th percentile on the total problems scale are identified as having high psychosocial difficulties [33]. In this study, the Spanish percentiles developed by Barriuso-Lapresa et al. were used [34].

The SDQ has adequate internal consistency and construct validity in Spanish school-aged children (internal consistency: Cronbach's alpha = 0.76; construct validity: root mean square error or approximation = 0.73 (95% CI = 0.068–0.077); comparative fit index = 0.93; goodness of fit index = 0.84) [32].

2.4. Data Analysis

Statistical analyses were conducted using IBM SPSS (version 25.0; IBM, Armonk, NY, USA) and JASP. Sample size was estimated using G*Power version 3.1.9.3. (https://doi.org/10.1016/j.paid.2016.06.069 (accessed on 10 January 2022). For descriptive purposes, frequency tables, mean, standard deviation, median and interquartile range were reported. Data were examined for normality using the Shapiro–Wilk test. As normality assumptions were not met for psychosocial measures, non-parametric bivariate analyses were used. Thus, Spearman correlations were conducted to examine the relationships between play performance domains, psychosocial problems and prosocial behavior. Differences in play performance among children with and without high psychosocial difficulties were analyzed using Student's *t* tests, and the differences in psychosocial problems and prosocial behavior among children with and without NDD-play were analyzed using Mann–Whitney U tests. Cohen's d and rank-biserial correlations were used to estimate effect sizes (small = 0.1, medium = 0.2 and large = 0.3) [27].

Finally, a linear regression model was performed to explore the predictive value of play performance factors over psychosocial problems. For all analyses, the alpha level was set to 0.05.

3. Results

3.1. Descriptive Results for Play and Psychosocial Problems

Descriptive findings for play performance and psychosocial problems are displayed in Table A1. Prevalence rates of NDD-play and high psychosocial difficulties according to the total scores on the MCP and SDQ scales were 10.6 and 7.8%, respectively.

3.2. Relationship between Psychosocial Problems and Play Performance

Small-to-large correlations were found between play performance factors and psychosocial problems (Table 2). All play factors were significantly associated with psychosocial problems and prosocial behavior except for "play environmental context" and for some psychosocial factors and "play preferences and interpersonal relationships". Children with more psychosocial problems and poorer prosocial behavior displayed poorer play performance. Among play factors, executive functions during play showed the strongest correlations with externalizing symptoms and prosocial behavior (rho = 0.311–0.620).

Table 2. Correlations between play and psychosocial factors (n = 142).

Psychosocial Factors	Play General Performance	Executive Functions	Environmental Context	Play Characteristics	Play Preferences and Interpersonal Relationships
Psychosocial general problems	0.678 ***	0.620 ***	0.198 *	0.528 ***	0.331 ***
Emotional symptoms	0.473 ***	0.323 ***	0.071	0.322 ***	0.459 ***
Conduct problems	0.494 ***	0.530 ***	0.148	0.373 ***	0.134
Hyperactivity	0.456 ***	0.537 ***	0.092	0.445 ***	0.020
Peer problems	0.465 ***	0.311 ***	0.175 *	0.280 ***	0.426 ***
Prosocial behavior	0.404 ***	0.457 ***	0.080	0.285 ***	0.256 **

* $p < 0.05$; ** $p < 0.01$; *** $p < 0.001$.

Children with NDD-play showed higher psychosocial problems and less prosocial behavior than children with typical play, with a significant and large effect size (rank-biserial correlations = 0.309–0.688; see Table 3), whether children with high psychosocial difficulties reported poorer play performance, also with large effect sizes (d = 0.714–1.913; see Table 4) except for the environmental context factor ($p > 0.05$). Overall, children with NDD-play were 10 times more likely to display high psychosocial difficulties (OR = 10.1, 95% CI = 2.6–38.9; see Table 5).

Table 3. Psychosocial factors according to play performance (n = 142).

Psychosocial Factors	Typical Play M (SD)	NDD-Play M (SD)	p Value	Rank-Biserial Correlation
Psychosocial general problems	8.0 (5.1)	15.0 (4.8)	<0.001	0.688
Emotional symptoms	2.0 (2.1)	4.0 (2.5)	0.001	0.493
Conduct problems	1.3 (1.4)	3.6 (2.3)	<0.001	0.588
Hyperactivity	3.7 (2.5)	5.4 (3.4)	0.049	0.309
Peer problems	0.9 (1.2)	2.0 (1.8)	0.011	0.382
Prosocial behavior	8.7 (1.5)	6.9 (7.5)	0.008	0.408

Table 4. Play performance according to psychosocial difficulties ($n = 142$).

Play Factors	No Psychosocial Difficulties M (SD)	High Psychosocial Difficulties M (SD)	p Value	Cohen's d
Play general performance	158.4 (11.5)	140.6 (7.3)	<0.001	1.580
Executive functions	43.5 (5.0)	33.9 (4.7)	<0.001	1.913
Environmental context	36.9 (4.0)	35.6 (3.1)	0.281	0.340
Play characteristics	42.1 (4.3)	38.4 (4.5)	0.007	0.862
Play preferences and interpersonal relationships	36.0 (4.2)	32.8 (6.7)	0.024	0.714

Table 5. Presence of psychosocial difficulties in children with typical and atypical play performance ($n = 142$).

	No Psychosocial Difficulties N (%)	High Psychosocial Difficulties N (%)	X^2	p Value
Play			15.363	<0.001
Typical	121 (92.4)	6 (54.5)		
NDD	10 (7.6)	5 (45.5)		

Play performance factors explained almost half of the variance in psychosocial problems (adjusted $R^2 = 0.477$, $p < 0.001$; see Table 6). Executive functioning during play accounted for most of the variance in psychosocial problems (B = −0.487 (95% CI = −0.626, −0.347)).

Table 6. Linear regression for psychosocial problems ($n = 142$).

Predictors	B	95% Confidence Interval Lower Limit	95% Confidence Interval Upper Limit	p Value
Executive functions	−0.487	−0.626	−0.347	<0.001
Environmental context	−0.108	−0.277	0.061	0.208
Play characteristics	−0.282	−0.456	−0.108	0.002
Play preferences and interpersonal relationships	−0.133	−0.291	0.025	0.099

4. Discussion

The main objective of this study was to examine comprehensively the relationship between several personal, environmental and activity-related aspects of play performance and psychosocial problems in typically developing children. Our findings show that play performance and mental health display a complex relationship according to the factors involved.

Most play performance factors and general performance showed significant and medium-to-large associations with mental health and prosocial behavior. Specifically, executive functioning and play characteristics were associated with internalizing and externalizing problems, but play preferences and interpersonal relationships only showed a significant relationship with internalizing problems and prosocial behavior. Influence of peer social play on mental health during early and middle childhood has been previously explored. For instance, both cross-sectional and longitudinal data show that better peer and parent play ability at a young age is a protective factor against later internalizing and externalizing problems for the general population [11,21].

The potential link between deficits in non-play related executive functioning and internalizing and externalizing problems have been reported in previous research [35,36] but not within the specific context of play performance. The strong relationships found in this work regarding executive functioning during play and internalizing and externalizing psychosocial problems suggest that higher cognitive aspects of play may have a relevant role on the development of psychosocial problems, thus expanding and contributing to support the hypothesis of Zhao and Gibson [21] regarding the mediating role of social cognition and self-regulatory skills on the influence of peer play over mental health outcomes during middle childhood.

Interestingly, the environmental context of play performance was the play-related factor that displayed a weaker association with mental health in this sample, except for psychosocial general problems and peer problems. These findings partially agree with the work of Hinkley et al. [37] and Fyfe-Johnson et al. [23], who reported that context of play participation was a strong predictor of mental health and of cognitive, behavioral and social skills. However, the small correlations found in this study may be explained due to the fact that all children came from a specific region of Spain and all were enrolled in public schools with alike characteristics; thus, it is possible that environmental opportunities were similar for most of the sample.

Our results also showed that children who performed an atypical play activity indicative of NDD reported higher internalizing and externalizing problems and poorer prosocial behavior, while children with high psychosocial difficulties displayed significantly worse play performance factors except for the environmental context. It must be noted that the prevalence of risk of NDD found in this sample is similar to that reported in recent research regarding undiagnosed neurodevelopmental difficulties in Spanish school-aged children [38]. This is in line with previous studies that have found that children with NDD display more psychosocial problems than typically developing children [39–41], which further supports the use of tailored and individual intervention strategies that assess all the personal, environmental and activity-related aspects of daily functioning [42]. Children with NDD or other developmental difficulties often face more activity limitations and participation restrictions than their typically developing peers, not only in play activities but in other occupations as relevant as self-care, education and instrumental activities [43–47].

Given the relationship between early play performance and later mental health outcomes in childhood, it could be that early restrictions in play participation have an additional impact on daily functioning through internalizing and externalizing problems. However, it must be noted that, given the cross-sectional nature of this study, it may be possible that psychosocial problems in middle childhood are partially responsible for a reduced ability to perform play activities, especially regarding executive functioning skills. Both externalizing and internalizing symptoms have been previously reported to be associated with executive functioning and general cognitive in children [35,36]. Interestingly in this sample, play performance was not equally associated with externalizing and internalizing symptoms, as play preferences and interpersonal relationships were strongly correlated with internalizing problems but not with externalizing problems, while executive functioning during play displayed the strongest correlations with externalizing symptoms. This finding contributes to understanding how different aspects of play performance may enhance or hinder psychosocial well-being in children. For instance, children with externalizing problems could benefit from play activities with high executive functions demands, but they also could be more easily frustrated by these kinds of activities. Moreover, as longitudinal research suggests that lack of peer play skills is a prime stressor that eventually results in an increased risk of mental health problems during childhood [21], findings from this study indicate that it could also be that the presence of psychosocial problems contribute to restricting participation of play activities and to worsening the child's performance in turn. In consequence, children showing externalizing symptoms, such as behavioral problems, may also display difficulties in executive functioning, while children with internalizing symptoms, such as anxiety or emotional and peer problems, could also display solitary play patterns, which may initiate a negative cycle that persists and worsens during late childhood and adolescence. Access to play should be guaranteed for all children, and thus it is necessary to detect those children at risk of restricted play participation to ensure that they are able to engage in those play activities that are beneficial for them.

Additionally, these findings suggest that typically developing school-age children face unmet needs regarding their play performance skills and psychosocial wellbeing. A high percentage of this sample was identified as having either atypical play associated with neurodevelopmental conditions or high psychosocial difficulties, which are two of the most prevalent problems during childhood and adolescence [38,48]. However, there is a systematic under-recognition of both mental and neurodevelopmental difficulties in children, which significantly limits prevention and treatment [38,49]. In this regard, schools may offer an excellent context to implement programs to enhance social and executive functioning development through playful interventions, as health professionals can identify and address performance and developmental difficulties early, thus preventing further, more pervasive, outcomes [50]. Accordingly, different school-based programs have been developed by psychologists and occupational therapists to promote different aspects of executive functioning and social skills, but also to improve mental health aspects through play activities, such as self-regulation [51–56].

Knowing which specific play-related factors correlate with psychosocial problems in children may help to tailor, play-based and evidence-driven interventions that comprehensively address the social and cognitive aspects of the proposed activities. However, occupational therapy-structured and evidence-based programs to promote mental health and development in schools are scarce in Spain although research indicates that they could be effective for promoting social play skills and self-regulation in typically developing school-aged children [57]. Using an interdisciplinary approach that includes both teachers and suitable health professionals may contribute to achieving adherence and positive outcomes, as teachers are able to identify social difficulties in children [58], and occupational therapists are experts regarding activity and performance analysis and play-based intervention [1,4,16]. In addition, poor parent–child play interactions and low playful environments have been found to be associated with psychosocial and behavioral problems in children [11,59]. Thus, enhancing family playfulness and involving parents using a family-centered approach may contribute to promote executive functioning and mental health in children, and to the generalization of those skills to other daily living contexts, such as home and community [58,60]. Mental health needs of children are usually unmet due to a lack of recognition or the unavailability of appropriate health care services [61,62]. As international recommendations advocate for a multitiered system of mental health support in schools [49,50], national policy makers can draw on research to implement context-specific and evidence-driven decisions. In the Spanish context, it is recommended that interdisciplinary, tailored, active and play-based methodologies to promote psychosocial and socio-emotional skills in mainstream schools be designed and carried out.

Limitations and Future Research

The present study has some limitations that should be acknowledged. First, two of the participating schools were selected using a nonrandom criterion. Although this decision was made to ensure the participation of children from rural areas, future studies should include larger samples of randomly selected children living in rural and urban settings. Second, the cross-cultural nature of this work did not allow causal relationships between play performance and psychosocial problems to be established. Thus, longitudinal studies should be conducted. Given the findings regarding executive functioning during play, it would be advisable to expand this line of research during early and middle childhood.

5. Conclusions

The findings of this study corroborate and expand the current understanding of the relationship between play performance aspects such as play characteristics and social interactions and executive functioning, as well as both psychosocial difficulties and social behavior. To our knowledge, the present study is the first to comprehensively assess play performance and psychosocial problems in school-aged Spanish children, but it has implications for international research. As executive functioning during play was the individual factor that accounted for most of the variance in psychosocial difficulties, it is possible that executive functions have a decisive role in both social cognition and self-regulation during play performance. However, social aspects of play performance may be more strongly associated with emotional and peer problems. Overall, it can be concluded that play performance and psychosocial behavior in children display a complex and intertwined relationship, where different play factors are specifically associated with either externalizing or internalizing symptoms. Identification and intervention programs could take these findings into account to design precise, tailored strategies that specifically adjust to the children's needs.

Author Contributions: Conceptualization, R.V.-D. and L.D.-L.; methodology, R.V.-D. and L.D.-L.; formal analysis, R.V.-D. and L.D.-L.; data curation, R.V.-D. and L.D.-L.; writing—original draft preparation, R.V.-D., L.D.-L. and R.M.-M.; writing—review and editing, L.D.-L., R.M.-M. and J.A.P.-S.; visualization, R.V.-D., L.D.-L., R.M.-M. and J.A.P.-S.; supervision, L.D.-L.; funding acquisition, J.A.P.-S. All authors have read and agreed to the published version of the manuscript.

Funding: This research received no external funding.

Institutional Review Board Statement: The study was conducted in accordance with the Declaration of Helsinki, and approved by the Research Ethics Committee of Principality of Asturias (protocol code 2022.082; date of approval 24 January 2022).

Informed Consent Statement: Informed consent was obtained from all subjects involved in the study.

Data Availability Statement: The data are not publicly available due to containing information that could compromise the privacy of research participants.

Acknowledgments: We thank all the parents who participated in this study. Additionally, we thank the nine participating schools for their support (CRA Llanes Número Uno, CRA Santana, CP Maliayo, CP El Pascón, CP Condado de Noreña, CP Hermanos Arregui, CP La Corredoria, CP Salvador Vega Berros, CEIP Xentiquina Lieres-Solvay).

Conflicts of Interest: The authors declare no conflict of interest.

Appendix A

Table A1. Descriptive results for the MCP and the SDQ (n = 142).

Play Performance and Psychosocial Problems	Mean (SD)	Median (IQR)
Play performance total score	157.0 (12.2)	157 (149.0–165.0)
Executive functions	42.7 (5.6)	43 (39.0–47.0)
Environmental context	36.8 (4.0)	37.0 (34.0–39.0)
Play characteristics	41.8 (4.4)	42.0 (39.0–45.0)
Play preferences and interpersonal relationships	35.7 (4.5)	36.0 (33.0–39.0)
Psychosocial problems total score	8.7 (5.5)	8.0 (4.0–12.0)
Emotional symptoms	2.2 (2.2)	2.0 (0.0–3.0)
Conduct problems	1.5 (1.6)	1.0 (0.0–2.0)
Hyperactivity	3.9 (2.7)	4.0 (2.0–5.0)
Peer problems	1.1 (1.3)	1.0 (0.0–1.8)
Prosocial behavior	8.5 (1.7)	9.0 (8.0–10.0)

References

1. Parham, L.D.; Fazio, L. *Play in Occupational Therapy for Children*, 2nd ed.; Mosby: St. Louis, MO, USA, 2008.
2. Eberle, S.G. The elements of play. Toward a philosophy and a definition of play. *Am. J. Play.* **2014**, *6*, 214–233.
3. Sutton-Smith, B. *The Ambiguity of Play*; Harvard University Press: Cambridge, MA, USA, 2009.
4. Mulligan, S.E. *Occupational Therapy Evaluation for Children: A Pocket Guide*; Lippincott Williams & Wilkins: Philadelphia, PA, USA, 2003.
5. Lynch, H.; Hayes, N.; Ryan, S. Exploring socio-cultural influences on infant play occupations in Irish home environments. *J. Occup. Sci.* **2016**, *23*, 352–369. [CrossRef]

6. Nielsen, L. Don't Downplay "Play": Reasons Why Health Systems Should Protect Childhood Play. *J. Med. Philos.* **2021**, *46*, 586–604. [CrossRef]
7. Nijhof, S.L.; Vinkers, C.H.; van Geelen, S.M.; Duijff, S.N.; Achterberg, E.J.M.; van der Net, J.; Veltkamp, R.C.; Grootenhuis, M.A.; van de Putte, E.M.; Hillegers, M.H.J.; et al. Healthy play, better coping: The importance of play for the development of children in health and disease. *Neurosci. Beiobehav. Rev.* **2018**, *95*, 421–429. [CrossRef]
8. Cohen, E.; Gadassi, R. The function of play for coping and therapy with children exposed to disasters and political violence. *Curr. Psychiatry Rep.* **2018**, *20*, 31. [CrossRef]
9. Yogman, M.; Garner, A.; Hutchinson, J.; Hirsh-Pasek, K.; Golinkoff, R.M.; Committee on Psychosocial Aspects of Child and Family Health; Council on Communications and Media. The power of play: A pediatric role in enhancing development in young children. *Pediatrics* **2018**, *142*, e20182058. [CrossRef]
10. American Occupational Therapy Association. Occupational therapy practice framework: Domain and process fourth edition. *Am. J. Occup. Ther.* **2020**, *74*, 7412410010.
11. Schneider, M.; Falkenberg, I.; Berger, P. Parent-Child Play and the Emergence of Externalizing and Internalizing Behavior Problems in Childhood: A Systematic Review. *Front. Psychol.* **2022**, *13*, 822394. [CrossRef]
12. Al-Yateem, N.; Rossiter, R.C. Unstructured play for anxiety in pediatric inpatient care. *J. Spec. Pediatr. Nurs.* **2017**, *22*, e12166. [CrossRef]
13. Chatterjee, S. Children's coping, adaptation and resilience through play in situations of crisis. *Child. Youth Environ.* **2018**, *28*, 119–145. [CrossRef]
14. Arbesma, M.; Bazyk, S.; Nochajski, S.M. Systematic review of occupational therapy and mental health promotion, prevention, and intervention for children and youth. *Am. J. Occup. Ther.* **2013**, *67*, 120–130. [CrossRef] [PubMed]
15. Wilkes-Gillan, S.; Bund, A.; Cordier, B.; Lincoln, M.; Chen, Y.-W. A Randomised Controlled Trial of a Play-Based Intervention to Improve the Social Play Skills of Children with Attention Deficit Hyperactivity Disorder (ADHD). *PLoS ONE* **2016**, *11*, e0160558. [CrossRef]
16. O'Brien, J.C.; Kuhaneck, H. *Occupational Therapy for Children and Adolescents*, 8th ed.; Elsevier: St. Louis, MO, USA, 2020.
17. Dodd, H.F.; Lester, K.J. Adventurous play as a mechanism for reducing risk for childhood anxiety: A conceptual model. *Clin. Child. Fam. Psychol. Rev.* **2021**, *24*, 164–181. [CrossRef] [PubMed]
18. García-Carrión, R.; Villarejo-Carballido, B.; Villardón-Gallego, L. Children and adolescents mental health: A systematic review of interaction-based interventions in schools and communities. *Front. Psychol.* **2019**, *10*, 918. [CrossRef] [PubMed]
19. Gibson, J.L.; Cornell, M.; Gill, T. A systematic review of research into the impact of loose parts play on children's cognitive, social and emotional development. *Sch. Ment. Health* **2017**, *9*, 295–309. [CrossRef] [PubMed]
20. Schwartz-Mette, R.A.; Shankman, J.; Dueweke, A.R.; Borowski, S.; Rose, A.J. Relations of friendship experiences with depressive symptoms and loneliness in childhood and adolescence: A meta-analytic review. *Psychol. Bull.* **2020**, *146*, 664–700. [CrossRef]
21. Zhao, Y.V.; Gibson, J.L. Evidence for Protective Effects of Peer Play in the Early Years: Better Peer Play Ability at Age 3 Years Predicts Lower Risks of Externalising and Internalising Problems at Age 7 Years in a Longitudinal Cohort Analysis. *Child Psychiatry Hum. Dev.* **2022**, 1–16. [CrossRef]
22. Bor, W.; Dean, A.J.; Najman, J.; Hayatbakhsh, R. Are child and adolescent mental health problems increasing in the 21st century? A systematic reivew. *Aust. N. Z. J. Psychiatry* **2014**, *48*, 606–615. [CrossRef]
23. Fyfe-Johnson, A.; Hazlehurst, M.F.; Perrins, S.P.; Bratman, G.N.; Thomas, R.; Garrett, K.A.; Hafferty, K.R.; Cullaz, T.M.; Marcuse, E.K.; Tandon, P.S. Nature and Child's Health: A Systematic Review. *Pediatrics* **2021**, *148*, e2020049155. [CrossRef]
24. Delgado-Lobete, L.; Montes-Montes, R.; Pértega-Díaz, S.; Santos-del-Riego, S.; Cruz-Valiño, J.M.; Schoemaker, M.M. Interrelation of individual, country and activity constraints in motor activities of daily living among typically developing children: A cross-sectional comparison of Spanish and Dutch populations. *Int. J. Environ. Res. Public Health* **2020**, *17*, 1705. [CrossRef]
25. Sociedad Asturiana de Estudios Económicos e Industriales. Población Oficial de Asturias, 1 de Enero de 2021. Available online: https://www.sadei.es/sadei/Resources/PX/Databases/Notas_prensa/02/Pob_oficial_2021.pdf (accessed on 10 January 2022).
26. IPREM. Indicador Público de Renta de Efectos Múltiples. Available online: http://www.iprem.com.es/ (accessed on 10 January 2022).
27. Gignac, G.E.; Szodorai, E.T. Effect size guidelines for individual differences researchers. *Pers. Individ. Diff.* **2016**, *102*, 74–78. [CrossRef]
28. Schneider, E.; Rosenblum, S. Development, reliability, and validity of the my child's play (MCP) questionnaire. *Am. J. Occup. Ther.* **2014**, *68*, 277–285. [CrossRef] [PubMed]
29. Romero-Ayuso, D.; Ruiz-Salcedo, M.; Barrios-Fernández, S.; Triviño-Juárez, J.M.; Maciver, D.; Richmond, J.; Muñoz, M.A. Play in Children with Neurodevelopmental Disorders: Psychometric Properties of a Parent Report Measure 'My Child's Play'. *Children* **2021**, *8*, 25. [CrossRef] [PubMed]
30. Goodman, R. The Strengths and Difficulties Questionnaire: A research note. *J. Child. Psychol. Psychiatry* **1997**, *38*, 581–586. [CrossRef]
31. Goodman, R. Psychometric properties of the strengths and difficulties questionnaire. *J. Am. Acad. Child Adolesc. Psychiatry* **2001**, *40*, 1337–1345. [CrossRef]

32. Rodríguez-Hernández, P.J.; Betancort, M.; Ramírez-Santana, G.M.; García, R.; Sanz-Álvarez, E.J.; De las Cuevas-Castresana, C. Psychometric properties of the parent and teacher versions of the Strength and Difficulties Questionnaire (SDQ) in a Spanish sample. *Int. J. Clin. Health Psychol.* **2012**, *12*, 265–279.
33. Goodman, A.; Lamping, D.L.; Ploubidis, G.B. When to use broader internalising and externalising subscales instead of the hypothesised five subscales on the Strengths and Difficulties Questionnaire (SDQ): Data from British parents, teachers and children. *J. Abnorm. Child Psychol.* **2010**, *38*, 1179–1191. [CrossRef]
34. Barriuso-Lapresa, L.M.; Hernando-Arizaleta, L.; Rajmil, L. Valores de referencia de la versión para padres del Cuestionario de Capacidades y Dificultades (SDQ) en población española, 2006. *Actas Esp. Psiquiatr.* **2014**, *42*, 43.
35. Blanken, L.M.; White, T.; Mous, S.E.; Basten, M.; Muetzel, R.L.; Jaddoe, V.W.V.; Wals, M.; Van Der Ende, J.; Verhulst, F.C.; Tiemeier, H. Cognitive functioning in children with internalising, externalising and dysregulation problems: A population-based study. *Eur. Child Adolesc. Psychiatry* **2017**, *26*, 445–456. [CrossRef]
36. Flouri, E.; Papachristou, E.; Midouhas, E.; Ploubidis, G.B.; Lewis, G.; Joshi, H. Developmental cascades of internalising symptosm, externalising problems and cognitive ability from early childhood to middle adolescence. *Eur. Psychiatry* **2019**, *57*, 61–69. [CrossRef]
37. Hinkley, T.; Brwon, H.; Carson, V.; Teychenne, M. Cross sectional associations of screen time and outdoor play with social skills in preschool children. *PLoS ONE* **2018**, *13*, e019700. [CrossRef] [PubMed]
38. Bosch, R.; Pagerols, M.; Rivas, C.; Sixto, L.; Bricollé, L.; Español-Martín, G.; Prat, R.; Ramos-Quiroga, J.A.; Casas, M. Neurodevelopmental disorders among Spanish school-age children: Prevalence and sociodemographic correlates. *Psychol. Med.* **2021**, *13*, 1–11. [CrossRef] [PubMed]
39. Miranda, A.; Berenguer, C.; Roselló, B.; Baixauli, I. Relationships between the social communication questionnaire and pragmatic language, socialization skills, and behavioral problems in children with autism spectrum disorders. *Appl. Neuropsychol. Child* **2020**, *9*, 141–152. [CrossRef] [PubMed]
40. Doering, S.; Lichtenstein, P.; Gillberg, C.; Kuja-Halkola, R.; Lundström, S. Internalizing and neurodevelopmental problems in young people: Educational outcomes in a large population-based cohort of twins. *Psychiatry Res.* **2021**, *298*, 113794. [CrossRef] [PubMed]
41. Helland, W.A.; Helland, T. Emotional and behavioural needs in children with specific language impairment and in children with autism spectrum disorder: The importance of pragmatic language impairment. *Res. Dev. Disabil.* **2017**, *70*, 33–39. [CrossRef]
42. World Health Organization. *International Classification of Functioning, Disability and Health for Children and Youth (ICF-CY)*; World Health Organization: Geneva, Switzerland, 2007.
43. Blanco-Martínez, N.; Delgado-Lobete, L.; Montes-Montes, R.; Ruiz-Pérez, N.; Ruiz-Pérez, M.; Santos-del-Riego, S. Participation in everyday activities of children with and without neurodevelopmental disorders: A cross-sectional study in Spain. *Children* **2020**, *7*, 157. [CrossRef]
44. Delgado-Lobete, L.; Montes-Montes, R.; Pértega-Díaz, S.; Santos-del-Riego, S.; Hartman, E.; Schoemaker, M.M. Motor performance and daily participation in children with and without probable developmental coordination disorder. *Dev. Med. Child Neurol.* **2022**, *64*, 220–227. [CrossRef]
45. De Schipper, E.; Lundequist, A.; Wilteus, A.L.; Coghill, D.; de Vries, P.J.; Granlund, M.; Holtmann, M.; Jonsson, U.; Karande, S.; Levy, F.; et al. A comprehensive scoping review of ability and disability in ADHD using the international classification of functioning, disability and health-children and youth version (ICF-CY). *Eur. Child Adolesc. Psychiatry* **2015**, *24*, 859–872. [CrossRef]
46. Magalhães, L.C.; Cardoso, A.A.; Missiuna, C. Activities and participation in children with developmental coordination disorder: A systematic review. *Res. Dev. Disabil.* **2011**, *32*, 1309–1316. [CrossRef]
47. De Schipper, E.; Lundequist, A.; Coghill, D.; de Vries, P.J.; Granlund, M.; Holtmann, M.; Jonsson, U.; Karande, S.; Levy, F.; Robison, J.E.; et al. Ability and Disability in Autism Spectrum Disorder: A Systematic Literature Review Employing the International Classification of Functioning, Disability and Health-Children and Youth Version. *Autism Res.* **2015**, *8*, 782–794. [CrossRef]
48. Patalay, P.; Gage, S.H. Changes in millennial adolescent mental health and health-related behaviours over 10 years: A population cohort comparison study. *Int. J. Epidemiol.* **2019**, *48*, 1650–1664. [CrossRef] [PubMed]
49. Schor, E.L. Developing a Structure of Essential Services for a Child and Adolescent Mental Health System. *Milbank Q.* **2021**, *99*, 62–90. [CrossRef] [PubMed]
50. Hoover, S.; Bostic, J. Schools as a Vital Component of the Child and Adolescent Mental Health System. *Psychiatr. Serv.* **2021**, *72*, 37–48. [CrossRef] [PubMed]
51. Low, S.; Cook, C.R.; Smolkowski, K.; Buntain-Ricklefs, J. Promoting social-emotional competence: An evaluation of the elementary version of Second Step®. *J. Sch. Psychol.* **2015**, *53*, 463–477. [CrossRef] [PubMed]
52. Bywater, T.; Hutchings, J.; Whitaker, C.; Evans, C.; Parry, L. The Incredible Years Therapeutic Dinosaur Programme to build social and emotional competence in Welsh primary schools: Study protocol for a randomised controlled trial. *Trials* **2011**, *12*, 39. [CrossRef]
53. Hagelskamp, C.; Brackett, M.A.; Rivers, S.E.; Salovey, P. Improving classroom quality with the RULER Approach to Social and Emotional Learning: Proximal and distal outcomes. *Am. J. Community Psychol.* **2013**, *51*, 530–543. [CrossRef]
54. Botella, C.; Mira, A.; Garcia-Palacios, A.; Quero, S.; Navarro, M.V.; Del Amo, A.R.L.; Molinari, G.; Castilla, D.; Moragrega, I.; Soler, C.; et al. Smiling is fun: A Coping with Stress and Emotion Regulation Program. *Stud. Health Technol. Inform.* **2012**, *181*, 123–127.

55. Bailey, R.; Jones, S.M. An Integrated Model of Regulation for Applied Settings. *Clin. Child Fam. Psychol. Rev.* **2019**, *22*, 2–23. [CrossRef]
56. Blackwell, A.L.; Yeager, D.C.; Mische-Lawson, L.; Bird, R.J.; Cook, D.M. Teaching Children Self-Regulation Skills within the Early Childhood Education Environment: A Feasibility Study. *J. Occup. Ther. Sch. Early Interv.* **2014**, *7*, 204–224. [CrossRef]
57. Romero-Ayuso, D.; Espinosa-García, B.; Gómez-Marín, E.; Gómez-Jara, N.; Cuevas-Delgado, C.; Álvarez-Benítez, I.; Triviño-Juárez, J.-M. A Pilot Study of Improving Self-Regulation and Social Interaction with Peers: An "Exciting School". *Children* **2022**, *9*, 829. [CrossRef]
58. Challita, J.; Chaparo, C.; Hinitt, J. Patterns of Social Skill Difficulties in Young Children with Reduced Social Competence: Parent and Teacher Perceptions. *J. Occup. Ther. Sch. Early Interv.* **2019**, *12*, 298–310. [CrossRef]
59. Menashe-Grinberg, A.; Atzaba-Poria, N. Mother-child and father-child play interaction: The importance of parental playfulness as a moderator of the links between parental behavior and child negativity. *Infant. Ment. Health J.* **2017**, *38*, 772–784. [CrossRef] [PubMed]
60. Smit, S.; Mikami, A.Y.; Normand, S. Effects of the Parental Friendship Coaching Intervention on Parental Emotion Socialization of Children with ADHD. *Res. Child Adolesc. Psychopathol.* **2022**, *50*, 101–115. [CrossRef]
61. Jensen, P.S.; Goldman, E.; Offord, D.; Costello, E.J.; Friedman, R.; Huff, B.; Crowe, M.; Amsel, L.; Bennett, K.; Bird, H.; et al. Overlooked and under-served: "action signs" for identifying children with unmet mental health needs. *Pediatrics* **2011**, *128*, 970–979. [CrossRef] [PubMed]
62. Brown, N.M.; Green, J.C.; Desai, M.M.; Weitzman, C.C.; Rosenthal, M.S. Need and unmet need for care coordination among children with mental health conditions. *Pediatrics* **2014**, *133*, e530–e537. [CrossRef] [PubMed]

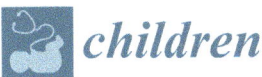

Article

Family Dysfunctional Interactive Patterns and Alexithymia in Adolescent Patients with Restrictive Eating Disorders

Chiara Coci [1], Livio Provenzi [1,2], Valentina De Giorgis [1], Renato Borgatti [1,2], Matteo Chiappedi [3,*], Martina Maria Mensi [1,2] and on behalf of the Mondino Foundation Eating Disorders Clinical and Research Group [†]

1. Department of Brain and Behavioral Sciences, University of Pavia, 27100 Pavia, Italy; chiara.coci01@universitadipavia.it (C.C.); livio.provenzi@mondino.it (L.P.); valentina.degiorgis@mondino.it (V.D.G.); renato.borgatti@mondino.it (R.B.); martina.mensi@mondino.it (M.M.M.)
2. Child Neurology and Psychiatry Unit, IRCCS Mondino Foundation, 27100 Pavia, Italy
3. Vigevano Child Neurology and Psychiatry Unit, ASST Pavia, 27100 Pavia, Italy
* Correspondence: matteo_chiappedi@asst-pavia.it
† Membership of the Mondino Foundation Eating Disorders Clinical and Research Group is provided in Acknowledgements.

Abstract: Adolescents diagnosed with Restrictive Eating Disorders (REDs) are at risk for alexithymia. REDs patients' families show dysfunctional interactive patterns, and childhood family environment influences alexithymia development. We aimed to assess the relationship between family dysfunctional interactive patterns and patients' alexithymia in a sample of adolescents diagnosed with REDs. Forty-five patients and their parents were enrolled. They participated in the clinical version of the Lausanne Triadic Play (LTPc), a standardized observational procedure to assess family functioning. We used the self-report questionnaire Toronto Alexithymia Scale (TAS-20) to assess patients' alexithymia. The TAS-20 provides a multi-factorial measure of patients' alexithymia: Difficulty in Identifying Feelings, DIF; Difficulty in Describing Feelings, DDF; Externally-oriented Thinking, EOT) and a total (TOT) score. DDF and EOT scores were significantly higher than DIF score. Patients' families showed dysfunctional interactive patterns, with a predominance of collusive alliance. Patients from families characterized by collusive alliance had higher TOT scores compared to counterparts from families exhibiting a different interactive dysfunctional pattern. In families characterized by a collusive triadic alliance, the dysfunctional interactive pattern was linked with the risk of alexithymia in patients with REDs. Assessment of family relationships should be included in the routine consultation with adolescent patients affected by REDs.

Keywords: alexithymia; adolescence; anorexia nervosa; family functioning; Lausanne Trilogue Play; restrictive eating disorders

Citation: Coci, C.; Provenzi, L.; De Giorgis, V.; Borgatti, R.; Chiappedi, M.; Mensi, M.M.; on behalf of the Mondino Foundation Eating Disorders Clinical and Research Group. Family Dysfunctional Interactive Patterns and Alexithymia in Adolescent Patients with Restrictive Eating Disorders. *Children* 2022, *9*, 1038. https://doi.org/10.3390/children9071038

Academic Editor: Gregory Neal Barnes

Received: 31 May 2022
Accepted: 10 July 2022
Published: 12 July 2022

Publisher's Note: MDPI stays neutral with regard to jurisdictional claims in published maps and institutional affiliations.

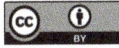

Copyright: © 2022 by the authors. Licensee MDPI, Basel, Switzerland. This article is an open access article distributed under the terms and conditions of the Creative Commons Attribution (CC BY) license (https://creativecommons.org/licenses/by/4.0/).

1. Introduction

Restrictive eating disorders (REDs) are a heterogeneous group of psychopathological conditions characterized by restricted oral intake associated with moderate to high levels of psychosocial and work impairment [1,2]. REDs' etiology is multi-factorial, depending on specific biological, psychological, environmental, familiar, socio-cultural risk factors, combined with an individual vulnerability, mainly expressed during adolescence [2–7]. It is necessary to look at these disorders with a broad and comprehensive view that considers the many variables involved in the development and maintenance of this complex disorder. Previous evidence indicates that adolescent patients diagnosed with REDs show a broad range of emotional dysfunctions, including poor emotion recognition and deficits in emotional information processing, a psychological feature called alexithymia [8–10]. This cognitive-affective deficit is characterized by three main dimensions: difficulty in identifying feelings, difficulty in describing feelings, and externally-oriented thinking. Difficulty in identifying feelings includes struggling in distinguishing emotions from physical sensations and being confused about which emotions are experienced. Difficulty in describing feelings is about struggling in sharing and describing emotional states to others. Finally, externally-oriented thinking concerns the preference to let things happen rather than reflect on their causes [11–13]. Alexithymia is identified as a personality trait that predisposes to the development of psychopathology [14], and previous studies have shown a clear prevalence in patients with eating disorders compared to the healthy population [10]. Alexithymia appears to be involved in the onset, maintenance, and even response to treatment, thus making it an important focus in patient care and therapeutic intake [15,16].

Moreover, dysfunctional interactive patterns have been described in REDs adolescents' families, identified especially in the maintenance mechanism [2,17–19]. The presence of dysfunctional interactive patterns can be assessed by using the clinical version of the Lausanne Trilogue Play (LTPc), a validated observational procedure that allows the analysis of families' triadic interactions [20]. In the LTPc, families are asked to take part in a videotaped four-phase semi-structured interactive game that replicates their everyday real-life functioning. By observing the quality of family members' interactive coordination, it is possible to characterize the type of family alliance. By using this instrument, previous studies have shown that families of adolescents with REDs present a deteriorated interaction quality, especially in the triadic phase, where families were required to act with greater coordination [21–23]. Moreover, Mensi and colleagues identified a distinctive REDs profile of family functioning, characterized by a collusive alliance in most of the families [21,24]. In other words, the various members of these families struggle to support each other to achieve the goal of the game, because of poor coordination [25].

Both alexithymia and dysfunctional interactional family patterns in adolescents have been independently correlated with REDs. At the same time, previous studies have identified a significant correlation between alexithymia in psychiatric patients and their parental bonding styles, supporting the idea that alexithymia may turn out to be the developmental response to a specific parenting style [26]. Despite this the relationship between each other have not been explored extensively, Mannarini and Kleinbub recently conducted a study assessing alexithymia and parental bonding in 32 Italian families consisting of an adolescent with anorexia, a sibling, and their parents [27]. They identified higher levels of alexithymia in patients than in other family members. Higher levels of alexithymia were also related to neglectful parenting styles [27]. Relying on what is known in the literature, we hypothesized that, in adolescents with REDs, high levels of alexithymia are associated with the presence of collusive alliance in their families. Indeed, the aim of the present study was to determine if there is a significant relationship between family dysfunctional interactive patterns and patients' alexithymia in a sample of adolescents diagnosed with REDs.

2. Materials and Methods
2.1. Participants

We enrolled 45 adolescent patients diagnosed with REDs during hospitalization at the Child Neurology and Psychiatry Unit of IRCCS Mondino Foundation in Pavia. All participants were Caucasian and lived in Italy. We included patients aged 12 to 18 years, with a diagnosis of REDs, including Anorexia Nervosa, ARFID, and Anorexia NAS according to the Diagnostic and Statistical Manual of Mental Disorders (DSM-5) criteria [28]. Adolescents were not eligible for the study if they presented any comorbid neurological disorder, intellectual disability or autism spectrum disorder, according to DSM-5 criteria, before the enrolment. The same exclusion criteria were also applied to parents. Furthermore, we excluded participants who had an insufficient understanding of the Italian language (Figure 1). To confirm appropriate RED diagnosis and exclude the presence of comorbidities, patients and their caregivers were interviewed using the DSM-based Kiddie Schedule for

Affective Disorders and Schizophrenia (K-SADS) [29]. The Structured Clinical Interview for DSM-5 Personality Disorders (SCID-5 PD) [30] was administered to the patients to evaluate the presence of any personality disorders. The absence of intellectual disability was assessed using the appropriate Wechsler intelligence scale according to patients' age [31,32].

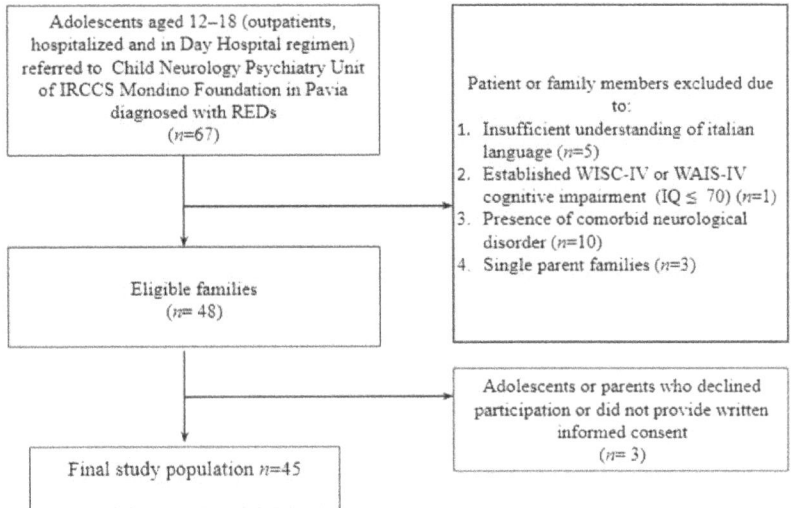

Figure 1. Flowchart of study population. IRCCS: Istituto di Ricovero e Cura a Carattere Scientifico (scientific hospitalization and treatment institute). REDs: Restrictive Eating Disorders.

All enrolled patients and their parents provided written informed consent to participate in the study. The study received the approval of the Ethics Committee of Policlinico San Matteo in Pavia (Protocol ID: P-20170016006). The authors assert that all procedures contributing to this work comply with the ethical standards of the relevant national and institutional committees on human experimentation and with the Helsinki Declaration of 1964 and its latter amendments. The dataset is available upon reasonable request to the corresponding author and it will be accessible through the Open Science online Zenodo repository.

2.2. Procedures

A trained child neuropsychiatrist interviewed parents and patients to collect sociodemographic and clinical data and performed a comprehensive clinical examination including medical and family history, and neurological and psychiatric assessments. Adolescent patients were asked to complete the self-report Toronto Alexithymia Scale (TAS-20) questionnaire [33,34], a validated scale for the measure of alexithymia [35]. To evaluate the presence of family dysfunctional interactive patterns, patients took part in the LTPc [20] with their parents. Every session was videotaped in a dedicated room, and subsequently coded off-line by two independent trained judges.

2.3. Measures

Toronto Alexithymia Scale (TAS-20) [33,36]

Each statement of TAS-20 is rated on a Likert scale from 1 (complete disagreement) to 5 (complete agreement). A total score (TOT) is obtained by summing the item ratings; a score between 61 and 100 indicates clinical alexithymia risk. Three subscales are also provided: difficulty in identifying feelings (DIF), difficulty in describing feelings (DDF), and externally-oriented thought (EOT), i.e., a tendency to focus on external events rather than their own internal affective state. Subscales do not present a clinical cut-off; however, higher scores reflect worse functioning in the specific subdomains of alexithymia.

Lausanne Trilogue Play—clinical version (LTPc) [20]

LTPc is a standardized and well-validated procedure to assess family functioning. The game is structured in four phases: in three phases, two members act together while the third one just observes, without taking part in the interaction (Phase I and Phase II: one parent plays with the patient and the other one assumes the role of observer; Phase IV: parents talk together, while the adolescent finishes the task independently), and in one phase the three members interact together (Phase III). The LTPc coding allows describing the interactive contribution of each family member and the overall family functioning through four functional level codes (i.e., participation, organization, focalization, affective contact) for each phase. A total family score ranging from 0 to 40 is obtained, identifying four types of family alliance: cooperative, in tension, collusive and disturbed [25]. Cooperative alliances (32–40) identify families that cooperate as a team, creating a positive atmosphere, and promoting the child's adaptation. Similarly, tension alliance (24–31) identifies a functional family model, although these families show greater difficulties in correcting each other's errors. In collusive alliances, (16–23) major complications in the parental system emerge: affective climate is constantly in tension and both parents and child struggle to support each other to achieve the goal, due to difficult coordination between the family members. Finally, in disturbed alliances (0–15) families are unable to complete the task due to the loss of family balance, the roles are confused, or one member is excluded from the triad.

2.4. Statistical Analysis

To assess the presence of significant differences among the TAS subscales (i.e., DIF, DDF, and EOT), a within-subject analysis of variance (ANOVA) was used on the entire sample of patients. Repeated contrasts were planned to test for pairwise mean differences in the case of a significant ANOVA test. As the collusive alliance has been previously described in families of adolescents with a diagnosis of RED, family dysfunctional interactive pattern was recoded dichotomously as collusive alliance (1 = yes, 0 = no). To test for the presence of a statistically significant difference in TAS TOT or in the TAS subscales (i.e., DIF, DDF, EOT) between triads divided by collusive alliance or non-collusive alliances, separate t-tests for independent samples were used. The analyses were conducted using SPSS 27 for Windows. A two-tailed $\alpha < 0.05$ criterion for statistical significance was adopted for all the analyses.

3. Results

Table 1 shows the descriptive statistics and clinical characteristics of the sample. At the study enrollment, patients had received individual psychotherapy, $n = 24$ (53%), family psychotherapy, $n = 2$ (4%), or parental couple psychotherapy, $n = 6$ (13%). Five families (11%) had received more than one intervention concurrently. While all the subjects received a diagnosis of RED, 21 (47%) also presented comorbidity for a depressive disorder, whereas other comorbidities included anxiety disorder, $n = 4$ (9%), obsessive-compulsive disorder, $n = 3$ (7%), personality disorder, $n = 2$ (4%), bipolar disorder, $n = 2$ (4%), and schizophrenia, $n = 1$ (2%).

Table 1. Descriptive statistics for the whole sample and split by collusive alliance.

		All (N = 45)		Collusive Alliance			
				Yes (N = 18)		No (N = 27)	
		N	%	N	%	N	%
Sex	Males	9	20.0	3	16.7	6	22.2
	Females	36	80.0	15	83.3	21	77.8
Socially withdrawn	No	40	88.9	16	88.9	24	88.9
	Yes	5	11.9	2	11.9	3	11.9
Academic retreat	No	37	82.2	12	66.7	25	92.6
	Yes	8	17.8	6	33.3	2	7.4
Self-harm behaviors	No	36	80.0	13	72.2	23	85.2
	Yes	9	20.0	5	27.8	4	14.8
Comorbid affective symptoms	No	24	53.3	8	44.4	16	59.3
	Yes	21	46.7	10	55.6	11	40.7
		Mean	SD	Mean	SD	Mean	SD
Demographic characteristics	Patients' age (years)	14.91	1.59	14.78	1.63	15.11	1.57
	Patients' weight (kg)	40.20	7.35	39.53	7.37	31.22	7.40
	Patients' BMI (kg/m^2)	15.88	2.50	16.52	2.33	15.45	2.57
	Fathers' age (years)	51.00	5.53	51.91	5.78	49.76	5.08
	Mothers' age (years)	48.25	5.41	48.43	5.69	48.00	5.16
TAS scores	DIF	22.84	7.47	25.33	6.82	21.19	7.54
	DDF	17.60	4.68	18.89	3.76	16.74	5.08
	EOT	21.20	4.41	22.72	3.79	20.19	4.57
	TOT	61.64	13.74	66.94	11.91	58.11	13.94

Abbreviations: BMI, Body Mass Index; TAS, Toronto Alexithymia Scale; DIF, Difficulty Identifying Feelings; DDF, Difficulty Describing Feelings; EOT, Externally-Oriented Thinking; TOT, Total score.

In the whole sample, a significant difference emerged for TAS subscales, $F(2,88) = 18.95$, $p < 0.001$, $\eta^2 = 0.30$: RED patients reported lower scores for the DDF subscale compared to DIF, $t(44) = 6.66$, $p < 0.001$, and EOT, $t(44) = 5.21$, $p < 0.001$ (Figure 2).

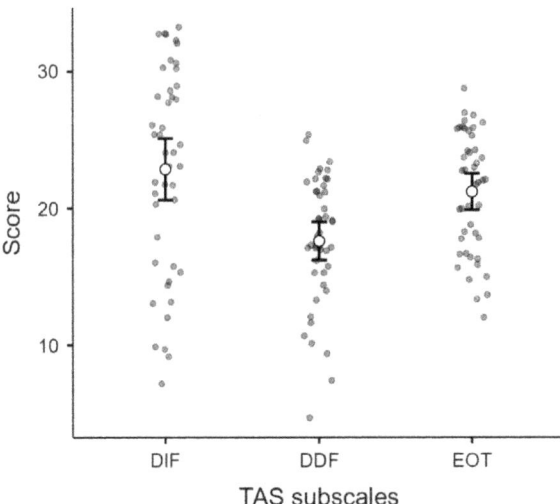

Figure 2. Distribution of TAS subscales scores in our sample. DIF, Difficulty Identifying Feelings; DDF, Difficulty Describing Feelings; EOT, Externally-Oriented Thinking.

Collusive alliance was the prevalent dysfunctional interactive pattern among the families included in the study (n = 18, 40%), followed by stressed alliance (n = 14, 31%)

and disordered alliance (n = 13, 29%). No families showed a cooperative alliance. A more comprehensive table including descriptive statistics for the sample by family alliance style is available in Supplementary Tables.

No differences emerged for socio-demographic characteristics and clinical variables by collusive alliance. Table 1 also reports the mean scores and standard errors for TAS TOT and subscales' scores for both groups, collusive alliance and other alliances. Adolescents with a family rated as collusive reported higher TOT scores compared to counterparts from families who did not show a collusive alliance, $t(43) = 1.88$, $p = 0.033$, $\eta^2 = 0.10$. Moreover, statistical trends emerged for specific TAS subscales: adolescents from collusive families tended to report higher scores in DIF, $t(43) = 1.88$, $p = 0.067$, $\eta^2 = 0.08$, and EOT, $t(43) = 1.95$, $p = 0.058$, $\eta^2 = 0.08$, compared to patients from non-collusive ones (Figure 3).

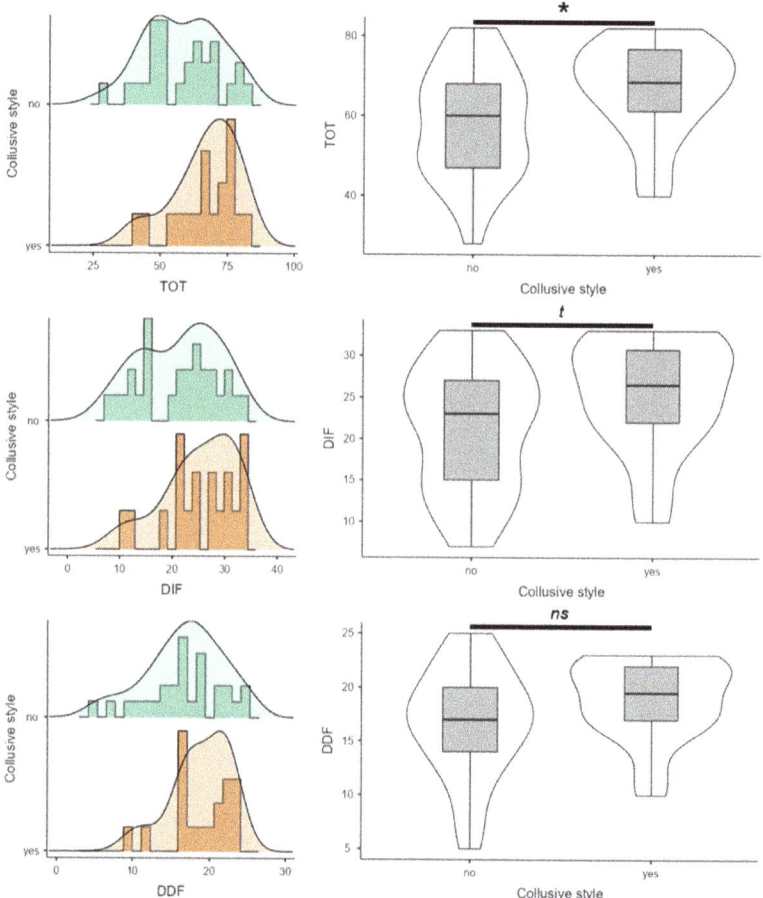

Figure 3. *Cont.*

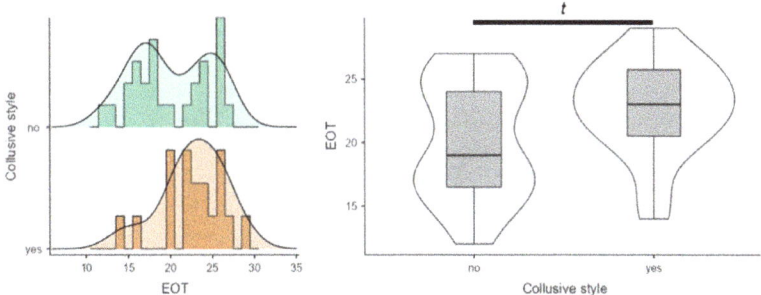

Figure 3. Comparison of TAS scores between collusive and non-collusive families. * = $p < 0.05$; t = tendency to statistical significance; ns = statistically not significant. DIF, Difficulty Identifying Feelings; DDF, Difficulty Describing Feelings; EOT, Externally-Oriented Thinking; TOT, Total Score.

4. Discussion

The aim of the current study was to explore the association between family dysfunctional interactive patterns and alexithymia in adolescent patients with REDs. Our results suggested that there may be a significant association between higher levels of alexithymia and the presence of family collusive alliance in adolescents diagnosed with REDs.

We found that, in our patients' sample, two specific subscales of alexithymia—DIF and EOT—showed higher scores when compared to the third DDF dimension. As shown by the effect size (i.e., $\eta^2 p = 0.30$) this difference was statistically robust. The presence of difficulties in recognizing emotions, and the tendency to adopt an externally-oriented style of thinking, could significantly interfere with patients' ability to recognize and express their inner suffering, leading to greater psychosomatic reactions. This finding confirms previous studies that highlighted how patients suffering from REDs may find specific difficulties in identifying their own and others' emotional states [10,12]. On the other hand, previous evidence of an association between EOT and REDs is mixed [12,37–40]. It is possible to speculate that while a specific difficulty in identifying feelings may be a core feature of alexithymia in these patients, the presence of an externally-oriented thinking style should not be considered as a feature or stable trait, but rather a potentially dysfunctional aspect that may be observed only in individual patients. We could hypothesize that environmental factors—e.g., the presence of specific dysfunctional interactive patterns in the family functioning—may facilitate the emergence of specific alexithymia features in these patients. Nonetheless, due to the cross-sectional nature of the present study, it cannot be excluded that in families of adolescents with REDs the risk of developing a collusive alliance pattern increases. Therefore, to better comprehend the causative association between patients' risk for alexithymia and family dysfunctional interactive patterns, future longitudinal studies are needed.

Furthermore, none of the families enrolled in this study exhibited an optimal interactive pattern, whereas a collusive alliance emerged as the prevalent dysfunctional interactive pattern in 40% of the sample. This finding confirms previous reports: Balottin and colleagues [21] reported a similar prevalence of the collusive alliance pattern in 12 out of 20 families of adolescent patients with REDs. Moreover, the present result further highlights that collusive alliance may be a common family dysfunctional pattern in adolescents diagnosed with REDs. In these families, parents are frequently unable to ensure proper guidance to their children by failing to respect proposed roles, and children seem to struggle to reach an independent role and to mature their own personal ideas [21,22].

Finally, we compared the levels of alexithymia recorded on the TAS scale between the group of families characterized by a collusive alliance, recognized in the literature as prevalent in REDs, and those that are not collusive. Thus, exploring the association between family functioning and patient's alexithymia, we were able to observe the presence of a significant correlation: adolescents from families exhibiting a collusive alliance had higher levels of alexithymia TOT score and the effect was medium ($\eta^2 = 0.10$). This kind of family alliance is characterized by difficulties in adhering to the assigned role during the LTPc procedure. Unlike the disordered alliance, a family structure is usually preserved, despite there often being significant open or hidden competition for control between parents. Within this interactive family style, it is easy to hypothesize that affective experiences are often poorly understood and only partially shared among family members, hindering the patient's development of emotional sensitivity, and contributing to the emergence of alexithymia traits. On the other hand, avoidance of emotional exploration and sharing inevitably aggravates family conflicts.

Moreover, exploring the TAS subscales, we found that adolescents from collusive families also showed a tendency to report greater DIF and EOT scores compared to families who did not exhibit the same interactive pattern. Notably, these are the subscales that emerged as specifically problematic in these patients. Despite this association not reaching statistical significance, the presence of a statistical tendency may suggest that these specific subscales or subdomains of the alexithymia construct should be specifically explored in future studies on the interactive patterns of families of adolescents with REDs.

A limitation of this study is the relatively small sample size. Of course, this was due to the need to include only families in which both parents were available to take part in the LTPc procedure. This limits the generalization of the present results and future replications are needed in larger samples. Nonetheless, the availability of observational measures of family interactive patterns is a strength of this study. Additionally, alexithymia was assessed with a self-report tool, and it is not free from the biases associated with self-reported measures. The lack of a comparison group with families of healthy adolescents is another limitation.

5. Conclusions

Families of adolescent patients diagnosed with REDs usually develop specific dysfunctional interactive patterns characterized by a collusive alliance. At the same time, these patients often manifest high levels of alexithymia with specific difficulties in identifying feelings and, in our sample, exhibiting externally-oriented thinking. Notably, this study further adds that there may be a significant association between the adolescent patients' risk for alexithymia and the presence of a specific pattern of family interactive dysfunction, namely collusive alliance. By highlighting a specific link between features of family functioning and the affective wellbeing of adolescent patients, these findings have critical implications for clinical practice. The detection of alexithymic traits and the study of family dynamics can support the clinician in the early identification of individuals predisposed to the development of REDs and thus enable the initiation of prompt and accurate treatment. Several studies suggest prioritizing a family-centered approach to the assessment and treatment of REDs [2,26,41,42]. By including a systematic evaluation of family interactive patterns in clinical practice, clinicians may identify relational risk factors linked with greater maladaptive emotional functioning, such as alexithymia. The clinical practice with adolescent patients with REDs may thus benefit from the assessment of both family functioning and alexithymia, promoting a family-centered approach in psychiatric settings.

Supplementary Materials: The following supporting information can be downloaded at: https://www.mdpi.com/article/10.3390/children9071038/s1, Tables with descriptive statistics for the sample by family alliance style.

Author Contributions: Conceptualization, M.M.M.; formal analysis and data curation, L.P.; investigation, Mondino Foundation Eating Disorders Clinical and Research Group; writing—original draft preparation, C.C. and M.C.; writing—review and editing, C.C., M.M.M., M.C., L.P.; visualization and supervision R.B., M.C., V.D.G., M.M.M.; project administration, M.M.M.; funding acquisition, R.B. All authors have read and agreed to the published version of the manuscript.

Funding: This research was funded by Italian Ministry of Health (Ricerca Corrente 2021).

Institutional Review Board Statement: The study received the approval of the Ethics Committee of Policlinico San Matteo in Pavia (Protocol ID: P-20170016006). The authors assert that all procedures contributing to this work comply with the ethical standards of the relevant national and institutional committees on human experimentation and with the Helsinki Declaration of 1964 and its latter amendments.

Informed Consent Statement: All enrolled patients and their parents provided written informed consent to participate in the study.

Data Availability Statement: Data are available upon reasonable request from Zenodo (http:10.5281/zenodo.49432).

Acknowledgments: We thank the Italian Ministry of Health for supporting the study (Ricerca Corrente 2021). Authors are thankful to the colleagues of the Child Neurology and Psychiatry Unit, to the patients and their parents who took part in this study. We thank Arianna Vecchio for her support with manuscript editing. Mondino Foundation Eating Disorders Clinical and Research Group: Giorgia Baradel, Renato Borgatti, Chiara Coci, Valentina De Giorgis, Marta Iacopelli, Martina Maria Mensi, Marika Orlandi, Livio Provenzi, Chiara Rogantini, Arianna Vecchio.

Conflicts of Interest: The authors declare no conflict of interest.

References

1. Hay, P.; Mitchison, D.; Collado, A.E.L.; González-Chica, D.A.; Stocks, N.; Touyz, S. Burden and Health-Related Quality of Life of Eating Disorders, Including Avoidant/Restrictive Food Intake Disorder (ARFID), in the Australian Population. *J. Eat. Disord.* **2017**, *5*, 21. [CrossRef] [PubMed]
2. Mensi, M.M.; Orlandi, M.; Rogantini, C.; Provenzi, L.; Chiappedi, M.; Criscuolo, M.; Castiglioni, M.C.; Zanna, V.; Borgatti, R. Assessing Family Functioning Before and After an Integrated Multidisciplinary Family Treatment for Adolescents With Restrictive Eating Disorders. *Front. Psychiatry* **2021**, *12*, 653047. [CrossRef] [PubMed]
3. Dell'Osso, L.; Abelli, M.; Carpita, B.; Pini, S.; Castellini, G.; Carmassi, C.; Ricca, V. Historical Evolution of the Concept of Anorexia Nervosa and Relationships with Orthorexia Nervosa, Autism, and Obsessive-Compulsive Spectrum. *Neuropsychiatr. Dis. Treat.* **2016**, *12*, 1651–1660.
4. Gutiérrez, T.; Espinoza, P.; Penelo, E.; Mora, M.; González, M.L.; Rosés, R.; Raich, R.M. Association of Biological, Psychological and Lifestyle Risk Factors for Eating Disturbances in Adolescents. *J. Health Psychol.* **2015**, *20*, 839–849. [CrossRef]
5. Lock, J.; La Via, M.C. Practice Parameter for the Assessment and Treatment of Children and Adolescents with Eating Disorders. *J. Am. Acad. Child Adolesc. Psychiatry* **2015**, *54*, 412–425. [CrossRef]
6. National Collaborating Centre for Mental Health (UK). *Eating Disorders: Core Interventions in the Treatment and Management of Anorexia Nervosa, Bulimia Nervosa and Related Eating Disorders*; British Psychological Society: Leicester, UK, 2004.
7. Rikani, A.A.; Choudhry, Z.; Choudhry, A.M.; Ikram, H.; Asghar, M.W.; Kajal, D.; Waheed, A.; Mobassarah, N.J. A Critique of the Literature on Etiology of Eating Disorders. *Ann. Neurosci.* **2013**, *20*, 157–161. [CrossRef]
8. Hatch, A.; Madden, S.; Kohn, M.; Clarke, S.; Touyz, S.; Williams, L.M. Anorexia Nervosa: Towards an Integrative Neuroscience Model. *Eur. Eat. Disord. Rev.* **2010**, *18*, 165–179. [CrossRef]
9. Oldershaw, A.; Treasure, J.; Hambrook, D.; Tchanturia, K.; Schmidt, U. Is Anorexia Nervosa a Version of Autism Spectrum Disorders? *Eur. Eat. Disord. Rev.* **2011**, *19*, 462–474. [CrossRef]
10. Westwood, H.; Tchanturia, K. Autism Spectrum Disorder in Anorexia Nervosa: An Updated Literature Review. *Curr. Psychiatry Rep.* **2017**, *19*, 41. [CrossRef]
11. Gaggero, G.; Bonassi, A.; Dellantonio, S.; Pastore, L.; Aryadoust, V.; Esposito, G. A Scientometric Review of Alexithymia: Mapping Thematic and Disciplinary Shifts in Half a Century of Research. *Front. Psychiatry* **2020**, *11*, 611489. [CrossRef]
12. Nowakowski, M.E.; McFarlane, T.; Cassin, S. Alexithymia and Eating Disorders: A Critical Review of the Literature. *J. Eat. Disord.* **2013**, *1*, 21. [CrossRef] [PubMed]
13. Taylor, G.J.; Bagby, R.M.; Parker, J.D.A.; Grotstein, J. *Disorders of Affect Regulation*; Cambridge University Press: Cambridge, UK, 1997.
14. Taylor, G.J.; Michael Bagby, R. New Trends in Alexithymia Research. *Psychother. Psychosom.* **2004**, *73*, 68–77. [CrossRef] [PubMed]
15. Treasure, J.; Schmidt, U. The Cognitive-Interpersonal Maintenance Model of Anorexia Nervosa Revisited: A Summary of the Evidence for Cognitive, Socio-Emotional and Interpersonal Predisposing and Perpetuating Factors. *J. Eat. Disord.* **2013**, *1*, 13. [CrossRef] [PubMed]
16. Pinna, F.; Sanna, L.; Carpiniello, B. Alexithymia in Eating Disorders: Therapeutic Implications. *Psychol. Res. Behav. Manag.* **2015**, *8*, 1–15. [CrossRef]
17. Anastasiadou, D.; Medina-Pradas, C.; Sepulveda, A.R.; Treasure, J. A Systematic Review of Family Caregiving in Eating Disorders. *Eat. Behav.* **2014**, *15*, 464–477. [CrossRef] [PubMed]
18. Lyke, J.; Matsen, J. Family Functioning and Risk Factors for Disordered Eating. *Eat. Behav.* **2013**, *14*, 497–499. [CrossRef] [PubMed]

19. Hibbs, R.; Rhind, C.; Leppanen, J.; Treasure, J. Interventions for Caregivers of Someone with an Eating Disorder: A Meta-Analysis. *Int. J. Eat. Disord.* **2015**, *48*, 349–361. [CrossRef]
20. Malagoli Togliatti, M.; Mazzoni, S. *Osservare, Valutare, e Sostenere La Relazione Genitori-Figli. Il Lausanne Trilogue Play Clinico [Observe, Evaluate, and Support the Parent-Child Relationship. The Clinical Lausanne Trilogue Play]*; Raffaello Cortina Editore: Milano, Italy, 2006.
21. Balottin, L.; Mannarini, S.; Mensi, M.M.; Chiappedi, M.; Gatta, M. Triadic Interactions in Families of Adolescents with Anorexia Nervosa and Families of Adolescents with Internalizing Disorders. *Front. Psychol.* **2017**, *7*, 2046. [CrossRef]
22. Mensi, M.M.; Balottin, L.; Rogantini, C.; Orlandi, M.; Galvani, M.; Figini, S.; Chiappedi, M.; Balottin, U. Focus on Family Functioning in Anorexia Nervosa: New Perspectives Using the Lausanne Trilogue Play. *Psychiatry Res.* **2020**, *288*, 112968. [CrossRef]
23. Balottin, L.; Mannarini, S.; Mensi, M.M.; Chiappedi, M.; Balottin, U. Are Family Relations Connected to the Quality of the Outcome in Adolescent Anorexia Nervosa? An Observational Study with the Lausanne Trilogue Play. *Clin. Psychol. Psychother.* **2018**, *25*, 785–796. [CrossRef]
24. Criscuolo, M.; Laghi, F.; Mazzoni, S.; Castiglioni, M.C.; Vicari, S.; Zanna, V. How Do Families of Adolescents with Anorexia Nervosa Coordinate Parenting? *J. Child Fam. Stud.* **2020**, *29*, 2542–2551. [CrossRef]
25. Fivaz-Depeursinge, E.; Corboz-Warnery, A. *The Primary Triangle: A Developmental Systems View of Mothers, Fathers and Infants*; Basic Books: New York, NY, USA, 1999.
26. Mannarini, S.; Balottin, L.; Palmieri, A.; Carotenuto, F. Emotion Regulation and Parental Bonding in Families of Adolescents with Internalizing and Externalizing Symptoms. *Front. Psychol.* **2018**, *9*, 1493. [CrossRef] [PubMed]
27. Mannarini, S.; Kleinbub, J.R. Parental-Bonding and Alexithymia in Adolescents with Anorexia Nervosa, Their Parents, and Siblings. *Behav. Sci.* **2022**, *12*, 123. [CrossRef] [PubMed]
28. American Psychiatric Association. *Diagnostic and Statistical Manual of Mental Disorders*, 5th ed.; American Psychiatric Association: Washington, DC, USA, 2013.
29. Kaufman, J.; Birmaher, B.; Rao, U.; Ryan, N. *K-SADS-PL DSM-5. Intervista Diagnostica per La Valutazione Dei Disturbi Psicopatologici in Bambini e Adolescenti. [Schedule for Affective Disorders and Schizophrenia for School-Aged Children: Present and Lifetime Version (K-SADS-PL) DSM-5]*; di Sogos, C., Di Noia, S.P., Fioriello, F., Picchiotti, G., Eds.; Erickson: Trento, Italy, 2019.
30. First, M.B.; Williams, J.B.W.; Janet, S.B.; Spitzer, R.L. *Structured Clinical Interview for DSM-5. Personality Disorders (SCID-5-PD)*; American Psychiatric Association: Washington, DC, USA, 2017.
31. Wechsler, D. *Wechsler Adult Intelligence Scale (WAIS-IV)*, 4th ed.; Giunti Organizzazioni Speciali: Firenze, Italy, 2008.
32. Wechsler, D. *Wechsler Intelligence Scale for Children (WISC-IV)*, 4th ed.; Giunti Organizzazioni Speciali: Firenze, Italy, 2003.
33. Bagby, R.M.; Parker, J.D.A.; Taylor, G.J. The Twenty-Item Toronto Alexithymia Scale-I. Item Selection and Cross-Validation of the Factor Structure. *J. Psychosom. Res.* **1994**, *38*, 23–32. [CrossRef]
34. Bressi, C.; Taylor, G.; Parker, J.; Bressi, S.; Brambilla, V.; Aguglia, E.; Allegranti, I.; Bongiorno, A.; Giberti, F.; Bucca, M.; et al. Cross Validation of the Factor Structure of the 20-Item Toronto Alexithymia Scale: An Italian Multicenter Study. *J. Psychosom. Res.* **1996**, *41*, 551–559. [CrossRef]
35. La Barbera, D.; Caretti, V.; Craparo, G. La Toronto Alexithymia Scale (TAS-20). In *Alessitimia. Valutazione e Trattamento*; Astrolabio Ubaldini: Roma, Italy, 2005; pp. 17–23.
36. Taylor, G.J.; Bagby, R.M.; Parker, J.D.A. The 20-Item Toronto Alexithymia Scale: IV. Reliability and Factorial Validity in Different Languages and Cultures. *J. Psychosom. Res.* **2003**, *55*, 277–283. [CrossRef]
37. Espina Eizaguirre, A.; Ortego Saenz de Cabezón, A.; Ochoa de Alda, I.; Joaristi Olariaga, L.; Juaniz, M. Alexithymia and Its Relationships with Anxiety and Depression in Eating Disorders. *Pers. Individ. Dif.* **2004**, *36*, 321–331. [CrossRef]
38. Gramaglia, C.; Ressico, F.; Gambaro, E.; Palazzolo, A.; Mazzarino, M.; Bert, F.; Siliquini, R.; Zeppegno, P. Alexithymia, Empathy, Emotion Identification and Social Inference in Anorexia Nervosa: A Case-Control Study. *Eat. Behav.* **2016**, *22*, 46–50. [CrossRef]
39. Montebarocci, O.; Codispoti, M.; Surcinelli, P.; Franzoni, E.; Baldaro, B.; Rossi, N. Alexithymia in Female Patients with Eating Disorders. *Eat. Weight Disord.* **2006**, *11*, 14–21. [CrossRef]
40. Torres, S.; Guerra, M.P.; Lencastre, L.; Roma-Torres, A.; Brandão, I.; Queirós, C.; Vieira, F. Cognitive Processing of Emotions in Anorexia Nervosa. *Eur. Eat. Disord. Rev.* **2011**, *19*, 100–111. [CrossRef]
41. Rogantini, C.; Provenzi, L.; Mensi, M.M. Prioritizing Family-Centered Mental Health Care for Pediatric Patients with Eating Disorders. *JAMA Pediatr.* **2020**, *175*, 324. [CrossRef] [PubMed]
42. Erriu, M.; Cimino, S.; Cerniglia, L. The Role of Family Relationships in Eating Disorders in Adolescents: A Narrative Review. *Behav. Sci.* **2020**, *10*, 71. [CrossRef] [PubMed]

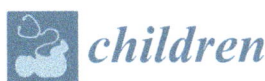

Article

Factors Affecting Psychological and Health-Related Quality-of-Life Status in Children and Adolescents with Congenital Heart Diseases

Hao-Chuan Liu [1,*], Chung-Hsien Chaou [2], Chiao-Wei Lo [3], Hung-Tao Chung [1] and Mao-Sheng Hwang [1]

1. Division of Cardiology, Department of Pediatrics, Chang Gung Memorial Hospital, Linkou Branch, Taoyuan City 333, Taiwan; hungtao@cgmh.org.tw (H.-T.C.); hms3013@cgmh.org.tw (M.-S.H.)
2. Department of Emergency Medicine, Chang Gung Memorial Hospital, Linkou Branch and Chang Gung University College of Medicine, Taoyuan City 333, Taiwan; shien@url.com.tw
3. Department of Pediatrics, Cathay General Hospital, Taipei Branch, Taipei City 106, Taiwan; bluesnowfalling@gmail.com
* Correspondence: sky@cgmh.org.tw

Abstract: Congenital heart disease (CHD), a severe cardiac defect in children, has unclear influences on young patients. We aimed to find the impacts of differently structure heart defects and various treatments on psychology and health-related quality of life (HRQoL) in CHD children and adolescents. CHD patients aged between 6 and 18 years old visited our hospital from 1 May 2018 to 31 September 2018, and their principal caregivers were asked to participate. We used two validated questionnaires, Children Depression Inventory-TW (CDI-TW) and Child Health Questionnaire—Parent Form 50 (CHQ-PF 50), to evaluate CHD patients' psychological and HRQoL conditions. Participants were grouped based on their cardiac defects and previous treatments. We analyzed the results via summary independent-samples t-test with post hoc Bonferroni correction and multivariant analysis. Two hundred and seventy-seven children and their principal caregivers were involved. There was no apparent depressive condition in any group. Single cardiac defect patients exhibited similar HRQoL to controls; simultaneously, those with cyanotic heart disease (CyHD), most multiple/complex CHDs children and adolescents, and those who received invasive treatments had poorer HRQoL. CyHD impacted the most on patients' psychological and HRQoL status. Patients with sole cardiac defect could live near-normal lives; on the other hand, CyHD had the worst effects on patients' psychology and HRQoL.

Keywords: congenital heart disease; children and adolescents; depression; health-related quality of life; questionnaire

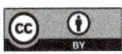

1. Introduction

Congenital heart disease (CHD) is the most common type of congenital disability. More than one million CHD children have been born worldwide. With advances in the treatment of congenital and acquired heart disease, the survival rate of CHD children has improved substantially over the years. More than 90% of CHD children could reach adulthood [1,2]. Due to the improving prenatal diagnosis and advanced treatments, the number of adults with CHDs (ACHDs) will eventually exceed the number of children with CHD in the future. Recent studies have shown elevated risks for physical disability, psychological distress, and social challenges in ACHD survivors [3,4]. Before CHD children reach adulthood, understanding their psychological condition is essential for medical and mental health professionals to provide adequate support and achieve more holistic care.

Many ACHDs have experienced significant emotional distress, including anxiety symptoms and depression [5]. Depression is increased significantly in ACHDs compared with controls [6]. This might be due to their cardiac defects which need long-term medical care, repeat hospitalization, and the uncertainty of future interventions. The relationship between depression and poor cardiovascular (CV) outcomes has been proposed for acquired heart disease patients [7]. Jackson et al. stated that chronic emotional distress might increase CV complications and premature mortality in ACHDs; however, emotional distress's prevalence and effect are still unknown in CHD children and adolescents [8].

Quality of life (QoL) is "an overall general well-being that comprises objective descriptors and subjective evaluations of physical, material, social, and emotional well-being together with the extent of personal developmental and purposeful activity, all weighted by a personal set of values" [9]. It includes physical and psychosocial components. Physical status indicates one's ability to perform various physical activities, self-care behaviors, and other tangible standards, whereas psychosocial status suggests one's function in school, social, and emotional domains [10]. Health-related quality of life (HRQoL) is one's QoL which is "affected by the presence of disease or treatment" [11]. Factors that cause poor QoL in CHD patients include higher frequency and severity of clinical symptoms, the severity of CHDs, the need for interventions, poor functional status, repeat hospitalizations, impaired general health status, and the number of inter-familial conflicts [12–15].

Premature morbidity and mortality are higher in many CHD survivors due to growing anxiety and depression with time. The depressed mood had been shown to correlate with poor QoL in ACHDs positively [5,13]. Identifying factors that cause depression and impaired QoL in younger CHD patients might improve their outcomes [16]. Previous studies usually divided patients into moderate and complex CHDs or whether they had cyanosis instead of more detailed CHD classifications and have had inconsistent results [5,12–15,17]. Given the heterogeneity of cardiac lesions in CHD, the variability in disease burden and lesion severity could be critical factors to different psychological and QoL outcomes. Our study uses a prospective method to evaluate disparate CHDs according to their hemodynamic characteristics and treatment methods. By using more precise classifications, we can obtain a more detailed cause of depression and HRQoL in young age CHD patients.

2. Materials and Methods

Three hundred and fifty patients with structural CHDs visited our hospital as in-patients or out-patients from 1 May to 31 September 2018, and one major caregiver each was asked about participation. Inclusion criteria were (1) confirmed diagnosis by either echocardiography, cardiac catheterization, or open-heart surgery; (2) aged between 6 and 18 years old; (3) no diagnosis with cardiomyopathies or simple congenital valvular regurgitations; (4) accompaniment by one major caregiver, such as a parent, who can read and write; and (5) both the patient and the caregiver being willing to join the study. Exclusion criteria: either the patient or the caregiver were (1) intellectually disabled, (2) unable to read or understand the questionnaire, or (3) unable to finish the questionnaire. Questionnaire of Children Depression Inventory-TW (CDI-TW) was given to the CHD patient or gone through with a research assistant if needed. Child Health Questionnaire—Parent Form 50 (CHQ-PF 50) was given to the caregiver simultaneously. We separated patients and their caregivers while filling out the questionnaire, if possible, to avoid untruthful answers. We reviewed their clinical data, including current age, gender, diagnosis, if the patient had been admitted to the intensive care unit (ICU), date and age of receiving operation, date of previous cardiac catheterization, and date of prior therapeutic cardiac catheterization. We categorized patients according to their management, i.e., admitted to ICU (ICU), received cardiac catheterization (CC), received therapeutic catheterization (TCC), and had operations (OP). The complexity of their CHD condition classified patients into simple CHDs (sCHD), which include pure atrial septal defect (pASD), pure ventricular septal defect (pVSD), pure right-side great arteries anomalies (pRGA), pure left-side great arteries anomalies (pLGA), and pure patent ductus arteriosus (pPDA); and multiple/complex CHD (mCHD), which include multiple/complex CHDs with atrial septal defect (mASD), with ventricular septal defect (mVSD), with right-side great arteries anomalies (mRGA), with left-side great arteries anomalies (mLGA), with venous return anomalies (mVR), or with patent ductus arteriosus (mPDA); and cyanotic heart diseases (CyHD).

2.1. Children Depression Inventory-TW

Children Depression Inventory-TW (CDI-TW) is a Chinese version of the Children Depression Inventory, the most widely validated tool used to evaluate children's depression [18]. The psychometrics in CDI-TW have been examined and validated on Taiwanese youth [19]. CDI-TW is a self-reported questionnaire with 27 different questions to assess various depressive symptoms. Each question has three options indicating different severity of depressive symptoms: 0, 1, and 2. The results are calculated and presented as other depressive aspects, including negative mood (NM), interpersonal problems (IP), ineffectiveness (IN), anhedonia (AN), and negative self-esteem (NE). Adding different aspects would generate a CDI-TW total score (CDI-TW score). A higher score means a more severe depressive condition. CDI total score of more than 20 is used as a cut-off score for detecting depressed patients [20]. We compare the results scores in each element and the total score with those of normal children with same-aged group in Taiwan. We also performed multivariant analysis for CDI-TW score to discover the correlation between CDI-TW and Child Health Questionnaire-parent Form 50 (CHQ-50PF).

2.2. Child Health Questionnaire—Parent Form 50

Child Health Questionnaire—Parent Form 50, a validated parent-proxy questionnaire, scores for 14 concepts (12 multi-item scales and two single items) using the major caregiver of 5 to 18 year-old patients. According to their latest four weeks' experience, they answered the questionnaire to explain patients' health-related quality of life (HRQoL) [21]. The evaluating concepts include physical functioning (PF), role/social-physical (RP), general health perceptions (GH), bodily pain (BP), role/social-emotional/behavioral (REB), parental impact-time (PT), parental impact-emotional (PE), self-esteem (SE), mental health (MH), behavior (BE), family activities (FA), family cohesion (FC), and change in health (CH). Previous reports have validated PF, RP, GH, and BP as a measure of physical health status; and REB, PE, SE, MH, BE, and FC scales are the best measurements for psychosocial conditions. A lower score indicates a more limited physical or psychosocial health condition. Physical summary score (PhS) and psychosocial summary score (PsS) are scored according to 11 concepts, but the scoring manual excluded FA and FC because they are still being worked on. At the same time, we calculated the Phs and PsS total scores according to the scoring manual, compared with scale norms from United States' general young population, and used PhS and PsS scores for further multivariant analysis.

2.3. Statistics

To understand the differences between our patients and the normal population, we compared different aspects of CDI-TW and CHQ-50PF with the aspects of healthy references. We analyzed continuous variables with a summary independent-samples t-test and performed Bonferroni correction as post hoc analysis. $p \leq 0.001$ was defined as statistically significant for these analyses. Furthermore, we analyzed the relationships between CDI-TW score, PhS, and PsS under different conditions to understand their effects on depression and HRQoL in CHD children and adolescents by performing multivariant analysis. The multivariant analysis also analyzed the relationships among PsS, PhS, and CDI-TW to understand the relationship between depressive mood and HRQoL in CHD children and adolescents. The statistical analysis was performed via IBM SPSS Statistics 25 (IBM Corp, New York, NY, USA) and SAS 9.4 (SAS Institute Inc., Cary, NC, USA). $p \leq 0.05$ was defined as statistically significant in the multivariant analysis.

3. Results

A total of 277 patients aged between 9–18 years old (or their major caregivers) completed and returned the questionnaires. The patients' mean age was 15.05 years old. Demographic results are shown in Table 1.

In the CDI-TW questionnaire, while comparing to the normative sample, all groups with pure, multiple/complex cardiac defects and various treatments showed no sign of significant depression in any aspect. However, CyHD children and adolescents had significantly negative attitudes toward their abilities and school performances (statistically significantly higher IN) than norms (Table 2).

In the CHQ-50PF questionnaire, CyHD children and adolescents showed significantly lower scores in almost all the aspects, including FA, PT, nearly all physical metrics (PF, RP, GH scales), and half of the psychosocial (REB, PE, and SE scales) health components. In other words, their physical and psychosocial status had deteriorated significantly, including most of the contributing factors. However, their mental health, general behavior, bodily pain, and family relationships were normal (significantly lower PhS and PsS but normal BP, MH, BE, and FC scales). All the sCHD children and adolescents were generally considered in poor health (lower GH); however, sASD and sVSD had less bodily pain than controls (higher BP) (Table 3). Major caregivers also considered that all the mCHD children and adolescents had poorer health (significantly lower GH). The questionnaire results showed that mVSD and mRGA children had similar scale distributions, with worse self-esteem, physical performance, family activity, parent time, and emotions. The decreased family activity, parent time, and emotions caused limitations in their daily lives and family relationships (statistically significantly lower SE, PF, FA, PT, and PE). In other mCHDs, mPDA had the third most abnormal scales compared to other mCHDs. In addition to health concerns (decreased GH), mASD children and adolescents had more behavioral problems (lower BE); their parents also felt much emotional stress about their health (significantly lower PE). However, they had less bodily pain than the standard samples (significantly lower BP). Groups of mVR had the least abnormal scales compared to the other mCHDs. Besides general health concerns, parents of mLGA and mPDA experienced more time limitations and emotional stress (significantly lower PT and PE). mPDA children and adolescents had less self-esteem than norms (significantly lower SE). Meanwhile, children and adolescents with mVR had fewer emotional problems in school (a considerably higher REB) than norms. Except for mVR children and adolescents, all the mCHD children and adolescents were impaired psychosocially (lower PsS score) compared to the normative sample. At the same time, mVSD and mRGA children and adolescents also had significantly worse physical condition (lower PhS score) related to HRQoL (Table 3).

For CHD children and adolescents who received treatments, ICU and OP groups were in worse psychosocial condition, and had physical limitations, poor general health, decreased self-esteem, immature behavior, interrupted family activity, limited parental time, and emotional stress (significantly lower PsS with lower PF, GH, SE, BE, FA, PT, and PE) compared to the normative sample; meanwhile, the CC group had similar results except a regular physical activity (normal PF). Furthermore, OP also were in significantly poorer psychosocial condition (lower PhS). The TCC group was considered to have poor health. Their parents experienced time limitations and emotional stress due to their health conditions (significantly lower GH, PT, and PE). All the treatment groups exhibited less bodily pain (significantly higher BPs) than norms (Table 3).

Table 1. Demographic data of children and adolescents with congenital heart disease.

	Simple Congenital Heart Diseases							Multiple/Complex Congenital Heart Disease						
	pASD	pVSD	pRGA	pLGA	pPDA	CyHD	mASD	mVSD	mRGA	mLGA	mVR	mPDA
Number	66	58	19	12	11	48	65	82	53	11	9	20
Mean age (year-old) (SD)	13.3 (3.2)	13.8 (3.3)	15.1 (2.7)	13.5 (3.4)	12 (3.8)	13.7 (3.0)	13.1 (3.5)	15.6 (2.8)	13.6 (3.1)	13.6 (3.9)	14.7 (3.2)	13.4 (4.2)
Male/female	25/41	31/27	9/10	9/3	5/6	24/24	28/37	42/40	29/24	6/5	4/5	11/9
Numbers had stayed in ICU (%)	38 (58%)	30 (52%)	2 (11%)	5 (42%)	2 (18%)	37 (77%)	50 (77%)	73(89%)	41 (77%)	9 (82%)	8 (89%)	19(95%)
Numbers had received catheterization (%)	46 (70%)	38 (66%)	13 (68%)	7 (58%)	9 (82%)	38 (79%)	55(85%)	73(89%)	49 (92%)	8 (72%)	8 (89%)	18 (90%)
Number had received therapeutic catheterization (%)	34 (52%)	4 (7%)	11 (58%)	6 (50%)	3 (27%)	5 (10%)	15(23%)	9 (11%)	7 (13%)	2 (18%)	1 (11%)	3 (15%)
Numbers had received operation(%)	13 (20%)	29 (50%)	0 (0%)	5 (42%)	0	43 (90%)	50 (77%)	79 (96%)	46 (87%)	11 (100%)	8 (89%)	20(100%)
Average age when operated (year-old) (range)	3.8 (0–14)	1.4 (0–9)	Nil	0	0	1.4 (0–13)	0.9 (0–6)	0.6 (0–12)	1.0 (0–12)	1.27 (0–14)	0.4 (0–2)	0.8 (0–14)
Average operation times within those had operation (range)	1 (1)	1.1 (1–3)	0	1.4 (1–2)	1 (1–1)	1.7 (1–4)	0.9 (1–2)	1.40 (1–4)	1.5 (1–4)	1.5 (1–2)	1.3 (1–3)	1.6 (1–4)

Abbreviations: Pure atrial septal defect (pASD), pure ventricular septal defect (pVSD), pure right-side great arteries anomalies (pRGA), pure left-side great arteries anomalies (pLGA), pure patent ductus arteriosus (pPDA), multiple/complex CHDs with atrial septal defect (mASD), multiple/complex CHDs with ventricular septal defect (mVSD), multiple/complex CHDs with right-side great arteries anomalies (mRGA), multiple/complex CHDs with left-side great arteries anomalies (mLGA), multiple/complex CHDs with venous return anomalies (mVR), multiple/complex CHDs with patent ductus arteriosus (mPDA), cyanotic heart diseases (CyHD).

Table 2. Children Depression Inventory-TW scores in children and adolescents with congenital heart disease.

	Norm (n = 1148)	Simple Congenital Heart Diseases						Multiple/Complex Congenital Heart Disease						Received Treatments			
		pASD (N = 66)	pVSD (N = 58)	pRGA (N = 19)	pLGA (N = 12)	pPDA (N = 11)	CyHD (N = 48)	mASD (N = 65)	mVSD (N = 82)	mRGA (N = 53)	mLGA (N = 11)	mVR (n = 9)	mPDA (N = 20)	ICU (N = 167)	CC (n = 207)	TCC (N = 80)	OP (N = 146)
CDI-TW Mean(SD)	9.98 (7.29)	9.24 (5.93)	8.79 (5.7)	7.79 (4.81)	9 (5.66)	10.91 (8.09)	11.81 (6.88)	9.74 (6.59)	9.63 (5.95)	10.17 (6.34)	12.18 (6.55)	7.67 (7.12)	9.95 (6.70)	9.8 (6)	9.64 (6.08)	9.29 (5.93)	10.02 (6.16)
NM Mean(SD)	2.21 (2)	1.76 (1.47)	1.9 (1.62)	1.47 (1.17)	2 (2.59)	2.55 (1.86)	2.19 (2.19)	1.83 (1.70)	1.76 (1.47)	1.92 (1.54)	2.09 (1.64)	1.78 (1.64)	1.75 (1.62)	1.84 (1.48)	1.86 (1.56)	1.79 (1.58)	1.87 (1.54)

Table 2. Cont.

		Simple Congenital Heart Diseases						Multiple/Complex Congenital Heart Disease							Received Treatments			
	Norm (n = 1148)	pASD (N = 66)	pVSD (N = 58)	pRGA (N = 19)	pLGA (N = 12)	pPDA (N = 11)	CyHD (N = 48)	mASD (N = 65)	mVSD (N = 82)	mRGA (N = 53)	mLGA (N = 11)	mVR (n = 9)	mPDA (N = 20)	ICU (N = 167)	CC (n = 207)	TCC (N = 80)	OP (N = 146)
IP Mean(SD)	0.77 (1.22)	0.77 (1)	0.66 (0.76)	0.26 (0.56)	0.92 (0.79)	1.55 (2.16)	1.04 (1.17)	1.05 (1.18)	0.82 (0.92)	0.77 (0.97)	1.73 (1.19)	0.89 (1.27)	1.20 (1.32)	0.83 (0.99)	0.85 (1.08)	0.88 (1.29)	0.87 (0.97)
IN Mean(SD)	1.9 (1.82)	2.08 (1.83)	1.59 (1.61)	1.79 (1.47)	1.92 (1.78)	1.64 (1.03)	2.77 (1.59) *	2.09 (1.70)	2.34 (1.69)	2.30 (1.69)	2.82 (1.47)	1.44 (1.24)	2.25 (1.55)	2.33 (1.72)	2.17 (1.73)	2.13 (1.68)	2.32 (1.73)
AN Mean(SD)	3.28 (2.66)	3.09 (2.43)	2.88 (2.54)	2.37 (2.19)	2.33 (2.1)	3 (2.93)	3.85 (2.95)	2.71 (2.49)	2.99 (2.57)	3.42 (2.71)	3.55 (2.42)	2.44 (2.3)	3.35 (2.28)	3.07 (2.49)	2.98 (2.44)	2.83 (2.24)	3.1 (2.57)
NE Mean(SD)	1.82 (1.82)	1.55 (1.25)	1.78 (1.33)	1.89 (1.33)	1.83 (1.59)	2.18 (1.78)	1.98 (1.62)	2.06 (1.55)	1.74 (1.23)	1.77 (1.35)	2.00 (1.61)	2 (1.66)	1.40 (1.23)	1.77 (1.38)	1.81 (1.41)	1.68 (1.35)	1.86 (1.43)
Depressed Patients & Number(%)	Nil	4 (6.06)	4 (6.90)	1 (5.26)	0	1 (9.09)	7 (14.58)	5 (7.69)	5 (6.10)	5 (9.43)	1 (9.09)	1 (11.11)	1 (5.00)	11 (6.59)	14 (6.76)	4 (5.00)	11 (7.53)

Abbreviations: CDI-TW total score (CDI-TW), negative mood (NM), interpersonal problems (IP), ineffectiveness (IN), anhedonia (AN), negative self-esteem (NE), pure atrial septal defect (pASD), pure ventricular septal defect (pVSD), pure right-side great arteries anomalies (pRGA), pure left-side great arteries anomalies (pLGA), pure patent ductus arteriosus (pPDA), multiple/complex CHDs with atrial septal defect (mASD), multiple/complex CHDs with ventricular septal defect (mVSD), multiple/complex CHDs with right-side great arteries anomalies (mRGA), multiple/complex CHDs with left-side great arteries anomalies (mLGA), multiple/complex CHDs with venous return anomalies (mVR), multiple/complex CHDs with patent ductus arteriosus (mPDA) cyanotic heart diseases (CyHD), patient had admitted to ICU (ICU), patients had received cardiac catheterization (CC), patients had received therapeutic catheterization (TCC), patients had received operations (OP). & Depressed patients are defined as CDI-TW more than 20. * $p \leq 0.001$.

Table 3. Child Health Questionnaire—Parent Form 50 scores in children and adolescents with congenital heart disease.

		Simple Congenital Heart Diseases						Multiple/Complex Congenital Heart Disease							Received Treatments			
	Norm (n = 391)	pASD (N = 66)	pVSD (N = 58)	pRGA (N = 19)	pLGA (N = 12)	pPDA (N = 11)	CyHD (N = 48)	mASD (N = 65)	mVSD (N = 82)	mRGA (N = 53)	mLGA (N = 11)	mVR (n = 9)	mPDA (N = 20)	ICU (N = 167)	CC (n = 207)	TCC (N = 80)	OP (N = 146)
PF Mean (SD)	96.1 (13.9)	96.75 (6.64)	94.01 (16.61)	98.82 (3)	86.88 (16.8)	96.45 (11.76)	82.02 (19.9) *	91.79 (14.58)	87.56 (18.11) *	84.88 (19.5) *	93.38 (12.94)	95 (9.05)	90.77 (18.14)	91.5 (16.03) *	92.68 (14.58)	94.26 (15.59)	90.62 (15.23) *
RP Mean (SD)	93.6 (18.6)	97.17 (8.71)	95.08 (17.74)	100 (0)	90.08 (15.31)	93.91 (20.2)	81.7 (22.71) *	90.90 (18.13)	86.83 (21.96)	85.66 (22.23)	84.68 (24.3)	98.11 (5.67)	81.48 (26.07)	90.6 (19.49)	91.93 (18.14)	94.31 (17.08)	89.82 (19.22)

Table 3. Cont.

	Norm (n = 391)	Simple Congenital Herat Diseases						Multiple/Complex Congenital Heart Disease							Received Treatments				
		pASD (N = 66)	pVSD (N = 58)	pRGA (N = 19)	pLGA (N = 12)	pPDA (N = 11)	CyHD (N = 48)	mASD (N = 65)	mVSD (N = 82)	mRGA (N = 53)	mLGA (N = 11)	mVR (n = 9)	mPDA (N = 20)	ICU (N = 167)	CC (n = 207)	TCC (N = 80)	OP (N = 146)
GH Mean (SD)	73 (17.3)	61.74 (14.77) *	61.98 (13.57) *	58.16 (12.72) *	50 (13.98) *	49.09 (20.23) *	50.21 (16.04) *	57.62 (13.7) *	53.54 (15.51) *	51.60 (14.7) *	50.45 (15.72) *	50.56 (9.17) *	50.50 (18.27) *	56.26 (15.28) *	56.98 (15.46) *	57.31 (16.36) *	55.31 (15.24) *
BP Mean (SD)	81.7 (19)	96.06 (10.21) *	90.52 (13.43) *	92.63 (14.08)	93.33 (16.14)	92.73 (9.05)	88.33 (15.89)	91.69 (15.67) *	91.22 (16.05) *	90.75 (15.17) *	86.36 (21.11)	86.67 (13.23)	93.00 (17.5)	92.34 (14.43) *	92.85 (13.51) *	94.38 (12.31) *	92.05 (14.52) *
FA Mean (SD)	89.7 (18.6)	84.72 (19.99)	86.57 (17.17)	84.65 (15.84)	77.78 (23.79)	78.79 (27.48)	76.48 (17.2) *	84.74 (17.87)	81.30 (18.23) *	79.80 (18.28) *	74.24 (22.03)	81.02 (14.45)	79.58 (22.98)	83.68 (18.89) *	83.35 (19.14) *	83.33 (22.36)	83.53 (17.69)
REB Mean (SD)	92.5 (18.6)	96.74 (7.87)	91.3 (20.61)	97.61 (6.07)	88.69 (16.68)	100 (0)	79.63 (23.85) *	89.78 (19.19)	85.33 (22.25)	84.09 (22.45)	79.61 (27.33)	100 (0) *	80.95 (27.9)	88.22 (21.07)	90.33 (19.14)	94.79 (14.24)	87.21 (21.13)
PT Mean (SD)	87.8 (19.9)	83.13 (22.65)	83.18 (26.45)	82.86 (22.8)	73.75 (24.94)	69.33 (27.37)	69.38 (26.35) *	79.44 (23.17)	76.05 (25.38) *	73.95 (25.35) *	66.42 (32.99)	76.26 (21.96)	72.58 (31.22) *	76.29 (26.53) *	77.77 (25.88) *	77.68 (25.65) *	76.1 (26.05) *
PE Mean (SD)	80.3 (19.1)	75.51 (19.82)	73.42 (27.42)	75.88 (22.72)	67.36 (24.48)	66.67 (25.28)	61.63 (25.19) *	67.82 (23.61) *	65.65 (24.16) *	65.57 (23.57) *	47.73 (33.14) *	64.81 (23.12)	54.17 (33.61)	67.61 (24.72) *	69.2 (24.75) *	68.85 (25.15) *	67.35 (25.02) *
SE Mean (SD)	79.8 (17.5)	73.04 (16.31)	74.78 (17.46)	77.63 (17.14)	74.31 (17.21)	79.92 (15.57)	68.58 (17.45) *	73.08 (18.85)	72.31 (18.13) *	70.36 (16.94) *	65.15 (16.7)	75.93 (18.61)	66.67 (19.78)	70.83 (17.1) *	72.1 (17.42) *	73.85 (16.82)	70.86 (17.33) *
MH Mean (SD)	78.5 (13.2)	81.36 (16.14)	79.22 (14.68)	78.68 (11.65)	75.42 (16.71)	76.82 (17.5)	74.27 (13.37)	76.00 (13.38)	77.13 (14.66)	75.47 (15.45)	70.45 (10.11)	76.11 (6.97)	71.75 (11.84)	77.57 (14.69)	78.07 (14.91)	79.44 (15.81)	77.4 (13.96)

Table 3. Cont.

	Norm (n = 391)	Simple Congenital Herat Diseases						Multiple/Complex Congenital Heart Disease								Received Treatments			
		pASD (N = 66)	pVSD (N = 58)	pRGA (N = 19)	pLGA (N = 12)	pPDA (N = 11)	CyHD (N = 48)	mASD (N = 65)	mVSD (N = 82)	mRGA (N = 53)	mLGA (N = 11)	mVR (n = 9)	mPDA (N = 20)	ICU (N = 167)	CC (n = 207)	TCC (N = 80)	OP (N = 146)
BE Mean (SD)	75.6 (16.7)	70.61 (16.58)	74.57 (15.74)	73.42 (13.75)	67.08 (18.02)	67.27 (19.67)	69.38 (13.98)	67.77 (16.3) *	70.24 (15.75)	70.19 (15.9)	66.82 (16.17)	69.44 (22.14)	68.25 (15.58)	69.28 (15.94) *	70.51 (16.16) *	69.69 (16.96)	70.14 (15.76) *
FC Mean (SD)	72.3 (21.6)	68.33 (22.94)	68.62 (22.1)	69.74 (20.98)	67.5 (26.5)	78.64 (15.83)	65.94 (22.64)	66.46 (23.21)	70.12 (21.76)	67.83 (21.54)	63.18 (23.9)	70.56 (19.44)	67.75 (25.26)	69.91 (22.57)	69.71 (22.63)	67.56 (23.15)	71.1 (22.23)
PhS Mean (SD)	53 (8.8)	54.14 (4.3)	52.14 (8.49)	53.82 (3.32)	48.4 (7.31)	50.36 (8.68)	45.03 (11.25) *	50.84 (8.36)	48.06 (10.45) *	47.00 (11.06) *	47.99 (10.38)	50.56 (4.41)	47.90 (11.87)	50.38 (9.24)	50.98 (8.57)	51.87 (8.63)	49.79 (8.99) *
PsS Mean (SD)	51.2 (9.1)	49.52 (8.96)	49.61 (10.01)	50.2 (7.58)	46.84 (7.86)	48.07 (9.73)	45.04 (8.36)	47.04 (9.09) *	47.10 (8.99) *	46.46 (8.73) *	41.20 (11.68)	48.19 (8.48)	43.22 (12.32) *	46.87 (9.36) *	47.68 (9.39) *	48.26 (9.32)	46.94 (9.08) *

Abbreviations: CDI-TW total score (CDI-TW), negative mood (NM), interpersonal problems (IP), ineffectiveness (IN), anhedonia (AN), negative self-esteem (NE), pure atrial septal defect (pASD), pure ventricular septal defect (pVSD), pure right-side great arteries anomalies (pRGA), pure left-side great arteries anomalies (pLGA), pure patent ductus arteriosus (pPDA), multiple/complex CHDs with atrial septal defect (mASD), multiple/complex CHDs with ventricular septal defect (mVSD), multiple/complex CHDs with right-side great arteries anomalies (mRGA), multiple/complex CHDs with left-side great arteries anomalies (mLGA), multiple/complex CHDs with venous return anomalies (mVR), multiple/complex CHDs with patent ductus arteriosus (mPDA), cyanotic heart diseases (CyHD), patient had admitted to ICU (ICU), patients had received cardiac catheterization (CC), patients had received therapeutic catheterization (TCC), patients had received operations (OP), physical functioning (PF), role/social-physical (RP), general health perceptions (GH), bodily pain (BP), role/social emotional/behavioral (REB), parental impact-time (PT), parental impact-emotional (PE), self-esteem (SE), mental health (MH), behavior (BE), family activities (FA), family cohesion (FC), change in health (CH), physical summary score (PhS), and psychosocial summary score (PsS). * $p \leq 0.001$.

Having CyHD and VSD significantly affected patients' depressive condition (CDI-TW) among all CHD patients in multivariant analysis (Table 4). The presence of CyHD caused a higher CDI-TW score compared to non-CyHD (beta: 5.62, SE: 2.0, p = 0.004); instead, having a VSD resulted in a lower CDI-TW score than not having a VSD (beta: −4.059, SE: 1.934, p = 0.037). The patients' physical condition (PhS score) was significantly related to CyHD. Having stayed in the ICU, and CHD children and adolescents only having ASD caused lower PhS total scores. Moreover, the factors of CyHD and having stayed in ICU also significantly caused significantly lower PsS scores. When evaluating the relationship between patients' depression, physical condition, and psychosocial condition, the depressive mood was significantly related to poorer psychosocial condition among CHD patients. (beta: −0.33, SE: 0.06, p < 0.0001) (Table 5).

Table 4. Multivariant analysis for the relationships between multiple factors and Children Depression Inventory-TW total score, physical summary score, or psychosocial summary score in Child Health Questionnaire—Parent Form 50.

	CDI-TW			PhS			PsS		
	Beta	(SE)	p-Value	Beta	(SE)	p-Value	Beta	(SE)	p-Value
Age	−0.099	0.162	0.539	0.111	0.144	0.441	−0.108	0.172	0.531
Male gender	−0.884	1.061	0.405	0.033	0.942	0.972	−0.765	1.128	0.498
ASD vs Non-ASD	1.535	2.260	0.498	−0.385	2.006	0.848	−1.481	2.402	0.538
pASD vs other CHDs	0.741	2.464	0.764	−4.756	2.187	0.031 *	0.652	2.619	0.804
VSD vs Non-VSD	−4.059	1.934	0.037*	−3.103	1.716	0.072	2.874	2.055	0.163
pVSD vs other CHD	4.130	2.927	0.159	−2.457	2.598	0.345	−3.582	3.111	0.251
RGA vs non-RGA	1.272	2.076	0.541	−3.058	1.843	0.098	−2.342	2.207	0.289
pRGA vs other CHDs	−1.077	3.369	0.749	−1.075	2.990	0.719	0.590	3.580	0.869
LGA vs Non-LGA	3.625	3.258	0.267	−3.877	2.892	0.181	−5.033	3.463	0.147
pLGA vs other CHDs	−2.350	4.592	0.609	−5.263	4.076	0.198	0.918	4.881	0.851
VR vs Non-VR	−4.357	6.266	0.488	2.473	5.561	0.657	7.609	6.660	0.254
PDA vs Non-PDA	−0.203	2.472	0.935	−2.826	2.194	0.199	−3.420	2.627	0.194
pPDA vs other CHDs	4.892	4.513	0.279	−4.475	4.005	0.265	−1.000	4.796	0.835
CyHD vs Non-CyHD	5.616	1.952	0.004 **	−7.411	1.727	0.000 ***	−4.487	2.074	0.031 *
ICU vs Non-ICU	1.423	1.860	0.445	−3.547	1.648	0.034 *	−3.977	1.977	0.045 *
TCC vs non-TCC	−0.537	1.584	0.735	−0.793	1.403	0.587	1.026	1.684	0.543
OP vs Non-OP	1.271	1.922	0.509	1.979	1.699	0.269	0.876	2.042	0.668

Abbreviation: CDI-TW total score (CDI-TW), physical summary score (PsS), psychosocial summary score (PhS), atrial septal defect (ASD), pure atrial septal defect (pASD), ventricular septal defect (VSD), pure ventricular septal defect (pVSD), congenital heart disease (CHD), right-side great arteries anomalies (RGA), pure right-side great arteries anomalies (pRGA), left-side great arteries anomalies (LGA), pure left-side great arteries anomalies (pLGA), venous return anomalies (VR), patent ductus arteriosus (PDA), pure patent ductus arteriosus (pPDA), cyanotic heart diseases (CyHD), the patient had admitted to ICU (ICU), patients had received therapeutic catheterization (TCC), patients had received operations (OP).* $p \leq 0.05$. ** $p \leq 0.01$. *** $p \leq 0.001$.

Table 5. Multivariant analysis for the relationship between physical summary score, and psychosocial summary score in Child Health Questionnaire—Parent Form 50.

	CDI-TW Score		
	Beta	(SE)	p-Value
PhS	0.01	0.06	0.852
PsS	−0.33	0.06	<0.0001 *

Abbreviation: CDI-TW total score (CDI-TW), physical summary score (PsS), psychosocial summary score (PhS), * $p \leq 0.001$.

4. Discussion

Our study presented the effects of detailed cardiac defects and management on psychological status and HRQoL in CHD children and adolescents. We also showed the relationships between depression, physical, and psychosocial conditions within those patients. Cyanotic heart disease children demonstrated "ineffectiveness," a depressive scale, and the worst HRQoL with impaired physical and psychosocial healthiness. Their health condition caused physical limitations and emotional changes, resulting in poor daily functioning and significantly impacting their personal lives, family lives, and school lives. Moreover, children and adolescents with CyHD had poorer self-esteem, their parents worried about their health more, and the disease impacted their parents' lives. Multiple/complex CHDs, such as mVSD and mRGA, and those who received interventions, also showed similar results. Among received treatment groups, those who underwent therapeutic catheterization had the best HRQoL without obvious physical and psychosocial impairments. Only their parents' lives were affected. On the contrary, those who received operations had significantly impaired physical and psychosocial status, along with CC and ICU stay groups. Their health condition afflicted their school and family lives, causing poorer self-esteem and more aggressive behavior. None of the groups showed depressive or mental health impairments in our study. Bodily pain was not seen in CHD children and adolescents and was even better or equal to the norms in most groups. Our results provide a more detailed overview and reflect the previous finding that more complex CHD, more hospital admissions, and more cardiac surgeries lead to poor QoL in CHD children and adolescents [22].

There was no difference between self-reporting and parent-proxy results regarding anxiety and depression in this study. For CDI-TW, a self-report questionnaire, there was no statistically significant difference in CDI-TW total score, a generally depressive symptom score, among CHD groups. Additionally, there was no statistically significant decreased MH, which represents a feeling of anxiety and depression, according to CHD-50PF, a parent-proxy report questionnaire. Varni et al. proved the reliability and validity of parent-proxy reporting in children [23,24]. The self and parent-proxy responses to the questionnaires are correlated [22]. Multiple reports have shown that the severity of CHD has positive relationships with depressive and psychological conditions [25,26]. Since a higher score in CDI-TW indicates a more severe depressive condition, almost all the scores in CDI-TW were high, including incredibly significantly higher IN, in CyHD, which is the most severe CHD.

Children's depressiveness and HRQoL is related to disease severity and condition after treatment. Simple CHDs had no depressive indicators and fewer QoL concerns. There were noticeable scale differences between sCHD and mCHD, except for mVR and those who received treatments. There were fewer significantly different scales using the CHQ-50PF in mVR, whose QoL scale scores were nearly the same as those of the sCHD groups. In our study, the most common disease in mVR was partial anomalous pulmonary venous return anomalies (PAPVR), classified as multiple cardiac defects, because it always has at least one more cardiac defect, i.e., an atrial defect. PAPVR children usually do not have heart symptoms or need to have them corrected at a very young age [8]. It was reasonable for mVR patients to have similar results to sCHDs. At the questionnaire age, they usually have no or only minimal heart symptoms. Children with venous return anomalies did not have a depressive condition. They had average general HRQoL, or even improved activity regarding their motions or behavior; however, their parents still believed their children's health was poor.

In children with more severe CHDs, such as CyHD, those who had multiple cardiac defects, and those who received treatments, their parents reported limited personal time, limited family activity, and experienced a great deal of emotional stress due to their children's condition. When taking care of CHD patients, parents bore more psychological stress, depression, and anxiety because of the uncertain future [27,28]. Parental mental health is crucial regarding HRQoL in CHD children [29]. More severe CHDs would cause worse parental health than sCHDs and worsen their HRQoL. In contrast, mVR, also known as mCHDs, had fewer impacts on parental mental health. When taking care of those mCHDs, parents had less or the same stress as those taking care of healthy children. Therefore, the parents have mental health status just like other ordinary parents.

Our results showed generally significantly decreased general heath in every group. There was no bodily pain or discomfort in CHD children and adolescents; surprisingly, CHD children felt less bodily pain/discomfort than average children. Instead of musculoskeletal pain, chest pain due to arrhythmia and heart failure were the most frequent painful sensations related to the heart in adult congenital heart disease patients. Generally, people regard CHDs as severe diseases in children due to their high mortality and morbidity. Parents usually suffer from much stress about their children's health. Even if the cardiac defect is not hemodynamically significant or has no severe symptoms before or after the surgery, parents still worry more about children's health. Due to parental concern, CHD children usually receive better care and even overprotection unrelated to the condition's severity [30,31]. In addition, their physical activity was usually limited [32,33]. Those factors would further decrease the chance of developing musculoskeletal pain or physical discomfort.

There was lower self-esteem in most CHD children and adolescents except in sCHD patients, relatively simple mCHD children, and TCC patients. Self-esteem is a personal characteristic that facilitates a positive perception of stress [34]. Poor self-esteem has been related to poor QoL and depression [35,36]. Lower self-esteem was previously found in CHD patients and correlated with disease severity, but improved after an operation [37,38]. Our results partially reflect previous results, though the poor self-esteem did not recover even received treatments, especially the open-heart surgery. That might have been caused by the relatively unstable condition of CHD children and the need for long-term following up. sCHDs, mASD, mLGA, mVR, and TCC children and adolescents presented good self-esteem in line with the normal population.

Cyanotic heart disease is the most severe structural cardiac defect that presents from birth. Disease severity and the perceived disease severity have been reported to be correlated with patients' depressiveness, psychosocial condition, and HRQoL [16,26,37,39–42]. CyHD children were aware of being different from other children due to regular and frequent hospital visits. The divergence between them and other children would affect their relationships and cause impaired psychosocial bonds. Strong friendship bonding could also be harder for them owing to their cyanotic appearance. These results affect their emotional, academic, cognitive, and behavioral functioning and lead to a more depressive mood and worse QoL. Besides disease severity, HRQoL is also impacted by the cardiac symptoms [15], and most evident cardiac symptoms need ICU treatment. In our multivariant analysis, having CyHD, the most severe CHD with the most prominent cardiac symptoms, was the main factor for a worse CDI-TW score, poor physical condition, and poor psychosocial status according to CHQ-50PF. Having previous ICU stays was also a factor for poor physical and psychosocial scores.

In our multivariant analysis, physical health was the factor that most affected CDI-TW total score, which indicates an individual's depressive status. Increased physical activity could reduce or prevent depressive symptoms and major depressive disorder [43,44]. Morgan et al. described that ceasing all forms of vigorous physical activity can cause an individual to develop depressive symptoms [45]. Exercise capacity was also shown to predict future mortality and morbidity in CHD patients [46]. With the importance of physical exercise, guidelines have included effective exercising in treatment guidelines for affective disorders [47]. Our results provide evidence that physical activity is essential and directly relates to the depressiveness in CHD children.

The strengths of this study included a sizeable total sample size, a high parent-patient paired response rate, an accurate disease classification, and using validated questionnaires with normative data across a wide age span. The study's limitations were a lack of broad geographic, racial, and ethnic diversity, a cross-sectional design, and a single medical center. In addition, CDI-TW could only pick up the most severely depressed patients and has poor sensitivity to subtle and non-clinical conditions. Moreover, CHQ-50PF is a generic instrument instead of a cardiac-specific tool like the Pediatric Cardiac Quality of Life Inventory (PCQLI) [48]. However, PCQLI does not have a validated Chinese translation. Furthermore, CHQ-50PF is a parent-proxy questionnaire that could cause a bias due to a potential difference between children and parent proxy reports [49]. Further investigations could focus on the impacts of QoL and depressive conditions on different CyHDs by using a cardiac-specific tool and insert more broad measurements for psychological functioning. Future analysis could also use a more detailed classification of age and gender to see the differences. Moreover, with the development of molecular biology, there are several new methods with which to understand people's genetics, such as whole-genome sequencing. With the new methods, one could also find the relationships between gene variants and different cardiac defects and related depressive and HRQoL conditions.

5. Conclusions

Our study showed impaired psychological condition and decreased HRQoL were more prevalent in children and adolescents who had CyHD, had received treatments, or had mCHD, except for those who were mVR. Among them, children and adolescents who received treatments, except for operations, had very few different physical status indicators from the normative sample. CyHD had the most impact on children's depressive mood and HRQoL. Simple CHD and mVR children could have a near-normal depressive and HRQoL status. Due to the advances in CHD treatments, there are rising numbers of CHD children reaching adolescence and adulthood, which is causing an increasing global burden [50]. Identifying the impaired HRQoL in CHD children might potentially improve the outcomes [16]. For better patient care, we should pay more attention to psychological and HRQoL condition in children with cyanotic heart diseases, in those with more complex congenital heart diseases, and in those who require management, since they are young, and encourage their families to let them live normal lives. For sCHD and mVR children and adolescents, we do not need to over-worry about their depressive and QoL conditions. We should treat them as near-normal children.

Supplementary Materials: The following supporting information can be downloaded at: https://www.mdpi.com/article/10.3390/children9040578/s1, The questionnaire and disease classification data are available in supplementary file.

Author Contributions: Conceptualization, H.-C.L. and C.-W.L.; formal analysis, C.-H.C. and H.-C.L.; writing—original draft, H.-C.L. and C.-W.L.; writing—review and editing, H.-C.L.; funding acquisition, H.-C.L., H.-T.C. and M.-S.H.; project administration, H.-C.L., H.-T.C. and M.-S.H. All authors have read and agreed to the published version of the manuscript.

Funding: This research was funded by Chang-Gung Memorial Hospital, Linkou branch, grant number CMRPG3G1331.

Institutional Review Board Statement: The study was conducted in accordance with the Declaration of Helsinki and approved by the Institutional Review Board (or Ethics Committee) of Chang Gung Memorial Hospital Linko branch (protocol code 201700458B0. Date of approval: 18 July 2017).

Informed Consent Statement: Informed consent was obtained from all subjects involved in the study. Written informed consent has been obtained from the patient(s) to publish this paper.

Data Availability Statement: The data used in this study are available in Supplementary Materials.

Acknowledgments: We also thank Lin Yu-Xuan for helping to collect the questionnaire from the patients.

Conflicts of Interest: The authors declare no conflict of interest. The funders had no role in the design of the study; in the collection, analyses, or interpretation of data; in the writing of the manuscript, or in the decision to publish the results.

References

1. Stout, K.K.; Daniels, C.J.; Aboulhosn, J.A.; Bozkurt, B.; Broberg, C.S.; Colman, J.M.; Crumb, S.R.; Dearani, S.F.; Fuller, S.; Gurvitz, M.; et al. 2018 AHA/ACC Guideline for the Management of Adults with Congenital Heart Disease. *J. Am. Coll. Cardiol.* **2019**, *73*, e81–e192. [CrossRef]
2. Bhatt, A.B.; Foster, E.; Kuehl, K.; Alpert, J.; Brabeck, S.; Crumb, S.; Davidson, W.R., Jr.; Ering, M.G.; Ghoshhajra, B.B.; Karamlou, T.; et al. Congenital heart disease in the older adult: A scientific statement from the American Heart Association. *Circulation* **2015**, *131*, 1884–1931. [CrossRef] [PubMed]
3. Chong, L.S.H.; Fitzgerald, D.A.; Craig, J.C.; Manera, K.E.; Hanson, C.S.; Celermajer, D.; Ayer, J.; Kasparian, N.A.; Tong, A. Children's experiences of congenital heart disease: A systematic review of qualitative studies. *Eur. J. Pediatr.* **2018**, *177*, 319–336. [CrossRef] [PubMed]
4. Lui, G.K.; Saidi, A.; Bhatt, A.B.; Burchill, L.J.; Deen, J.F.; Earing, M.G.; Gewitz, M.; Ginns, J.; Kay, J.D.; Kim, Y.Y.; et al. Diagnosis and Management of Noncardiac Complications in Adults with Congenital Heart Disease: A Scientific Statement from the American Heart Association. *Circulation* **2017**, *136*, e348–e392. [CrossRef] [PubMed]
5. Jackson, J.L.; Leslie, C.E.; Hondorp, S.N. Depressive and Anxiety Symptoms in Adult Congenital Heart Disease: Prevalence, Health Impact and Treatment. *Prog. Cardiovasc. Dis.* **2018**, *61*, 294–299. [CrossRef]
6. Kessler, R.C.; Bromet, E.J. The epidemiology of depression across cultures. *Annu. Rev. Public Health* **2013**, *34*, 119–138. [CrossRef]
7. Gan, Y.; Gong, Y.; Tong, X.; Sun, H.; Cong, Y.; Dong, X.; Wang, Y.; Xu, X.; Yin, X.; Deng, J.; et al. Depression and the risk of coronary heart disease: A meta-analysis of prospective cohort studies. *BMC Psychiatry* **2014**, *14*, 371. [CrossRef]
8. Alsoufi, B.; Cai, S.; Van Arsdell, G.S.; Williams, W.G.; Caldarone, C.A.; Coles, J.G. Outcomes After Surgical Treatment of Children with Partial Anomalous Pulmonary Venous Connection. *Ann. Thorac. Surg.* **2007**, *84*, 2020–2026. [CrossRef] [PubMed]
9. Felce, D.; Perry, J. Quality of life: Its definition and measurement. *Res. Dev. Disabil.* **1995**, *16*, 51–74. [CrossRef]
10. Cassidy, A.R.; Ilardi, D.; Bowen, S.R.; Hampton, L.E.; Heinrich, K.P.; Loman, M.M.; Sanz, J.H.; Wolfe, K.R. Congenital heart disease: A primer for the pediatric neuropsychologist. *Child Neuropsychol.* **2018**, *24*, 859–902. [CrossRef]
11. Ebrahim, S. Clinical and public health perspectives and applications of health-related quality of life measurement. *Soc. Sci. Med.* **1995**, *41*, 1383–1394. [CrossRef]
12. Landolt, M.A.; Valsangiacomo Buechel, E.R.; Latal, B. Health-related quality of life in children and adolescents after open-heart surgery. *J. Pediatr.* **2008**, *152*, 349–355. [CrossRef] [PubMed]
13. Drakouli, M.; Petsios, K.; Giannakopoulou, M.; Patiraki, E.; Voutoufianaki, I.; Matziou, V. Determinants of quality of life in children and adolescents with CHD: A systematic review. *Cardiol. Young* **2015**, *25*, 1027–1036. [CrossRef] [PubMed]
14. Denniss, D.L.; Sholler, G.F.; Costa, D.S.J.; Winlaw, D.S.; Kasparian, N.A. Need for Routine Screening of Health-Related Quality of Life in Families of Young Children with Complex Congenital Heart Disease. *J. Pediatr.* **2019**, *205*, 21–28. [CrossRef] [PubMed]
15. Bertoletti, J.; Marx, G.C.; Hattge, S.P., Jr.; Pellanda, L.C. Health-related quality of life in adolescents with congenital heart disease. *Cardiol. Young* **2015**, *25*, 526–532. [CrossRef] [PubMed]
16. Uzark, K.; Jones, K.; Slusher, J.; Limbers, C.A.; Burwinkle, T.M.; Varni, J.W. Quality of life in children with heart disease as perceived by children and parents. *Pediatrics* **2008**, *121*, e1060–e1067. [CrossRef]
17. Lee, J.S.; Cinanni, N.; Cristofaro, N.D.; Lee, S.; Dillenburg, R.; Adamo, K.B.; Mondal, T.; Barrowman, N.; Shanmugam, G.; Timmons, B.W.; et al. Parents of Very Young Children with Congenital Heart Defects Report Good Quality of Life for Their Children and Families Regardless of Defect Severity. *Pediatr. Cardiol.* **2020**, *41*, 46–53. [CrossRef]
18. Kovacs, M. Rating scales to assess depression in school-aged children. *Acta Paedopsychiatr.* **1981**, *46*, 305–315.
19. Chen, S.H. *Children's Depression Inventory—Taiwan Version Technical Manual*, 1st ed.; Psychological Publishing Co.: New Taipei City, Taiwan, 2008.
20. Bang, Y.R.; Park, J.H.; Kim, S.H. Cut-Off Scores of the Children's Depression Inventory for Screening and Rating Severity in Korean Adolescents. *Psychiatry Investig.* **2015**, *12*, 23–28. [CrossRef]
21. HealthActCHQ. *The CHQ Scoring and Interpretation Manual*; HealthActCHQ: Boston, MA, USA, 2013.
22. Wray, J.; Franklin, R.; Brown, K.; Cassedy, A.; Marino, B.S. Testing the Pediatric Cardiac Quality of Life Inventory in the United Kingdom. *Acta Paediatr.* **2013**, *102*, e68–e73. [CrossRef]
23. Varni, J.W.; Limbers, C.A.; Burwinkle, T.M. Parent proxy-report of their children's health-related quality of life: An analysis of 13,878 parents' reliability and validity across age subgroups using the PedsQL 4.0 Generic Core Scales. *Health Qual. Life Outcomes* **2007**, *5*, 2. [CrossRef] [PubMed]
24. Sprangers, M.A.; Aaronson, N.K. The role of health care providers and significant others in evaluating the quality of life of patients with chronic disease: A review. *J. Clin. Epidemiol.* **1992**, *45*, 743–760. [CrossRef]
25. Amedro, P.; Dorka, R.; Moniotte, S.; Guillaumont, S.; Fraisse, A.; Kreitmann, B.; Borm, B.; Bertet, H.; Barrea, C.; Ovaert, C.; et al. Quality of Life of Children with Congenital Heart Diseases: A Multicenter Controlled Cross-Sectional Study. *Pediatr. Cardiol.* **2015**, *36*, 1588–1601. [CrossRef]
26. DeMaso, D.R.; Calderon, J.; Taylor, G.A.; Holland, J.E.; Stopp, C.; White, M.T.; Bellinger, D.C.; Rivkin, M.J.; Wypij, D.; Newburger, J.W. Psychiatric Disorders in Adolescents with Single Ventricle Congenital Heart Disease. *Pediatrics* **2017**, *139*, e20162241. [CrossRef]
27. Wray, J.; Cassedy, A.; Ernst, M.M.; Franklin, R.C.; Brown, K.; Marino, B.S. Psychosocial functioning of parents of children with heart disease-describing the landscape. *Eur. J. Pediatr.* **2018**, *177*, 1811–1821. [CrossRef] [PubMed]

28. Cohen, M.; Mansoor, D.; Gagin, R.; Lorber, A. Perceived parenting style, self-esteem and psychological distress in adolescents with heart disease. *Psychol. Health Med.* 2008, *13*, 381–388. [CrossRef] [PubMed]
29. Dulfer, K.; Duppen, N.; Van Dijk, A.P.J.; Kuipers, I.M.; Van Domburg, R.T.; Verhulst, F.C.; der Ende, J.V.; Helbing, W.A.; Utens, E.M.W.J. Parental mental health moderates the efficacy of exercise training on health-related quality of life in adolescents with congenital heart disease. *Pediatr. Cardiol.* 2015, *36*, 33–40. [CrossRef]
30. Garson, A., Jr.; Benson, R.S.; Ivler, L.; Patton, C. Parental reactions to children with congenital heart disease. *Child Psychiatry Hum. Dev.* 1978, *9*, 86–94. [CrossRef] [PubMed]
31. Ong, L.; Nolan, R.P.; Irvine, J.; Kovacs, A.H. Parental overprotection and heart-focused anxiety in adults with congenital heart disease. *Int. J. Behav. Med.* 2011, *18*, 260–267. [CrossRef] [PubMed]
32. Muller, J.; Amberger, T.; Berg, A.; Goeder, D.; Remmele, J.; Oberhoffer, R.; Ewert, P.; Hager, A. Physical activity in adults with congenital heart disease and associations with functional outcomes. *Heart* 2017, *103*, 1117–1121. [CrossRef]
33. Werner, H.; Latal, B.; Valsangiacomo Buechel, E.; Beck, I.; Landolt, M.A. Health-related quality of life after open-heart surgery. *J. Pediatr.* 2014, *164*, 254–258.e1. [CrossRef] [PubMed]
34. Lazarus, R.S.; Folkman, S. *Stress, Appraisal, and Coping*; Springer Publishing Company: New York, NY, USA, 1984; p. 460.
35. Sowislo, J.F.; Orth, U. Does low self-esteem predict depression and anxiety? A meta-analysis of longitudinal studies. *Psychol. Bull.* 2013, *139*, 213–240. [CrossRef]
36. Ernst, M.M.; Marino, B.S.; Cassedy, A.; Piazza-Waggoner, C.; Franklin, R.C.; Brown, K.; Wray, J. Biopsychosocial Predictors of Quality of Life Outcomes in Pediatric Congenital Heart Disease. *Pediatr. Cardiol.* 2018, *39*, 79–88. [CrossRef]
37. Cohen, M.; Mansoor, D.; Langut, H.; Lorber, A. Quality of life, depressed mood, and self-esteem in adolescents with heart disease. *Psychosom. Med.* 2007, *69*, 313–318. [CrossRef]
38. Wray, J.; Sensky, T. How does the intervention of cardiac surgery affect the self-perception of children with congenital heart disease? *Child Care Health Dev.* 1998, *24*, 57–72. [CrossRef]
39. Moon, J.R.; Song, J.; Huh, J.; Kang, I.-S.; Park, S.W.; Chang, S.-A.; Yang, J.-H.; Jun, T.-G. The Relationship between Parental Rearing Behavior, Resilience, and Depressive Symptoms in Adolescents with Congenital Heart Disease. *Front. Cardiovasc. Med.* 2017, *4*, 55. [CrossRef] [PubMed]
40. Kasmi, L.; Calderon, J.; Montreuil, M.; Geronikola, N.; Lambert, V.; Belli, E.; Bonnet, D.; Kalfa, D. Neurocognitive and Psychological Outcomes in Adults with Dextro-Transposition of the Great Arteries Corrected by the Arterial Switch Operation. *Ann. Thorac. Surg.* 2018, *105*, 830–836. [CrossRef]
41. Wang, Q.; Hay, M.; Clarke, D.; Menaham, S. The prevalence and predictors of anxiety and depression in adolescents with heart disease. *J. Pediatr.* 2012, *161*, 943–946. [CrossRef] [PubMed]
42. Vitaro, F.; Boivin, M.; Bukowski, W.M. The role of friendship in child and adolescent psychosocial development. In *Handbook of Peer Interactions, Relationships, and Groups*; Bukowski, W.M., Laursen, B., Rubin, K.H., Eds.; The Guilford Press: New York, NY, USA, 2009; pp. 568–585.
43. Rebar, A.L.; Stanton, R.; Geard, D.; Short, C.; Duncan, M.J.; Vandelanotte, C. A meta-meta-analysis of the effect of physical activity on depression and anxiety in non-clinical adult populations. *Health Psychol. Rev.* 2015, *9*, 366–378. [CrossRef]
44. Currier, D.; Lindner, R.; Spittal, M.J.; Cvetkovski, S.; Pirkis, J.; English, D.R. Physical activity and depression in men: Increased activity duration and intensity associated with lower likelihood of current depression. *J. Affect. Disord.* 2020, *260*, 426–431. [CrossRef]
45. Morgan, J.A.; Olagunju, A.T.; Corrigan, F.; Baune, B.T. Does ceasing exercise induce depressive symptoms? A systematic review of experimental trials including immunological and neurogenic markers. *J. Affect. Disord.* 2018, *234*, 180–192. [CrossRef] [PubMed]
46. Diller, G.P.; Giardini, A.; Dimopoulos, K.; Gargiulo, G.; Muller, J.; Derrick, G.; Giannakoulas, G.; Khambadkone, S.; Lammers, A.E.; Picchio, F.M.; et al. Predictors of morbidity and mortality in contemporary Fontan patients: Results from a multicenter study including cardiopulmonary exercise testing in 321 patients. *Eur. Heart J.* 2010, *31*, 3073–3083. [CrossRef]
47. National Institute for Health and Care Excellence (NICE). *Depression in Children and Young People: Identification and Management*; NICE: London, UK, 2019.
48. Marino, B.S.; Shera, D.; Wernovsky, G.; Tomilnson, R.S.; Aguirre, A.; Gallagher, M.; Lee, A.; Gho, C.J.; Stern, W.; Davis, L.; et al. The development of the pediatric cardiac quality of life inventory: A quality of life measure for children and adolescents with heart disease. *Qual. Life Res.* 2008, *17*, 613–626. [CrossRef] [PubMed]
49. Marino, B.S.; Tomlinson, R.S.; Drotar, D.; Claybon, E.S.; Aguirre, A.; Ittenbach, R.; Welkom, J.S.; Helfaer, M.A.; Wernovsky, G.; Shea, J.A. Quality-of-life concerns differ among patients, parents, and medical providers in children and adolescents with congenital and acquired heart disease. *Pediatrics* 2009, *123*, e708–e715. [CrossRef] [PubMed]
50. Zimmerman, M.S.; Smith, A.G.C.; Sable, C.A.; Echko, M.M.; Wilner, L.B.; Olsen, H.E.; Atalay, H.T.; Awasthi, A.; Bhutta, Z.A.; Boucher, J.L.; et al. Global, regional, and national burden of congenital heart disease, 1990–2017: A systematic analysis for the Global Burden of Disease Study 2017. *Lancet Child Adolesc. Health* 2020, *4*, 185–200. [CrossRef]

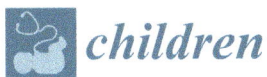

Article

The Psychometric Properties and Cutoff Score of the Child and Adolescent Mindfulness Measure (CAMM) in Chinese Primary School Students

Xin Chen [1,2], Kaixin Liang [1,2], Liuyue Huang [1,2], Wenlong Mu [3], Wenjing Dong [1,2], Shiyun Chen [4], Sitong Chen [5] and Xinli Chi [1,2,*]

[1] School of Psychology, Shenzhen University, Shenzhen 518061, China; ccchenxin19@163.com (X.C.); liangkaixin2020@email.szu.edu.cn (K.L.); 1910481006@email.szu.edu.cn (L.H.); dongwj1997@126.com (W.D.)
[2] Center for Mental Health, Shenzhen University, Shenzhen 518061, China
[3] School of Economics and Management, Wuhan University, Wuhan 430072, China; mu.w@whu.edu.cn
[4] Department of Psychology and Human Development, Institute of Education, University College London, London WC1E 6BT, UK; shiyun.chen.21@ucl.ac.uk
[5] Institute for Health and Sport, Victoria University, Melbourne 8001, Australia; sitong.chen@live.vu.edu.au
* Correspondence: xinlichi@szu.edu.cn

Abstract: To date, the Child and Adolescent Mindfulness Measure (CAMM) has been translated into several languages, including Chinese. This study aimed to explore the reliability and validity of the Chinese version of the CAMM and to identify the appropriate cutoff score among Chinese primary school students. A total of 1283 participants (52.2% males; 11.52 ± 0.78 years of age) completed a series of questionnaires to evaluate their mental health, including mindfulness, subjective well-being, positive youth development (PYD), depression, and anxiety. Item analysis, Confirmatory Factor Analysis (CFA), Exploratory Structural Equation Modeling (ESEM), criterion-related validity analysis, Receiver Operating Characteristic (ROC) analysis, and reliability analysis were performed. The results show that the Chinese version of the CAMM had acceptable item–scale correlation (r = 0.405–0.775, $p < 0.001$) and was the best fit for the two-factor ESEM model (χ^2 = 168.251, $p < 0.001$, df = 26, TLI = 0.910, CFI = 0.948, RMSEA = 0.065, SRMR = 0.033) among Chinese primary school students. Additionally, the total score of the Chinese version of the CAMM was significantly associated with subjective well-being and PYD (r = 0.287–0.381, $p < 0.001$), and negatively associated with depression, and anxiety (r = −0.612−−0.542, $p < 0.001$). Moreover, a cutoff score of 22 or higher revealed a significant predictive power for all the included criteria. Finally, the Chinese version of the CAMM had good internal consistency (Cronbach's α = 0.826, McDonald's ω = 0.826). Altogether, the Chinese version of the CAMM had satisfactory psychometric properties, and it can be applied to Chinese children.

Keywords: Child and Adolescent Mindfulness Measure (CAMM); reliability; validity; cutoff; primary school students; Chinese

1. Introduction

Mindfulness, an important predictor of people's physical and mental health, has received a considerable amount of attention from researchers, practitioners, and the general public in the last 10 years. In the Buddhist scriptures, mindfulness is written in Pali as sammā sati, which means maintaining a clear and proper awareness of goals in the present moment [1]. As the concept of mindfulness has been gradually introduced into the field of psychology, Kabat-Zinn [2] described it as an awareness that emerges from paying attention to the present moment in a conscious and non-judgmental way. Baer [3] noted that mindfulness is a psychological process that observes the ongoing streams of internal and external stimuli without judgment. Based on these descriptive definitions,

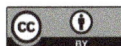

the current study defines mindfulness as perceiving and accepting the present moment without judgment.

The development of research on mindfulness has elicited the need to identify tools to measure it. The Child and Adolescent Mindfulness Measure (CAMM) [4] is one of the few available tools for measuring mindfulness in children and adolescents, including awareness of the present moment and a non-judgmental, non-avoidant stance toward thoughts and feelings. The CAMM, a 10-item scale, is applicable to children and adolescents ranging in age from 10 to 17, and it has been validated and used in children and adolescents in many countries, such as The Netherlands [5], Australia [6], Spain [7,8], Italy [9], Canada [10], Turkey [11], Chile [8], France [12], Iran [13], Greece [14], and China [15]. The reliability and validity of the Chinese version of the CAMM was found to be satisfactory among junior high school students [15]. However, the scale has not been validated in primary school students whose cognitive and emotion regulation capabilities are different from those of junior high school students; thus, the differences in the characteristics of these types of students may lead to differences in the mindfulness measurements. As the social attention on children's mental health increases, it is urgent to test the applicability of the Chinese version of the CAMM in primary school students to provide a simplified and effective tool in order to promote mindfulness-related research in Chinese children.

The findings from most CAMM studies conducted in other countries are consistent with the result from the original study conducted in an English-speaking population, which concluded that the CAMM consists of a reliable single factor. However, the Chinese version of the CAMM displayed a two-factor structure among Chinese middle school students; those factors are awareness and non-judgment (observing the present without judgment), and acceptance (accepting all the thoughts and feelings that arise) [15]. To examine the construct validity of the scale, most CAMM validation studies adopted Exploratory Factor Analysis (EFA) and Confirmatory Factor Analysis (CFA) for the psychometric analysis. It is important to note that the use of Exploratory Structural Equation Modeling (ESEM) is limited. The ESEM framework, which allows items to load on multiple factors, can be used in both an exploratory and confirmatory manner [16] to adequately consider more possible models. Therefore, the current study established one/two-factor models in CFA/ESEM frameworks to provide more evidence for the examination of the construct validity of the Chinese version of the CAMM.

Previous studies have shown that mindfulness is associated with positive outcomes among children, such as self-regulation of emotions [17,18], subjective well-being [19], psychological resilience [20], prosociality behaviors and empathy [21,22], and interpersonal relationships [18]. Mindfulness is also related to better concentration [17,23,24], cognitive flexibility [25], and academic outcomes [21,23,24]. Furthermore, mindfulness is connected with fewer children's ruminations and intrusive thoughts [18], depression and anxiety [17,24], physical and verbal aggression, and other problem behaviors [23,26–28]. Hence, both negative and positive criteria were used to examine the criterion-related validity of the Chinese version of the CAMM.

Additionally, despite widespread use of the CAMM scale worldwide, to date, no optimal cutoff score has been proposed. Obtaining a cutoff score for the scale makes it easier to classify the participants into either a high level of mindfulness or a low level of mindfulness. It may also facilitate the ability to interpret and compare the research outcomes, thus increasing the opportunities to further explore cultural differences between different populations.

The current study aimed to examine the construct validity, criterion-related validity, cutoff score, and internal consistency of the Chinese version of the CAMM in primary school students in China.

2. Methods

2.1. Study Participants and Procedure

With the support of the Educational Science Research Institute of Shenzhen, the current study was conducted in Shenzhen, China in March 2021. The targeted participants were grade 5 and grade 6 students from 8 primary schools, who had the ability to read and understand Chinese well and were competent to finish a series of online questionnaires. Before collecting the data, all the participants and their guardians were informed of the main purpose of the study. The students who disagreed with participating in the survey and those whose guardians or teachers disagreed with them participating in the survey were excluded. With the assistance of teachers and school staff in the local schools, and with the class as a unit, participants got together to complete the online questionnaires anonymously in computer rooms, which took about 20 min. The questionnaires that were not submitted within the allotted time, were not complete, or gave excessive repetitive responses were eliminated.

2.2. Measurement

2.2.1. Mindfulness

The Chinese version of the CAMM was used to assess each individual's level of mindfulness. This instrument consists of 10 items assessed on a 5-point Likert scale ranging from 0 (never) to 4 (always). All items are scored in reverse, with higher total scores indicating higher levels of mindfulness. The instrument was validated and administered to Chinese youth in previous research [15].

2.2.2. Subject Well-Being

The World Health Organization—Five Well-being Index (WHO-5) uses 5 items to measure children's subjective well-being [29]. Each item is assessed on a 6-point Likert scale ranging from 0 (none) to 5 (always), with higher total scores indicating higher levels of subjective well-being.

2.2.3. Positive Youth Development (PYD)

This study used the Five Cs of Positive Youth Development—Very Short Form (PYD-VSF) to measure PYD [30]. The adapted 16-item Chinese version of the PYD-VSF has been demonstrated to have acceptable reliability and validity in Chinese youth [31]. Each item was rated on a 5-point Likert scale from 1 (not at all) to 5 (very much), with higher total scores indicating better positive development.

2.2.4. Depression Symptoms

Depression symptoms were measured using the Chinese version of the 9-item Patient Health Questionnaire (PHQ-9). This instrument consists of 9 items assessed on a 4-point Likert scale ranging from 0 (never) to 3 (nearly every day), with higher total scores reflecting more severe depression symptoms. The severity of depression symptoms can be classified based on the total PHQ-9 scores: 0–4, minimal; 5–9, mild; 10–14, moderate; 15–19, moderately severe; and 20–27, severe. Previous studies show that the Chinese PHQ-9 version is appropriate to Chinese youth [32,33].

2.2.5. Anxiety Symptoms

The 7-item Generalized Anxiety Disorder Scale (GAD-7) can be used to measure anxiety symptoms [34]. The Chinese version of the GAD-7 has been validated and used in the Chinese population [35]. It consists of seven items, each of which is rated on a 4-point Likert scale from 0 (not at all) to 3 (nearly every day), with a higher total score indicating more severe anxiety symptoms. The severity of anxiety can be classified as minimal (0–4), mild (5–9), moderate (10–14), and severe (15–21).

2.3. Statistical Analyses

First, the total score data of the Chinese version of the CAMM were used for item analysis in SPSS version 26.0 software, including item–total correlation and the independent samples T-test for the high-score group and the low-score group (both were 27%).

Second, the construct validity of the Chinese version of the CAMM was examined. The maximum likelihood (ML) estimation was used for the Kaiser-Meyer-Olkin (KMO) test and the Bartlett's test to ensure the feasibility of the factor analysis. According to previous studies, the data were used to establish one-factor models and two-factor models in the CFA and ESEM frameworks, which were run via Mplus version 8.3 software with robust maximum likelihood (MLR) estimation and target oblique rotation. In the ESEM models, cross-loadings were allowed but they tended to be zero [36]. The two-factor models were established based on existing research in China [15]. Factor 1 is awareness and non-judgment, including items 1, 2, 3, 6, 7, and 8. Factor 2 is acceptance, including items 4, 5, 9, and 10. The best model was then selected based on the chi-square test value, the degree of freedom, and several model fit indices: Root Mean Square Error of Approximation (RMSEA), Bentler's Comparative Fit Index (CFI), the Tucker–Lewis Index (TLI), and standardized root mean square residual (SRMR). For an adequate model fit, the indices' criteria should meet the CFI and the TLI > 0.90, and RMSEA and SRMR < 0.05, with <0.08 being satisfactory [37,38].

Third, this study estimated the coefficients of correlation between mindfulness and each criterion according to previous studies [6,7,9,11,17,19,24] to test the criterion validity, particularly, subjective well-being, PYD, depression, and anxiety.

Fourth, Receiver Operating Characteristic (ROC) analysis was performed to define the appropriate cutoff score for the Chinese version of the CAMM in relation to the above-mentioned variables, which served as the external criteria. Dichotomous variables were created out of the total WHO-5, PHQ-9, and GAD-7 scores, using the cutoff score of 10 to assess subjective well-being, depression, and anxiety, respectively [29,32,35]. Moreover, according to the mean total score, the participants were categorized based on the cutoff score of 60 for PYD. After identifying the cutoff points, the participants with a total score above the given cutoff value were considered to be cases with a high level of mindfulness. Those with a total score below the given cutoff value were regarded as having a low level of mindfulness. The Youden index was used to determine the optimal cutoff score and to reduce the risk of misclassification.

Finally, the reliability of the scale was examined by its internal consistency, indicated by Cronbach's α and McDonald's ω.

3. Results

3.1. Participant Characteristics and Reliabilities of Measurements

In total, 1584 students initially received the survey invitation and 131 students refused to participate in the current study. After excluding invalid data, the final sample consisted of 1283 children aged 10–14 years (mean age = 11.52 years, SD = 0.78). Participant information is detailed in Table 1, including gender (male 52.2%, female 47.8%); grade (grade 5 50.3%, grade 6 49.7%); and sibling, paternal, and maternal education. The reliabilities of the WHO-5, PYD-VSF, PHQ-9, and GAD-7 in the current study were greater than 0.900.

Table 1. Participant characteristics and reliabilities of measurements.

Characteristics	n	%
Gender		
Male	670	52.2
Female	613	47.8
Grade		
Grade 5	645	50.3
Grade 6	638	49.7

Table 1. Cont.

Characteristics	n	%		
Sibling				
Only child	329	25.6		
Non-only child	954	74.4		
Paternal education				
Junior middle school or below	264	20.6		
High school or equivalent	341	26.6		
Bachelor or equivalent	479	37.3		
Master or above	47	3.7		
Unclear	152	11.8		
Maternal education				
Junior middle school or below	320	24.9		
High school or equivalent	329	25.6		
Bachelor or equivalent	468	36.5		
Master or above	32	2.5		
Unclear	134	10.4		
Measurements	**M**	**SD**	**α**	**ω**
WHO-5	21.11	6.65	0.935	0.936
PYD-VSF	59.37	10.69	0.906	0.909
PHQ-9	4.12	4.97	0.911	0.907
GAD-7	2.69	4.12	0.931	0.931

Note. n: number of subjects. M: total mean score. SD: standard deviation of total score. α: Cronbach's α. ω: McDonald's ω. WHO-5: The World Health Organization—Five Well-being Index. PYD-VSF: the Five Cs of Positive Youth Development–Very Short Form. PHQ-9: the 9-item Patient Health Questionnaire. GAD-7: the 7-item Generalized Anxiety Disorder Scale.

3.2. Item Analysis

The item–scale correlation coefficient ranged from 0.405 to 0.775 ($p < 0.001$), which is greater than 0.400. Moreover, there was a significant difference between the high-score and low-score groups ($p < 0.001$). Therefore, all 10 items were retained. Independent sample T-test results showed that there was no difference in the level of mindfulness between males and females ($p = 0.626$), or between grade 5 and grade 6 ($p = 0.492$).

3.3. Construct Validity

The KMO value of the data was 0.877 ($p < 0.001$), and the value of the Bartlett's test was 3966.650 ($p < 0.001$), which indicated the feasibility of factor analysis. There were two factors that showed initial eigenvalues greater than 1, specifically 4.090, and 1.356. The variance rates were 40.896% and 13.561%, and the cumulative variance rate was 54.457%. The CFA and ESEM results indicated that (see Table 2), in comparison to the one-factor model, the two-factor model had a better imitative effect for the Chinese version of the CAMM regardless of which frameworks were used. The model fit indices of the two-factor ESEM model were superior to those of the two-factor CFA model, presenting a preferable psychometric quality in both the previous Chinese study [15] and the current study. The standardized factor loadings of the two-factor CFA model and the two-factor ESEM model are shown in Figures 1 and 2, respectively. The factor loading of the two-factor ESEM model ranged from 0.376 to 0.780, and the correlation coefficient of the two factors is 0.546 ($p < 0.001$), which is lower than that of the two-factor CFA model. Therefore, the Chinese version of the CAMM was the best fit for the two-factor ESEM model, with satisfactory construct validity among Chinese primary school students.

Table 2. Test of goodness of fit of the original and Chinese versions of the CAMM for children and adolescents.

	χ^2	df	TLI	CFI	RMSEA	SRMR
			≥0.90	≥0.90	≤0.08	≤0.08
The original English study by Greco and Bear, 2011 ($n = 332$)						
One-factor CFA	—	—	0.87	0.90	0.07	0.06
The Chinese study by Liu et al., 2019 ($n = 309$)						
One-factor CFA	205.75 **	35	0.72	0.78	0.13	0.08
Two-factor CFA	99.47 **	34	0.89	0.92	0.08	0.05
The current study ($n = 1283$)						
One-factor CFA	446.231 ***	35	0.808	0.850	0.096	0.066
One-factor ESEM	446.230 ***	35	0.808	0.850	0.096	0.066
Two-factor CFA	308.995 ***	34	0.867	0.900	0.079	0.056
Two-factor ESEM	168.251 ***	26	0.910	0.948	0.065	0.033

Note. ** $p < 0.01$; *** $p < 0.001$. n: number of subjects. CAMM: the Child and Adolescent Mindfulness Measure. CFA: Confirmatory Factor Analysis. ESEM: Exploratory Structural Equation Modeling. TLI: Tucker–Lewis Index. CFI: Bentler's Comparative Fit Index. RMSEA: Root Mean Square Error of Approximation. SRMR: standardized root mean square residual.

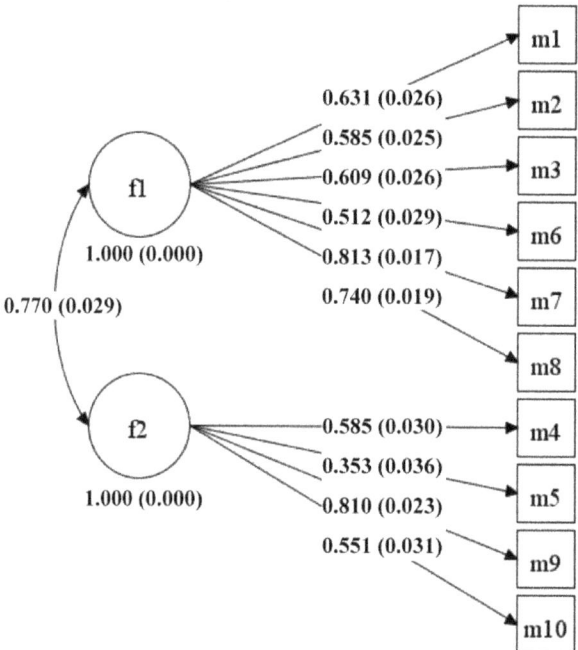

Figure 1. Diagrams of the two-factor CFA standardized model of the Chinese version of the CAMM for primary school students ($n = 1283$). f1 and f2 are the two factors of the Chinese version of the CAMM; m1–m10 are items 1–10.

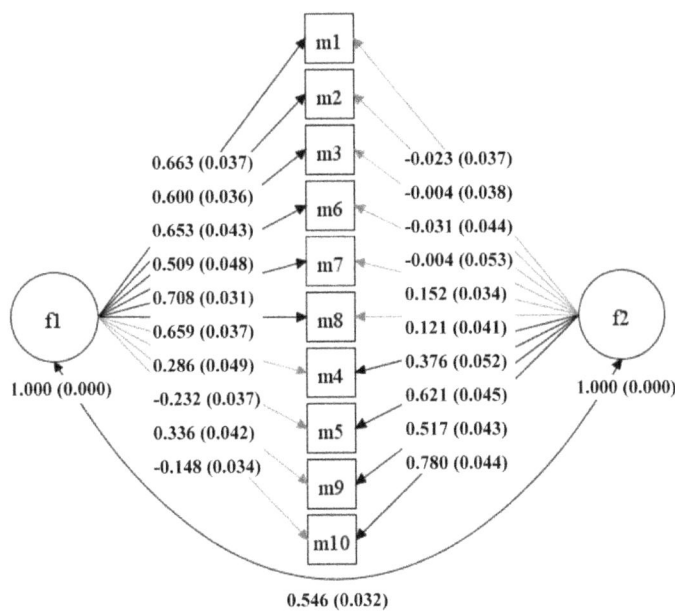

Figure 2. Diagrams of the two-factor ESEM standardized model of the Chinese version of the CAMM for primary school students (n = 1283).

3.4. Criterion-Related Validity

In this study, subjective well-being, PYD, depression, and anxiety were used as the criteria. As shown in Table 3, after controlling for gender and grade, the total score and factor scores of the Chinese version of the CAMM were significantly positively correlated with subjective well-being and PYD; they were significantly negatively correlated with depression and anxiety. These findings indicate that the scale had an acceptable criterion-related validity.

Table 3. The correlation coefficients of the total scores and factor scores of the Chinese version of the CAMM and six criteria (n = 1283).

	Total	Factor 1	Factor 2
Subjective well-being	0.381 ***	0.482 ***	0.129 ***
PYD	0.287 ***	0.390 ***	0.060 *
Depression	−0.612 ***	−0.679 ***	−0.335 ***
Anxiety	−0.542 ***	−0.613 ***	−0.281 ***

Note. * p < 0.05; *** p < 0.001. PYD: positive youth development.

3.5. Cutoff Score

To identify the appropriate cutoff score of the Chinese version of the CAMM, the ROC curve and Youden index were used to determine the predictive validity of the scale for subjective well-being, PYD, depression, and anxiety. The value of the Youden index provided the best tradeoff between sensitivity and specificity [39]. According to the Youden index values presented in Table 4, a cutoff score of 22 or higher was optimal for the children in the current study.

Table 4. Sensitivity, specificity, and Youden index for a selection of best cutoff points of the Chinese version of the CAMM for children.

	Subjective Well-Being				PYD		
Cutoff≥	Sensitivity	Specificity	Youden Index	Cutoff≥	Sensitivity	Specificity	Youden Index
20.5	0.8312	0.4182	0.2494	20.5	0.8906	0.2752	0.1658
21.5	0.7928	0.4727	0.2656	21.5	0.8587	0.3232	0.1819
22.5	*0.7460*	*0.5273*	*0.2732*	22.5	0.8252	0.3856	0.2108
23.5	0.7076	0.5455	0.2530	23.5	0.7948	0.4288	0.2236
24.5	0.6641	0.5909	0.2550	24.5	0.7538	0.4752	0.2290
25.5	0.6002	0.6182	0.2184	*25.5*	*0.6960*	*0.5392*	*0.2352*
26.5	0.5541	0.6636	0.2178	26.5	0.6429	0.5776	0.2205
	Anxiety				Depression		
Cutoff≥	Sensitivity	Specificity	Youden Index	Cutoff≥	Sensitivity	Specificity	Youden Index
20.5	0.8467	0.7229	0.5696	20.5	0.8758	0.6959	0.5717
21.5	0.8075	0.7711	0.5786	*21.5*	*0.8388*	*0.7568*	*0.5955*
22.5	*0.7600*	*0.8193*	*0.5793*	22.5	0.7912	0.8041	0.5952
23.5	0.7217	0.8313	0.5530	23.5	0.7507	0.8108	0.5615
24.5	0.6750	0.8313	0.5063	24.5	0.7048	0.8378	0.5427
25.5	0.6142	0.8916	0.5057	25.5	0.6414	0.8784	0.5198
26.5	0.5658	0.9036	0.4694	26.5	0.5912	0.8919	0.4831

Note. Estimates in italic typeface are the suggested optimal cutoffs. PYD: positive youth development.

3.6. Internal Consistency

The internal consistency of the Chinese version of the CAMM among primary school students was indicated by Cronbach's α and McDonald's ω. The Cronbach's α of the scale had a value of 0.826; the Cronbach's α values for factor 1 and factor 2 were 0.815 and 0.689, respectively. The McDonald's ω of the scale had a value of 0.826; the McDonald's ω was 0.707 for both factor 1 and factor 2.

4. Discussion

Overall, this study explored the reliability and validity of the Chinese version of the CAMM in Chinese primary school students so as to enrich the tools used to measure mindfulness in China. The analytical results showed that the Chinese version of the CAMM had acceptable item–scale correlation and satisfactory discrimination. The two-factor ESEM model had the best fit indexes among the Chinese primary school students. After controlling for gender and grade, the scores of the scale were significantly positively correlated with subjective well-being and PYD; they were significantly negatively correlated with depression and anxiety. The optimal cutoff score of the Chinese version of the CAMM was 22 or higher for children. The scale also had good internal consistency and composite reliability. In summary, the Chinese version of the CAMM has satisfactory psychometric quality and it can be applied to Chinese children to measure the level of mindfulness.

Specifically, different from the results obtained from studies conducted in other countries, the Chinese version of the CAMM was more aligned with the two-factor model than the one-factor model for both the CFA and ESEM frameworks. To explain the difference, the original version of the CAMM was adapted from three of the four facets found on the Kentucky Inventory of Mindfulness Skills [40], namely, assessing mindfulness in the dimensions of observing, acting with awareness, and accepting without judgment [6]. These dimensions are similar to the two dimensions of the Chinese version of the CAMM: "awareness and non-judgment" and "acceptance". Additionally, the descriptive definitions of mindfulness [4,5] commonly emphasized non-judgment and acceptance [41]. To measure non-judgmental acceptance, operational definitions of mindfulness were proposed. Bishop et al. [42] regarded mindfulness as a state-like quality containing two dimensions: self-regulation to attention and orientation to one's experience. Thus, for both the descriptive definition and the operational definition, the concept of mindfulness has a two-dimensional structure that is similar to the two dimensions of the Chinese version of the CAMM. Furthermore, the results may also reveal a cultural difference. Compared with people in other countries, the Chinese people attach more importance to academic performances, so children have to avoid distractions and focus on their studies. Thus, acceptance is important in the Chinese context and has become an independent dimension of the Chinese version of the CAMM. The Dutch version of the CAMM [5] and the Persian version of the CAMM [13] also found two-factor structures, and their factor names were similar to those in the Chinese version of the CAMM. The two dimensions of the Dutch version of the CAMM are "present moment awareness" and "avoidance of thoughts and feelings". The two dimensions of the Persian version of the CAMM are "present-moment non-judgmental awareness" and "suppressing or avoiding thoughts and feelings". Consequently, the two-dimensional structure result obtained in the current study is acceptable.

It is worth noting that the current study's result indicated that the Chinese version of the CAMM had better goodness of fit when using the ESEM than when using the CFA. The ESEM models showed a better imitative effect than that of the CFA models. Given that mindfulness tends to be a multi-construct, a certain degree of association could be present between the items and the non-target, but conceptually related factors, that is, some cross-loadings between factors, should be expected. In the ESEM model, cross-loadings were allowed. In the CFA model, cross-loading was specified at zero, which was more restrictive than that in the ESEM model [16]. Thus, the ESEM framework can adequately consider more possible models, reducing biases and avoiding unsatisfactory representations of the construct [16,43–45].

The current study also found that there was no difference in the level of mindfulness between males and females, which is similar to previous studies [6,9,12]. Evaluation of the criterion-related validity found that, after adjusting for gender and grade, there was a higher level of mindfulness, subjective well-being, and PYD, and a lower level of depression and anxiety, which is similar to the results reported in previous studies [7,9,11]. Not only did these results validate that the scale had a satisfactory criterion-related validity, but they also indicated that mindfulness could act as a strong predictor of children's mental health [19,24]. Since many mental disorders begin in childhood or adolescents [46,47], children and adolescents are at severe risk of developing psychological distress and mental illness [47–49]. Given the enormous personal and societal burdens of mental illness, it might be profitable to begin mental health predictions and interventions in childhood. The development of mindfulness-related research may increase the chance of mindfulness practices, thus promoting children's mental health.

In the current study, an optimal cutoff score of 22 or higher revealed a significant predictive power for subjective well-being, PYD, depression, and anxiety among children. Determining a valid cutoff point with significant predictive power is meaningful; thus, it is possible to classify the participants into a high or low level of mindfulness easily. However, it is important to note that very few studies on the CAMM cutoff score have been conducted in other countries. Therefore, the proposed cutoff score must be interpreted with caution, and more studies on the cutoff score are needed to confirm the cutoff score's predicting ability.

This study has some limitations that must be considered. Firstly, the participants originated from the general Chinese population, so the cohort may have contained people without clinical depression or anxiety, which may have limited the reliability of the result of the cutoff score. Future studies can carry out similar investigations among both the general population and patients with clinical depression or anxiety to provide further evidence in order to confirm an optimal cutoff score. Moreover, only certain types of reliability and validity analyses were performed in the current study. It is necessary to investigate the cross-time stability of the scale. Despite these limitations, this study is the first to examine the construct validity of the CAMM using an ESEM framework, and it identified an optimal cutoff score among children, which provides a reference value for future studies investigating the effect of multiple mindfulness measurement tools and interventions. In short, the Chinese version of the CAMM, with satisfactory psychometric properties, is suitable for primary school students in China.

Author Contributions: Conceptualization, X.C. (Xin Chen) and X.C. (Xinli Chi); data curation, X.C. (Xinli Chi); formal analysis, X.C. (Xin Chen); funding acquisition, X.C. (Xinli Chi); investigation, K.L. and L.H.; methodology, X.C. (Xin Chen), K.L., L.H., W.M. and W.D.; project administration, S.C. (Sitong Chen) and X.C. (Xinli Chi); resources, X.C. (Xin Chen) and X.C. (Xinli Chi); software, X.C. (Xin Chen); supervision, S.C. (Sitong Chen) and X.C. (Xinli Chi); validation, X.C. (Xin Chen); visualization, X.C. (Xin Chen); writing—original draft, X.C. (Xin Chen); writing—review and editing, X.C. (Xin Chen), K.L., L.H., W.M., W.D., S.C. (Shiyun Chen), S.C. (Sitong Chen) and X.C. (Xinli Chi). All authors have read and agreed to the published version of the manuscript.

Funding: The research was funded by the Natural Science Foundation of Guangdong Province (General Program), grant number 2021A1515011330, and the Shenzhen Humanities & Social Sciences Key Research Bases of Center for Mental Health, Shenzhen University.

Institutional Review Board Statement: The study was conducted according to the guidelines of the Declaration of Helsinki and approved by the Shenzhen University Ethics Committee (No. 2020005; ethic approval date is 12 March 2020).

Informed Consent Statement: Online consent forms were obtained from the participants and their guardians.

Data Availability Statement: The data presented in this study are available on request from the corresponding author.

Acknowledgments: The authors express their sincere gratitude to the adolescents who participated in this study and thank all the people who promoted this research.

Conflicts of Interest: The authors declare no conflict of interest.

References

1. Mahinda, V. *Note of Abhidhamma (No.1)*; Yunnan Buddihist Association: Kunming, China, 2009; p. 294.
2. Kabat-Zinn, J. Mindfulness-based interventions in context: Past, present, and future. *Clin. Psychol. Sci. Pract.* **2003**, *10*, 144–156. [CrossRef]
3. Baer, R.A. Mindfulness training as a clinical intervention: A conceptual and empirical review. *Clin. Psychol. Sci. Pract.* **2003**, *10*, 125. [CrossRef]
4. Greco, L.A.; Baer, R.A.; Smith, G.T. Assessing mindfulness in children and adolescents: Development and validation of the Child and Adolescent Mindfulness Measure (CAMM). *Psychol. Assess.* **2011**, *23*, 606. [CrossRef] [PubMed]
5. Bruin, E.I.; Zijlstra, B.J.; Bögels, S.M. The meaning of mindfulness in children and adolescents: Further validation of the Child and Adolescent Mindfulness Measure (CAMM) in two independent samples from the Netherlands. *Mindfulness* **2013**, *5*, 422–430. [CrossRef]
6. Kuby, A.K.; McLean, N.; Allen, K. Validation of the Child and Adolescent Mindfulness Measure (CAMM) with non-clinical adolescents. *Mindfulness* **2015**, *6*, 1448–1455. [CrossRef]
7. Viñas, F.; Malo, S.; González, M.; Navarro, D.; Casas, F. Assessing mindfulness on a sample of Catalan-speaking Spanish adolescents: Validation of the Catalan version of the child and adolescent mindfulness measure. *Span. J. Psychol.* **2015**, *18*, E46. [CrossRef]
8. García-Rubio, C.; Rodríguez-Carvajal, R.; Langer, A.I.; Paniagua, D.; Steinebach, P.; Andreu, C.I.; Vara, M.D.; Cebolla, A. Validation of the Spanish version of the child and adolescent mindfulness measure (CAMM) with samples of Spanish and Chilean children and adolescents. *Mindfulness* **2019**, *10*, 1502–1517. [CrossRef]
9. Chiesi, F.; Dellagiulia, A.; Lionetti, F.; Bianchi, G.; Primi, C. Using item response theory to explore the psychometric properties of the Italian version of the Child and Adolescent Mindfulness Measure (CAMM). *Mindfulness* **2016**, *8*, 351–360. [CrossRef]
10. Dion, J.; Paquette, L.; Daigneault, I.; Godbout, N.; Hébert, M. Validation of the French version of the Child and Adolescent Mindfulness Measure (CAMM) among samples of French and indigenous youth. *Mindfulness* **2017**, *9*, 645–653. [CrossRef]
11. Sünbül, Z.A. Psychometric Evaluation of Child and Adolescent Mindfulness Measure (CAMM) with Turkish Sample. *Online Submiss.* **2018**, *7*, 56–59.
12. Roux, B.; Franckx, A.C.; Lahaye, M.; Deplus, S.; Philippot, P. A french validation of the child and adolescent mindfulness measure (CAMM). *Eur. Rev. Appl. Psychol.* **2019**, *69*, 83–89. [CrossRef]
13. Mohsenabadi, H.; Shabani, M.J.; Assarian, F.; Zanjani, Z. Psychometric properties of the child and adolescent mindfulness measure: A psychological measure of mindfulness in youth. *Iran. J. Psychiatry Behav. Sci.* **2020**, *14*, e79986. [CrossRef]

14. Theofanous, A.; Ioannou, M.; Zacharia, M.; Georgiou, S.N.; Karekla, M. Gender, age, and time invariance of the child and adolescent mindfulness measure (CAMM) and psychometric properties in three Greek-speaking youth samples. *Mindfulness* **2020**, *11*, 1298–1307. [CrossRef]
15. Liu, X.; Chi, X.; Zhang, J.; Duan, W.; Wen, Z. Validation of Child and adolescent Mindfulness Measure (CAMM) in Chinese Adolescents. *Psychol. Explor.* **2019**, *39*, 250–256.
16. Asparouhov, T.; Muthén, B. Exploratory structural equation modeling. *Struct. Equ. Model. Multidiscip. J.* **2009**, *16*, 397–438. [CrossRef]
17. Campion, J.; Rocco, S. Minding the mind: The effects and potential of a school-based meditation programme for mental health promotion. *Adv. Sch. Ment. Health Promot.* **2009**, *2*, 47–55. [CrossRef]
18. Mendelson, T.; Greenberg, M.T.; Dariotis, J.K.; Gould, L.F.; Rhoades, B.L.; Leaf, P.J. Feasibility and preliminary outcomes of a school-based mindfulness intervention for urban youth. *J. Abnorm. Child Psychol.* **2010**, *38*, 985–994. [CrossRef] [PubMed]
19. Gao, L.; Geng, Y.; Liu, X. Mindfulness and Subjective Well-being among Junior School Students: Mediating Role of Self-esteem. *China J. Health Psychol.* **2014**, *22*, 1749–1752.
20. Bluth, K.; Eisenlohr-Moul, T.A. Response to a mindful self-compassion intervention in teens: A within-person association of mindfulness, self-compassion, and emotional well-being outcomes. *J. Adolesc.* **2017**, *57*, 108–118. [CrossRef] [PubMed]
21. Schonert-Reichl, K.A.; Oberle, E.; Lawlor, M.S.; Abbott, D.; Thomson, K.; Oberlander, T.F.; Diamond, A. Enhancing cognitive and social–emotional development through a simple-to-administer mindfulness-based school program for elementary school children: A randomized controlled trial. *Dev. Psychol.* **2015**, *51*, 52. [CrossRef]
22. Rodríguez-Ledo, C.; Orejudo, S.; Cardoso, M.J.; Balaguer, Á.; Zarza-Alzugaray, J. Emotional intelligence and mindfulness: Relation and enhancement in the classroom with adolescents. *Front. Psychol.* **2018**, *9*, 2162. [CrossRef]
23. Semple, R.J.; Lee, J.; Rosa, D.; Miller, L.F. A randomized trial of mindfulness-based cognitive therapy for children: Promoting mindful attention to enhance social-emotional resiliency in children. *J. Child Fam. Stud.* **2010**, *19*, 218–229. [CrossRef]
24. Lu, S.; Huang, C.C.; Rios, J. Mindfulness and academic performance: An example of migrant children in China. *Child. Youth Serv. Rev.* **2017**, *82*, 53–59. [CrossRef]
25. Oberle, E.; Schonert-Reichl, K.A.; Lawlor, M.S.; Thomson, K.C. Mindfulness and Inhibitory Control in Early Adolescence. *J. Early Adolesc.* **2012**, *32*, 565–588. [CrossRef]
26. Singh, N.N.; Lancioni, G.E.; Singh Joy, S.D.; Winton, A.S.; Sabaawi, M.; Wahler, R.G.; Singh, J. Adolescents with conduct disorder can be mindful of their aggressive behavior. *J. Emot. Behav. Disord.* **2007**, *15*, 56–63. [CrossRef]
27. Lee, J.; Semple, R.J.; Rosa, D.; Miller, L. Mindfulness-based cognitive therapy for children: Results of a pilot study. *J. Cogn. Psychother.* **2008**, *22*, 15–28. [CrossRef]
28. Haydicky, J.; Wiener, J.; Badali, P.; Milligan, K.; Ducharme, J.M. Evaluation of a mindfulness-based intervention for adolescents with learning disabilities and co-occurring ADHD and anxiety. *Mindfulness* **2012**, *3*, 151–164. [CrossRef]
29. Allgaier, A.; Pietsch, K.; Frühe, B.; Prast, E.; Sigl-Glöckner, J.; Schulte-Körne, G. Depression in pediatric care: Is the WHO-Five Well-Being Index a valid screening instrument for children and adolescents? *Gen. Hosp. Psychiatry* **2012**, *34*, 234–241. [CrossRef] [PubMed]
30. Geldhof, G.J.; Bowers, E.P.; Boyd, M.J.; Mueller, M.K.; Napolitano, C.M.; Schmid, K.L.; Lerner, J.V.; Lerner, R.M. Creation of short and very short measures of the five Cs of positive youth development. *J. Res. Adolesc.* **2014**, *24*, 163–176. [CrossRef]
31. Huang, L.; Liang, K.; Chen, S.; Kang, W.; Chi, X. Validity and reliability of the Chinese version of the 5Cs Positive Youth Development Scale—Very Short Form. *Chin. Ment. Health J.* **2022**, in press.
32. Bian, C.; He, X.; Qian, J.; Wu, W.; Li, C. The reliability and validity of a modified patient health questionnaire fore screening depressive syndrome in general hospital outpatients. *J. Tongji Univ. (Med. Sci.)* **2009**, *30*, 136–140. [CrossRef]
33. Hu, X.; Zhang, Y.; Liang, W.; Zhang, H.; Yang, S. Reliability and validity of patient health questionnaire Depression Scale (PHQ-9) in adolescents. *Sichuan Ment. Health* **2014**, *27*, 357–360. [CrossRef]
34. Spitzer, R.L.; Kroenke, K.; Williams, J.B.; Löwe, B. A brief measure for assessing generalized anxiety disorder: The GAD-7. *Arch. Intern. Med.* **2006**, *166*, 1092–1097. [CrossRef] [PubMed]
35. He, X.; Li, C.; Qian, J.; Cui, H.; Wu, W. Reliability and validity of generalized anxiety disorder scale in general hospital outpatients. *Shanghai Arch. Psychiatry* **2010**, *22*, 200–203. [CrossRef]
36. Browne, M.W. An Overview of Analytic Rotation in Exploratory Factor Analysis. *Multivar. Behav. Res.* **2001**, *36*, 111–150. [CrossRef]
37. Hu, L.T.; Bentler, P.M. Cutoff criteria for fit indexes in covariance structure analysis: Conventional criteria versus new alternatives. *Struct. Equ. Model. Multidiscip. J.* **1999**, *6*, 1–55. [CrossRef]
38. Wen, Z.; Hau, K.T.; Herbert, W.M. Strucutal equation model testing: Cutoff criteria for goodness of fit indices and Chi-square test. *Acta Psychol. Sin.* **2004**, *36*, 186–194.
39. Youden, W.J. Index for rating diagnostic tests. *Cancer* **1950**, *3*, 32–35. [CrossRef]
40. Baer, R.A.; Smith, G.T.; Allen, K.B. Assessment of mindfulness by self-report: The Kentucky Inventory of Mindfulness Skills. *Assessment* **2004**, *11*, 191–206. [CrossRef] [PubMed]
41. Duan, W. Disagreements of Studies on Mindfulness: Conceptualization and Measurements. *Adv. Psychol. Sci.* **2014**, *22*, 1616–1627. [CrossRef]

42. Bishop, S.R.; Lau, M.; Shapiro, S.; Carlson, L.; Anderson, N.D.; Carmody, J.; Segal, Z.V.; Abbey, S.; Speca, M.; Devins, G. Mindfulness: A proposed operational definition. *Clin. Psychol. Sci. Pract.* **2004**, *11*, 230. [CrossRef]
43. Neff, K.D.; Tóth-Király, I.; Yarnell, L.M.; Arimitsu, K.; Castilho, P.; Ghorbani, N.; Guo, H.X.; Hirsch, J.K.; Hupfeld, J.; Hutz, C.S.; et al. Examining the factor structure of the Self-Compassion Scale in 20 diverse samples: Support for use of a total score and six subscale scores. *Psychol. Assess.* **2019**, *31*, 27. [CrossRef] [PubMed]
44. Mai, Y.; Wen, Z. Exploratory Structural Equation Modeling (ESEM): An integration of EFA and CFA. *Adv. Psychol. Sci.* **2014**, *21*, 934–939. [CrossRef]
45. Asparouhov, T.; Muthén, B.; Morin, A.J.S. Bayesian structural equation modeling with cross-loadings and residual covariances: Comments on Stromeyer et al. *J. Manag.* **2015**, *41*, 1561–1577. [CrossRef]
46. Kessler, R.C.; Angermeyer, M.; Anthony, J.C.; DE Graaf, R.; Demyttenaere, K.; Gasquet, I.; DE Girolamo, G.; Gluzman, S.; Gureje, O.; Haro, J.M.; et al. Lifetime prevalence and age-of-onset distributions of mental disorders in the World Health Organization's World Mental Health Survey Initiative. *World Psychiatry* **2007**, *6*, 168–176.
47. Patton, G.C.; Coffey, C.; Romaniuk, H.; Mackinnon, A.; Carlin, J.B.; Degenhardt, L.; Olsson, C.A.; Moran, P. The prognosis of common mental disorders in adolescents: A 14-year prospective cohort study. *Lancet* **2014**, *383*, 1404–1411. [CrossRef]
48. Hou, J.; Chen, Z. *The Interannual Evolution of Adolescents' Mental Health Status in 2009 and 2020*; Report on National Mental Health Development in China (2019–2020); Social Sciences Academic Press: Beijing, China, 2021; pp. 188–202.
49. Zhou, H.; Li, D.; Song, Y.; Zong, C.; Wu, J.; Lu, H. Epidemiologic study of anxiety state in adolescents in China. *J. Shanghai Jiaotong Univ. (Med. Sci.)* **2007**, *27*, 1379–1388.

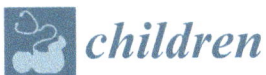

Article

Generalization Task for Developing Social Problem-Solving Skills among Young People with Autism Spectrum Disorder

Saray Bonete [1,2,*], Clara Molinero [1] and Adrián Garrido-Zurita [1]

[1] Departament of Psychology, Universidad Francisco de Vitoria, 28223 Pozuelo de Alarcón, Spain; c.molinero.prof@ufv.es (C.M.); adrian.garrido@centta.es (A.G.-Z.)
[2] HUM-129 Behavior Analysis Group, Universidad de Granada, 18071 Granada, Spain
* Correspondence: s.bonete.prof@ufv.es; Tel.: +34-913510303

Abstract: This study aims to examine the usefulness of an ad hoc worksheet for an Interpersonal Problem-Solving Skills Program (SCI-Labour) the effectiveness of which was tested by Bonete, Calero, and Fernández-Parra (2015). Data were taken from 44 adolescents and young adults with Autism Spectrum Disorder (ASD) (age M = 19.73; SD = 3.53; 39 men and 5 women; IQ M = 96.27, SD = 15.98), compared to a matched group (in age, sex, and nonverbal IQ) of 48 neurotypical participants. The task was conceived to promote the generalization of interpersonal problem-solving skills by thinking on different possible scenarios in the workplace after the training sessions. The results show lower scores in the worksheet delivered for homework (ESCI-Generalization Task) in the ASD Group compared to neurotypicals in total scores and all domains (Problem Definition, Quality of Causes, and Solution Suitability) prior to program participation. In addition, after treatment, improvement of the ASD Group was observed in the Total Score ESCI-Generalization Task and in the domains of Problem Definition, Quality of Causes, Number or Alternatives and Consequences, Time, and Solution Suitability. This is a valuable task in furthering learning within the SCI-Labour Program and may be a supplementary material in addressing the difficulties of interpersonal skills within this population, both in the workplace and in daily life. In conclusion, this task may provide useful information for identifying key difficulties among this population and could be implemented in a clinical setting as a complement to the SCI-Labour Program.

Keywords: Autism Spectrum Disorder; adolescents; social problem-solving skills; interpersonal skills; treatment; assessment; generalization

Citation: Bonete, S.; Molinero, C.; Garrido-Zurita, A. Generalization Task for Developing Social Problem-Solving Skills among Young People with Autism Spectrum Disorder. *Children* **2022**, *9*, 166. https://doi.org/10.3390/children9020166

Academic Editor: Matteo Alessio Chiappedi

Received: 17 December 2021
Accepted: 26 January 2022
Published: 28 January 2022

Publisher's Note: MDPI stays neutral with regard to jurisdictional claims in published maps and institutional affiliations.

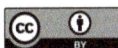

Copyright: © 2022 by the authors. Licensee MDPI, Basel, Switzerland. This article is an open access article distributed under the terms and conditions of the Creative Commons Attribution (CC BY) license (https://creativecommons.org/licenses/by/4.0/).

1. Introduction

Autism Spectrum Disorder (ASD) is a neurodevelopmental disorder characterized by deficits in social interaction and communication, restrictive patterns, and repetitive behaviors, interests or activities [1]. Numerous studies have found poor performance in social cognition and other skills that are involved in it (theory of mind, recognition of emotions, executive functioning, cognitive flexibility, and planning and inhibitory control [2–6]. These, along with verbal and nonverbal communication deficits, result in the lack of skills to deal with interpersonal conflicts, hindering social inclusion which increases as they reach adulthood [7–9].

There are many interventions for the development of socialization skills from early childhood to adulthood, some based on evidence-based practices [10–12]. There are at least three theoretical proposals in which social skills interventions could be classified: the *social skills to solve conflicts* approach [13] conceiving social skills as being domain-specific skills; *the social problem-solving process* [14,15], which considers that social problems are solved through a cognitive–emotional–behavioral process, and *interpersonal skills* framework as phases of the problem-solving process [16,17]. All these skills must be developed before adulthood, and in the absence of this development, psychological problems may arise [18].

During the course of training, changes are evaluated in a number of ways [19] using different assessment tools, such as questionnaires and self-report instruments, behavioral rating scales, lab-based behavioral observations, and performance tasks and expressive techniques [20]. Some problem-solving tasks are based on images, while others use comics, vignette sequences, etc. Working with ASD populations, different tasks have been used to assess performance and the improvement of social problem-solving skills [2,21–29]. However, problems tend to persist in maintaining these skills and with generalization to daily routines [30–34].

The goal of this study is to evaluate a performance task using a social problem-solving worksheet (ESCI-Generalization Task) applied during an intervention focused on interpersonal skills. Bonete et al. (2015) tested the ESCI-Labour Program effectiveness in a previous study. The theorical background of both the program and the task is based on the *interpersonal skills* approach [17,35], for which there is a lack of research in the ASD population [36]. The original study [23] programmed generalization based on the Train and Hope technique and Train Sufficient Examplers [31]. With this purpose, a mediational approach was used, and homework tasks were required. In this task, a social situation was described and a series of questions had to be answered. Each question was focused on a particular phase of the problem-solving process, the same phases participants were being trained with during the intervention. The first aim was to assess the validity of the ESCI-Generalization Task, discriminating between participants with ASD and neurotypicals. It was hypothesized that neurotypicals would score higher than the ASD Group prior to any training, and these differences would be smaller after the treatment. The second aim was to evaluate the potential utility of the ESCI-Generalization Task as an outcome measure of the effects of a manualized program for people with ASD in the context of an open clinical trial. We hypothesized that improvements in the ESCI-Generalization Task would be observed post-training, compared with pretreatment.

2. Materials and Methods

2.1. Participants

The sample was taken from data collected for a wider study examining the preliminary effectiveness of the Interpersonal Problem-Solving Skills for Workplace Adaptation [23]. The ASD Group was composed of 44 participants (39 men and 5 women) with ASD (ASD Group) aged between 16 and 30 years of age (M = 19.73; SD = 3.53) and with a global IQ within the limits of normality (M = 96.27; SD = 15.98) measured by the Reynolds Intellectual Screening Test [37]. The Comparison Group (CG) was the same as in the original study, recruited to match the ASD Group on sex, age, and nonverbal IQ [23]. It was composed of 48 subjects (42 men and 6 women) also aged 16 to 30 (M = 19.41; SD = 3.20) and with an IQ of M = 103.75; SD = 12.79. All participants were student volunteers with neurotypical development. All participants from the ASD Group had a confirmed diagnosis by gold standard measures [38,39] without any comorbidity or major psychiatric disorders, such as attention deficit hyperactivity disorder, obsessive compulsive disorder, or other disorders (See [23] for a full description of the sample). Intervention was implemented with the ASD Group exclusively who were asked to complete a worksheet after each session as homework. Only 37 participants from the ASD Group submitted the Pre ESCI-Generalization Task (completed after session 3), and 39 participants from the ASD Group submitted the Post ESCI-Generalization Task (completed after session 10). The CG only filled the Post ESCI-Generalization Task (session 10).

2.2. Intervention: SCI-Labour Program

The original SCI-Labour Program is a 10-week (90 min session once a week) interpersonal problem-solving training program [16] adapted for young people with ASD in the context of workplace adaptation. The SCI-Labour sessions were delivered in a small group format. A mediational approach was adopted through sequential training in a cognitive and metacognitive process; that is, each session developed one of the steps necessary to obtain the complete image of an interpersonal problem. Sessions 1 and 2 were introductory sessions: (I) introduction session and description of ASD characteristics and (II) conversational skills. The following sessions focused on a particular phase of the problem-solving process: (1) detecting and defining a social problem, (2) considering different perspectives, (3) looking for causes, (4) generating solutions, (5) considering consequences and (6) choosing the most adequate one, (7) making an action plan, (8) evaluating actions, and (9) facing failure. Each phase was based on exposure to typical interpersonal conflicts using social vignettes, videos, and scripts. These social situations were used to illustrate a problem and how it could be addressed using a cognitive process. Each session started with a personal problem (without social content), leading to a person-to-person problem, and to a group problem. A previous study confirmed the feasibility and effectiveness of using an open trial [23].

2.3. Target Measure: Social Problem-Solving Generalization Worksheet (ESCI-Generalization Task)
2.3.1. Procedure

A performance task was designed to consolidate the skills developed in training with the SCI-Labour Program by practicing the content acquired after each session. The explicit aim was to promote generalization of the sequence of phases to solve an interpersonal problem by thinking of different possible scenarios in the workplace after training sessions. Over the course of the program, participants were asked to practice dealing with interpersonal conflicts at home using scripts [23]. This was an ad hoc homework task for the program, inspired by the material published by Paradiz [40]. Each worksheet describes an interpersonal conflict in a short story. The person must answer different questions following the sequence of steps of the social problem-solving process. Each question refers to a step which was addressed in a particular session. The worksheet template used for all the different scenarios is included in Appendix A.

The worksheet was introduced after the second session. In order to promote generalization, continuous practice was required [30,41]. Every week, participants were asked to analyze two scripts with different interpersonal conflicts: a *training task*, in which participants completed the cells of the worksheet referring to the social problem-solving skills trained during that session and a *generalization task* for which participants tried to complete the total sequence of steps for the adequate solution of that specific conflict. In the analysis, the generalization task after session 3 was used as the baseline (ESCI-Generalization Task Pre), while session 10 was taken as the Post-test to evaluate changes over time (ESCI-Generalization Task Post). Table 1 provides an overview of the scripts of social conflicts, session by session, used as generalization tasks of the program.

Different scenarios are described in each situation. However, the scripts for each session were selected from slightly different situations that were addressed during each treatment group session. In general, the worksheet was always the same: a short script followed by questions: (1) What clues do I use to detect there is a problem? (2) What is the problem? (3) What are the "main character's" thoughts and feelings? (4) What do you think that the other person is thinking and feeling? (5) Point out as many possibilities as you can imagine, (6) List the different alternatives you can think as solutions, (7) Write at least one possible consequence that follows each alternative, and (8) Choose the solution that you think is most adequate to face this social situation.

In this study, only the task performance of scenarios Pre (session 3) and Post (session 10) were analyzed. These two situations were considered equivalent as they both addressed problems of shift work and how the decisions of others may affect performance at work.

2.3.2. Response Coding

Each question of the ESCI-Generalization Task refers to a particular phase of the interpersonal problem-solving process (see Figure A1). Answers were coded into 10 categories: *Problem Definition* (PD), *Theory of Mind* (ToM), *Number of Causes* (CAUS), *Quality of Causes* (CAUS-QLTY), *Number of Alternatives* (ALT), *Quality of Alternatives* (ALT-QLTY), *Content of*

Alternatives (ALT-CONT), *Number of Consequences* (CONSQ), *Time* (T), and *Solution Suitability* (SS). These items were based on definitions used in previous research examining interpersonal problem-solving skills [28,42–44]. A *Total score* was also calculated as the sum of the nine primary outcomes, except *Content of Alternatives* (ALT-CONT). This category, *Content of Alternatives* (ALT-CONT), was generated as a qualitative variable, exploring differences in the type of solutions generated, to see if the training also improved this aspect of social problem-solving skills. A description of each category rating is provided in Table 2.

Table 1. Scripts of the ESCI-Generalization Task after each treatment session.

Variables	Task
Session 2	There was no generalization task for homework
Session 3 *	Carlos has left home late in the morning and has missed the bus, so he will arrive late to work. When he arrives to the office, he sees that his supervisor looks angry.
Session 4	Pedro has been working in a library for two weeks. The first days, the manager explained to him all the tasks that he had to do. Among them was to send the letters that the manager always left sealed on top of the table. Today, Pedro found five letters with the address written on them and prepared to send, but they are open. The manager had left, so Pedro decided to send them anyways. When the manager arrived and realized, he becomes very angry and told him off because the letters were for important people and they were incomplete, he shouldn't have sent them. Pedro is very sad; he thinks that his boss has no reason to be angry like this.
Session 5	German works for a company, every employee works at their desk. Today, German takes a cup of coffee over to the boss' desk. When he gives it to him, his hand trembles and the coffee falls onto his boss computer keyboard. The boss draws back abruptly, German can see the discomfort in his boss' face."
Session 6	Sonia works as a doorman for the cultural center for her neighbourhood. The manager of the cultural center has asked her to write up a document with the detailed timetable of the center's activities. It took two days to finish it and she is very proud of how it looks with very pretty colors and writing. However, when she shows it to the manager, he tells her seriously that he doesn't like how it's done, and she will have to it all over.
Session 7	Julia works restocking a supermarket. Alongside her colleague, she makes sure all is done in the "Home" section. But her colleague, who has been working for the company longer than she has, most times isn't very careful about placing the price labels, making the work slower and making it difficult for Julia to find what is missing.
Session 8	Felipe has been working as an electrician in a company for a short time. The boss asks him every day to stay a little longer after he finishes his shift. This is starting to become a problem for Felipe.
Session 9	Patricia works as a secretary. She has all documents filed in alphabetic order, but her boss doesn't like how it's done, and asks her to do it in a way that seems absurd to her.
Session 10 *	Jacinto is a security guard. He has finished his shift, but his supervisor, who is the one who must substitute him, hasn't arrived.

*: Coded and analyzed homework tasks.

Table 2. Description of dimensions of social problem-solving skills coded in the ESCI-Generalization Task.

Categories	Description
Problem Definition (PD)	Indicating if the problem was clearly stated (2 points), vaguely understood (1 point), or not understood at all (0 points). Maximum score: 2
Theory of Mind (ToM)	Score based on the understanding of emotions (1 point) and thoughts (1 point) about the principal actor and the other person involved. Maximum score: 4
Number of Causes (CAUS)	Number of causes attributed to the problem. 1 point was given for every plausible cause, relevant to the situation. Maximum score: 10
Quality of Causes (CAUS-QLTY)	The causes listed were categorized into "proximal" (refers to a cause with a recent effect) or "distant" (refers to a cause with a delayed effect). For coding, when a proximal and a distant cause are selected, the maximum score is given; if only a proximal or distant cause is selected, 1 point is given. Maximum score: 2
Number of Alternatives (ALT)	Participants were asked to list possible actions (plausible and relevant) for the principal actors to solve the scenario. Each plausible and relevant solution scores 1 point. Maximum score: 8
Quality of Alternatives (ALT-QLTY)	This score is the sum of four different subdomains exploring different aspects of the provided alternatives. A maximum of 8 for each of the 7 possible alternatives. Maximum score: 56 Activity (ACT): A solution is considered active if the main actor actually executes (2 points), but it is passive if action means to solve the problem through a third party not directly involved in the social problem (1 point). Relevancy (RELV): This scores if the action directly solves the issue (2 points) or is a step in a sequence of actions, indirectly solving the problem (1 point). Perspective (PERSP): 2 points if the participant took the other person involved into perspective and considered them affected by the action. Quality of Action (A-QLTY): 2 points when the action showed social sensitivity (coded in PERSP), and practical effectiveness (coded in RELV)
Number of Consequences (CONSQ)	Participants were required to list consequences to each alternative action that were plausible and relevant to the situation. 1 point for each option. Maximum score: 8
Time (T)	This task measured whether participants consider the duration of the consequence. This task was measured by whether it had short- (ST) or long-term (LG) consequences. 2 points for each option if both types of consequence were considered up to 8 consequences. Maximum score: 16
Solution Suitability (SS)	From the list of alternative actions, participants were to select the most appropriate and socially adequate actions regarding the situation. Maximum score: 2
Total ESCI-Generalization Task	With the sum of the responses of the subject in the previous dimensions, this task provides a total score. Maximum score: 108

An extra category was evaluated qualitatively, *Content of Alternatives* (ALT-CONT), according to 6 topics: (1) Search for help; (2) Verbal aggression; (3) No confrontation; (4) Compromise; (5) Negotiation/Agreement; and (6) Other, in order to analyze its frequency and if any changes appear after treatment.

2.3.3. Coding Reliability

In coding the worksheets, the lead author (SB) trained two raters (blind study hypothesis) until interjudge reliability was established between them and the lead author in the coding of 20% of the total homework tasks. Checkers were considered in agreement when they gave the same rating to each category. Interrater reliability was calculated as ([Number of Agreement/Total Number of Codes] × 100). Reliability was considered acceptable once both raters achieved >80% of agreement in 28 aleatory selected worksheets. After that, all samples were coded by the same rater (blinded to group condition). The lead author did not rate any task.

2.4. Statistic Design

Data analyses were performed using the Statistical Package for the Social Sciences 22.0 (SPSS).

Given the features of the sample and the use of nominal variables, nonparametric measures were used. ESCI-Generalization Task validity was confirmed if the Total ESCI-Task discriminated between participants in the ASD Group and CG. Chi-squared tests were conducted comparing both groups in *Problem Definition* (PD), *Quality of Causes* (CAUS-QLTY), and *Solution Suitability* (SS) scores. The Mann–Whitney U test for independent samples was used to compare the ASD Group and CG scores in the main categories: ToM, CAUS, CAUS-QLTY, ALT, ALT-QLTY, CONSQ, T, and *Total Generalization task* score. Effect sizes were reported. As a complementary analysis, a logistic regression model was also calculated to evaluate predictive validity. The ESCI-*Total Generalization task* score was the independent variable (for the ASD Group the Post score was used), and the assigned group (ASD Group vs. CG) was the dependent variable. A qualitative analysis was presented when categorizing possible alternatives based on Content of Alternatives.

In order to examine the potential utility of the ESCI-Generalization Task to measure change after treatment, the Wilcoxon signed-rank test was used to compare pre- and post-treatment means in the ASD Group (n = 32 participants who complete Pre and Post) for the same categories.

3. Results

3.1. Differences between ASD Group Pre and Post-Treatment and Comparison Group

Examining the categorical variables, the comparison of the Pre-ASD Group and CG of the representative values of the contingency table and the differences between the groups is provided in Table 3. The CG showed fewer incorrect responses and more complete responses in Problem Definition (χ^2 (2) = 17.41, p < 0.001), Quality of Causes (χ^2 (2) = 27.96, p < 0.001), and Solution Suitability (χ^2 (2) = 30.21, p < 0.001).

Table 3. Contingency table of Chi Squared test in the categorical variables between Pre-ASD Group and CG.

Variables		Pre-ASD Group N (37)		CG N (48)		χ^2 (df = 2)	p	r
		N (%)	Res	N (%)	Res			
PD	Incorrect	5 (13.5%)	2.8 *	0 (0%)	−2.8 *	17.41	0.000	0.45
	Partial	28 (75.7%)	4.9 *	25 (52.1%)	−4.9 *			
	Complete	4 (10.8%)	−7.8 *	23 (47.9%)	7.8 *			
CAUS-QLTY	Incorrect	12 (32.4%)	4.6 *	5 (10.4%)	−4.6 *	27.96	0.000	0.57
	Partial	22 (59.5%)	7.2 *	12 (25%)	−7.2 *			
	Complete	3 (8.1%)	−11.8 *	31 (64.6%)	11.8 *			
SS	Incorrect	23 (62.2%)	10.8 *	5 (10.4%)	−10.8 *	30.21	0.000	0.60
	Partial	7 (18.9%)	0.9	7 (14.6%)	−0.9			
	Complete	7 (18.9%)	−11.7 *	36 (75%)	11.7 *			

Note. PD: Problem Definition; CAUS-QLTY: Quality of Causes; SS: Solution Suitability; N: Number of participants; %: Percentage in groups; *Res*: Untyped waste; * (significant corrected residuals = −1.96 < 1.96); p: level of significance; χ^2: Chi Squared; and r: Effect size.

Comparing the Post-ASD Group and CG (Table 4), the CG showed fewer incorrect responses in Problem Definition (χ^2 (2) = 16.38, p < 0.001) and more complete responses in Quality of Causes (χ^2 (2) = 18.79, p < 0.001) and Solution Suitability (χ^2 (2) = 8.32, p < 0.05). The comparison also revealed that a greater number of the Post-ASD Group participants offered completed responses than the Pre-ASD Group (comparing Tables 3 and 4).

Table 4. Contingency table of Chi Squared test in the categorical variables between Post-ASD Group and CG.

Variables		Post-ASD Group N (39)		CG N (48)		χ^2 (df = 2)	p	r
		N (%)	Res	N (%)	Res			
PD	Incorrect	5 (12.8%)	2.8 *	0 (0%)	−2.8 *	16.38	0.000	0.43
	Partial	6 (15.4%)	−7.9 *	25 (52.1%)	7.9 *			
	Complete	28 (71.8%)	5.1 *	23 (47.9%)	−5.1 *			
CAUS-QLTY	Incorrect	18 (47.4%)	7.8*	5 (10.4%)	−7.8 *	18.79	0.000	0.46
	Partial	11 (28.9%)	0.8	12 (25%)	−0.8			
	Complete	9 (23.7%)	−8.7 *	31 (64.6%)	8.7 *			
SS	Incorrect	14 (35.9%)	5.5 *	5 (10.4%)	−5.5 *	8.32	0.016	0.31
	Partial	5 (12.8%)	−0.4	7 (14.6%)	0.4			
	Complete	20 (51.3%)	−5.1 *	36 (75%)	5.1 *			

Note. PD: Problem Definition; CAUS-QLTY: Quality of Causes; SS: Solution Suitability; N: Number of participants; %: Percentage in groups; Res: Untyped waste; * (significant corrected residuals = −1.96 < 1.96); p: level of significance; χ^2: Chi Squared; and r: Effect size.

For the rest of the main variables, the Mann–Whitney U test showed significantly lower scores in the Pre-ASD Group in Number of Causes ($U = 436.5$, $z = −4.07$, $r = 0.44$), Number of Alternatives ($U = 360$, $z = −4.76$, $r = 0.52$), Quality of Alternatives ($U = 248.5$, $z = −5.68$, $r = 0.62$), Number of Consequences ($U = 351.5$, $z = −4.83$, $r = 0.52$), Time ($U = 190.5$, $z = −6.26$, $r = 0.68$), and Total ESCI-Generalization Task ($U = 187$, $z = −6.22$, $r = 0.67$) with a large effect size (see Table 5). No significant differences were found in ToM.

Table 5. Descriptive statistics and Mann–Whitney U test in the variables between the Pre-ASD Group (n = 37), Post-ASD Group (n = 39), and the Comparison Group (n = 48).

Variables	ASD Group N (37)			CG N (48)			U	z	r
	Md	M	DT	Md	M	DT			
ToM									
Pre	2	2.67	0.97	2	2.62	0.89	865.5	−0.22	0.02
Post	2	1.92	1.24	2			636.5 **	−2.83	0.31
Number of causes									
Pre	1	1.27	1.36	3	3.04	2.19	436.5 ***	−4.07	0.44
Post	1	1.02	1.11	3			389.5 ***	−4.75	0.51
Number of alternatives									
Pre	2	2.19	1.70	4	4.02	1.31	360 ***	−4.76	0.52
Post	3	2.92	1.69	4			576 **	−3.13	0.32
Quality of alternatives									
Pre	2	7.78	7.16	4	16.04	5.94	248.5 ***	−5.68	0.62
Post	10	9.51	6.85	15.5			447 ***	−4.18	0.45
Number of consequences									
Pre	7	2.10	1.95	15.5	1.51	1.51	351.5 ***	−4.83	0.52
Post	3	2.84	1.88	4			503.5 ***	−3.75	0.41
Time									
Pre	1	1.24	1.46	4	1.60	1.60	190.5 ***	−6.26	0.68
Post	2	2.28	1.99	4			433 ***	−4.36	0.47
Total ESCI-Task									
Pre	19	19.56	12.71	38.5	38.85	10.55	187 ***	−6.22	0.67
Post	23	21.27	14.50	38.5			355 ***	−5.48	0.59

Note. ***: $p < 0.001$; **: $p < 0.01$. Md: Median; M: Mean; DT: Typical deviation; U: Mann–Whitney U Statistic N: Number of participants; z: Normal distribution; and r: Effect size.

When examining the difference from the CG and Post-ASD Group, the Mann–Whitney U test showed significantly higher scores in the Post-ASD Group in the categories of Number of Consequences ($U = 503.5$, $z = −3.75$, $r = 0.41$), Time ($U = 433$, $z = −4.36$, $r = 0.47$), and in Total ESCI-Generalization Task with a large effect size ($U = 355$, $z = −548$, $r = 0.59$). The CG scored higher in Number of Alternatives ($U = 576$, $z = −3.13$, $r = 0.32$), Quality of Alternatives

($U = 447$, $z = -4.18$, $r = 0.45$), Number of Consequences ($U = 503.5$, $z = -3.75$, $r = 0.41$), Time ($U = 433$, $z = -4.36$, $r = 0.47$), and Total ESCI-Task ($U = 355$, $z = -5.48$, $r = 0.59$) (see Table 5).

Regarding effect size differences (comparing the performance of the Pre-ASD Group and CG against the Post-ASD Group and CG), it was observed that effect sizes decreased from large to medium in the variables Number of Alternatives, Number of Consequences, and Time according to Cohen's Criteria (1988) (see Table 5). The Mann–Whitney U test showed significant differences between the ASD Group pre- and post-treatment scores and the CG.

Concerning the predictive validity of the ESCI-Generalization Task, the logistic regression model was statistically significant, χ^2 (2, $N = 92$) = 51.53, $p < 0.001$. The model explained between 45.7% (Cox and Snell R square) and 61.3% (Nagelkerke R squared), generating an odds ratio of 1.08 for the Post-ASD Group. Thus, for every unit of increase in the *Total ESCI-Generalization Task*, the probability of having an ASD diagnosis was reduced by a factor of 1.08.

The qualitative analyses of the Content of Alternatives based on frequencies of answers showed that both the ASD Group and CG used mostly nonconfrontational and compromise actions.

3.2. ASD Group Differences before and after Treatment

Comparing Pre- and Postintervention outcomes in the ASD Group, Table 6 shows more correct responses in the categories Problem Definition (χ^2 (2) = 32.20, $p < 0.001$), Quality of Causes (χ^2 (2) = 7.85, $p < 0.05$), and Solution Suitability (SS) (χ^2 (2) = 8.73, $p < 0.05$) after treatment.

Table 6. Contingency table of Chi Squared test in the categorical variables between Pre- and Post-ASD Group.

Variables		Pre-ASD Group N (37)		Post-ASD Group N (39)		χ^2	p	r
		N (%)	Res	N (%)	Res			
PD	Incorrect	5 (13.5%)	0.1	5 (12.8%)	−0.1	32.20	0.000	0.65
	Partial	28 (75.7%)	11.4 *	6 (15.4%)	−11.4 *			
	Correct	4 (10.8%)	−11.6 *	28 (71.8%)	11.6			
CAUS-QLTY	Incorrect	12 (32.4%)	−2.8 *	18 (47.4%)	2.8	7.85	0.020	0.32
	Partial	22 (59.5%)	5.7 *	11 (28.9%)	−5.7 *			
	Complete	3 (8.1%)	−2.9 *	9 (23.7%)	2.9 *			
SS	Incorrect	23 (62.2%)	5 *	14 (35.9%)	−5 *	8.73	0.013	0.34
	Partial	7 (18.9%)	1.2	5 (12.8%)	−1.2			
	Complete	7 (18.9%)	−6.1 *	20 (51.3%)	6.1 *			

Note. PD: Problem Definition; CAUS-QLTY: Quality of Causes; SS: Solution Suitability; N: Number of participants; %: Percentage in groups; Res: Untyped waste; * (significant corrected residuals = −1.96 < 1.96); p: level of significance; χ^2: Chi Squared; and r: Effect size.

The Wilcoxon signed-rank test showed significant increases after training in Number of Alternatives ($Z = -2.15$, $p = 0.05$, $r = 0.47$), Number of Consequences ($Z = -2.07$, $p = 0.05$, $r = 0.23$), Time ($Z = -2.69$, $p = 0.01$, $r = 0.30$), and *Total ESCI-Generalization Task* ($Z = -2.00$, $p = 0.05$, $r = 0.10$), although the effect size was small. There were no significant differences in Number of Causes and Quality of Alternatives (see Table 7). The Theory of Mind (ToM) category scored lower in Post ($Z = -3.34$, $p = 0.01$, and $r = 0.38$).

Table 7. Descriptive statistics of the quantitative variables and Wilcoxon signed-rank test between the Pre-ASD Group and the Post-ASD Group.

Categories	Pre-ASD Group N (32)			Post-ASD Group N (32)			Z	r
	Md	M	DT	Md	M	DT		
ToM	2	2.69	0.93	2	1.84	1.32	−3.34 **	0.38
Number of causes	1	1.21	1.43	1	1.09	1.17	−0.05	0.00
Number of alternatives	2	2.15	1.76	3	2.90	1.75	−2.15 *	0.24
Quality of alternatives	7	7.40	7.06	10	9.50	6.76	−1.53	0.17
Number of consequences	2	2.19	2.04	3	2.90	2.01	−2.07 *	0.23
Time	1	1.22	1.47	2	2.41	2.08	−2.69 **	0.30
Total ESCI-Task	19	19.22	13.24	23	24.12	13.51	−2.00 *	0.10

Note. **: $p < 0.01$; *: $p < 0.05$. Md: Median; M: Mean; DT: Typical deviation; N: Number of participants; Z: Normal distribution; and r: Effect size.

4. Discussion

In examining whether the *ESCI-Generalization Task* is useful for the evaluation of interpersonal conflict resolution skills among those with ASD, the aim was to determine if its application enhanced this learning process of interpersonal skills. This study also aimed to explore the effectiveness of this task in assessing changes after training and differences between neurotypicals and participants with ASD.

To ensure the validity of the *ESCI-Generalization Task*, raters were trained to reliably code.

The results of the analysis of the Pre-ASD Group and CG confirmed the hypothesis; higher scores were seen from the CG in all dimensions except for the ToM category [45,46]. These results indicate that for these variables, the *ESCI-Generalization Task* does effectively discriminate between the two groups and detects differences in the categories of the interpersonal problem-solving process.

Comparing the Post-ASD Group and CG, there was a decrease in the effect size (compared to the mean differences test with Pre-ASD and CG) in the variables of Number of Alternatives, Quality of Alternatives, Number of Consequences, and Time, indicating that the scores of the ASD Group, after intervention, are closer to those of the CG, as was the case with the scores for the different variables presented in the original study [23]. Significantly, there was an improvement not only in Number of Alternatives and Consequences but also in Quality of the Alternatives (based on the four aspects described) and the richness of the consequences, as there were improvements in the explanation of short-and long-term consequences. In general terms, one of the novelties of the *ESCI-Generalization Task* (as with other tasks of this type) is the quantification of the quality of the answers in aspects related to the kindness, efficacy, and relevance of the social responses to obtain an objective score.

With regards to post-treatment changes, the *ESCI-Generalization Task* proved to be a sensitive tool for measuring change after intervention. After training, the ASD Group showed great improvement in Problem Definition (71.8% of participants compared with 10.8% of participants in pretreatment) with enriched definitions. Although the Number of Causes showed nonsignificant changes, there was a clear improvement in Quality of Causes, 23.7% of participants included close and distant causes compared to 8.1% in pretreatment. Concerning the Number of Alternatives, the ASD Group significantly improved after training, even though the effect size was small. This is in line with the results of other studies in which generating solutions was one of the areas of change [30,47].

However, no improvements were found in the ASD Group after training in Quality of Alternatives; this category was composed of various aspects, such as Perspective of others, Activity, and Relevancy and Quality of Action, in which participants can show variability. In fact, standard deviation scores revealed that variability between subjects was as high as the mean scores. Individual changes were masked. For clinical purposes, computing the Reliable Change Index (RCI) [48] would be useful to observe individual changes.

As expected, in post-treatment, the ASD Group scored significantly higher in Number of Consequences and Time. This suggests that in addition to proposing a higher number of consequences in evaluating alternative solutions to a social problem, they learned to visualize to some extent the short-term and/or long-term consequences. In this regard, no studies were found that noted whether those with ASD distinguish between short- or long-term consequence when proposing solutions to interpersonal problems [21]. Looking at enrichment of the Solution Suitability chosen by participants, at post-treatment, 51.3% of the participants chose as the most appropriate action one with the higher score in the different aspects examined (*activity*, *relevance*, *perspective*, and *quality*) compared to only 18.9% at pretreatment. Finally, the Total ESCI-Generalization Task showed significant differences between the Pre-ASD and Post-ASD Groups, indicating a slight improvement. It could have positive ramifications on the use of the *ESCI-Generalization Task* as a measurement tool for outcomes with ASD sample groups. Contrary to expectations, for the Theory of Mind dimension, the average score of the ASD Group after training was lower than before, with no improvements in relation to the CG. Our interpretation is that the specific interpersonal situation described after session 10 (Post) might have presented a totally new challenge. Subjects had to try again to answer what thoughts or emotions the main character and the other person might have. Competence in Theory of Mind for the ASD population, as many studies have shown, may appear impaired or not [49]. A number of studies reported that ASD populations passed second-order tests of ToM successfully [4]. Our study was focused on young people, some of whom may have trained this precise ability during their childhood. This could explain the absence of changes and the similarities between groups. The original study showed similar upgrades in the rest of the outcome variables of the program [23]. It was expected that trained skills generalize to real-world life in the daily life. Programming generalization through exposure to different scenarios [30] in which social problem-solving skills play a role may have been mediating for improvements, although this variable was not controlled. Future studies could deepen in this controlling the possible practice effect of training with a structured task.

Among the limitations of the study is the size of the sample. Not all participants completed all the training sessions, nor did they all complete each assigned session task. This study represents only a preliminary step toward the validation of the *ESCI-Generalization Task*. It would have been interesting to analyze the rest of the worksheets (continuous probes of generalization) that participants completed after each session. Collecting maintenance data three months after the intervention would have enriched results consistency. Although the groups were homogeneous in verbal IQ, not all individuals with ASD have competent writing or reading comprehension skills, which may play a role in the general level of performance on tasks or specific variables. Someone unable to express the interpersonal situation in writing might find it very difficult to carry out the task. Finally, the complexity of the coding of tasks made the interpreting and correcting process more difficult. In this case, a double-blind coding was carried out with two trained people showing 80% agreement in their coding, but this is clearly limited and insufficient for extension to clinical use.

With regards to future lines of research, it may be interesting to explore if improvements in the ASD Group persist, that is, if a few years after the intervention they obtain similar competence when doing the worksheet with a different scenario. Studies have shown that although people with ASD can be taught tools to improve their social problem-solving skills, there is little evidence these improvements remain or can be generalized to other contexts [34,50–52]. Recent studies indicate that social skills training curricula are insufficient to improve the development of meaningful friendships among these individuals, interactional aspects of the program, and generalization tasks.

This study showed how the ASD Group improved its performance compared to the CG, but only the ASD Group that received training. Another study could assess the differences of learning achievement when both groups were compared in the training program. Another interesting possible line of research would be to validate the *ESCI-Generalization Task* in a wider neurotypical sample and to verify its cross-cultural validity. Finally, it would be interesting to obtain evidence about the effectiveness of this task, change its themes when applied to everyday situations and thus achieve better generalization skills, and to evaluate the use of this scheme and the acquired skills in the long term and under interactional conditions [53].

5. Conclusions

The *ESCI-Generalization Task* is a measurement tool for social problem-solving skills which, to some extent, show psychometric properties. The tool measures changes after treatment and distinguishes social problem-solving skills among those with ASD from neurotypicals. The results suggest that it is useful for detecting general changes among the sample, as progress is seen in solving interpersonally conflicting situations, particularly in the resolution phases of Problem Definition, Quality of Causes, Number or Alternatives and Consequences, Time, and Suitability of the Chosen Alternative. The *ESCI-Generalization Task* may also provide useful information in identifying key difficulties among this population in both working and everyday situations, generating an individualized profile for each person. In addition, this task can be implemented in the clinical field as a complement to the training program in the resolution of interpersonal problems and in order to further the learning of interpersonal skills and examining changes. This pilot study provides preliminary support for the *ESCI-Generalization Task* as part of a battery of assessment tools for various aspects of socialization.

Author Contributions: Conceptualization, S.B. and C.M.; methodology, C.M. and A.G.-Z.; validation, S.B.; formal analysis, C.M. and A.G.-Z.; writing—original draft preparation, S.B., C.M. and A.G.-Z. All authors have read and agreed to the published version of the manuscript.

Funding: This project was partially funded by the University of Granada FPU 'Plan Propio' grant and the Universidad Francisco de Vitoria.

Institutional Review Board Statement: This study was conducted according to the guidelines of the Declaration of Helsinki and approved by the Ethics Committee of the University of Granada (Code: 75, Date: 4 December 2009).

Informed Consent Statement: Written informed consent was obtained from all subjects involved in the study.

Data Availability Statement: The data presented in this study are available on request from the corresponding author. The data are not publicly available due to data protection policy.

Acknowledgments: We thank the adolescents and adults who participated in this study and the professionals from the following associations who cooperated in the study: Asociación Asperger Madrid, Asociación Asperger Granada, Centro Hans Asperger Sevilla, Asociación Aspeger ASPALI, and Asociación Asperger Valencia. We would like to thank Linda Adeyemo for her participation in the research project. This project was approved by the Ethics Committee of the University of Granada.

Conflicts of Interest: The authors declare no conflict of interest. The funders had no role in the design of the study; in the collection, analyses, or interpretation of data; in the writing of the manuscript, or in the decision to publish the results.

Appendix A

SITUATION: Jacinto is vigilant, he has finished his shift, but his supervisor, who is the one who has to replace him in the post, does not arrive

On what clues do I base myself to detect that there is a problem?_____

_____

_____

What is the problem?:_____

Steps: Write your answers	
What are Jacinto's thoughts and feelings?	What do you think that the other person (_____) is thinking and feeling?
CAUSES OF THE INTERPERSONAL PROBLEM. Points out as many possibilities as you can imagine.	
List the different alternatives you can think as SOLUTIONS.	Write at least one possible CONSEQUENCE that follows of each alternative
Choose the SOLUTION that you think is MOST ADEQUATE in this case to face this social situation: -	

Figure A1. Worksheet ESCI-Generalization Task for Session 10 (Post) adapted from Bonete [54].

References

1. American Psychiatric Association. *Diagnostic and Statistical Manual of Mental Disorders*, 5th ed.; American Psychiatric Publishing: Washington, DC, USA, 2013.
2. Stichter, J.P.; Herzog, M.J.; Visovsky, K.; Schmidt, C.; Randolph, J.; Schultz, T.; Gage, N. Social Competence Intervention for Youth with Asperger Syndrome and High-functioning Autism: An Initial Investigation. *J. Autism Dev. Disord.* **2010**, *40*, 1067–1079. [CrossRef] [PubMed]
3. Berenguer-Forner, C.; Miranda-Casas, A.; Pastor-Cerezuela, G.; Rosello-Miranda, R. Comorbidity of autism spectrum disorder and attention deficit with hyperactivity. A review study. *Rev. Neurol.* **2015**, *60*, S37–S43. [PubMed]

4. Bowler, D.M. Theory of Mind in Asperger's Syndrome Dermot M. Bowler. *J. Child Psychol. Psychiatry* **1992**, *33*, 877–893. [CrossRef] [PubMed]
5. Kennedy, D.P.; Adolphs, R. Perception of emotions from facial expressions in high-functioning adults with autism. *Neuropsychologia* **2012**, *50*, 3313–3319. [CrossRef]
6. Robinson, S.; Goddard, L.; Dritschel, B.; Wisley, M.; Howlin, P. Executive functions in children with Autism Spectrum Disorders. *Brain Cogn.* **2009**, *71*, 362–368. [CrossRef]
7. Hillier, A.; Fish, T.; Cloppert, P.; Beversdorf, D. Outcomes of a Social and Vocational Skills Support Group for Adolescents and Young Adults on the Autism Spectrum. *Focus Autism Other Dev. Disabil.* **2007**, *22*, 107–115. [CrossRef]
8. Symes, W.; Humphrey, N. Peer-group indicators of social inclusion among pupils with autistic spectrum disorders (ASD) in mainstream secondary schools: A comparative study. *Sch. Psychol. Int.* **2010**, *31*, 478–494. [CrossRef]
9. Walsh, E.; Holloway, J.; Lydon, H. An Evaluation of a Social Skills Intervention for Adults with Autism Spectrum Disorder and Intellectual Disabilities preparing for Employment in Ireland: A Pilot Study. *J. Autism Dev. Disord.* **2017**, *48*, 1727–1741. [CrossRef]
10. Chan, R.W.S.; Leung, C.N.W.; Ng, D.C.Y.; Yau, S.S.W. Validating a Culturally-sensitive Social Competence Training Programme for Adolescents with ASD in a Chinese Context: An Initial Investigation. *J. Autism Dev. Disord.* **2017**, *48*, 450–460. [CrossRef]
11. Gates, J.A.; Kang, E.; Lerner, M.D. Efficacy of group social skills interventions for youth with autism spectrum disorder: A systematic review and meta-analysis. *Clin. Psychol. Rev.* **2017**, *52*, 164–181. [CrossRef]
12. Wong, C.; Odom, S.L.; Hume, K.; Cox, A.W.; Fettig, A.; Kucharczyk, S.; Schultz, T.R. *Evidence-Based Practices for Children, Youth, and Young Adults with Autism Spectrum Disorder*; The University of North Carolina, Frank Porter Graham Child Development Institute, Autism Evidence-Based Practice Review Group: Chapel Hill, CA, USA, 2013.
13. Goldstein, A.P. Social skills training. In *Response to Aggression: Methods of Control and Prosocial Alternatives*; Pergamon Press: New York, NY, USA, 1981; pp. 159–218.
14. D'Zurilla, T.J.; Goldfried, M.R. Problem solving and behavior modification. *J. Abnorm. Psychol.* **1971**, *78*, 107–126. [CrossRef] [PubMed]
15. Heppner, P.P.; Krauskopf, C.J. An Information-Processing Approach to Personal Problem Solving. *Couns. Psychol.* **1987**, *15*, 371–447. [CrossRef]
16. Calero, M.D.; García-Martín, M.B.; Bonete, S. Programa de entrenamiento en habilidades de resolución de problemas interpersonales para niños. In *ESCI: Solución de Conflictos Interpersonales*; García-Martín, M.B., Calero, M.D., Eds.; Manual Moderno: Bogotá, Colombia, 2019.
17. Pelechano, V. Inteligencia social y habilidades interpersonales [Social Intelligence and Interpersonal Skills]. *Análisis Y Modif. Conducta* **1984**, *10*, 393–420.
18. Nolen-Hoeksema, S.; Aldao, A. Gender and age differences in emotion regulation strategies and their relationship to depressive symptoms. *Pers. Individ. Differ.* **2011**, *51*, 704–708. [CrossRef]
19. Matson, J.L.; Wilkins, J. A critical review of assessment targets and methods for social skills excesses and deficits for children with autism spectrum disorders. *Res. Autism Spectr. Disord.* **2007**, *1*, 28–37. [CrossRef]
20. Merrel, K.W. Assessment of Children's Social Skills: Recent Developments, Best Practices, and New Directions. *Except. A Spec. Educ. J.* **2001**, *9*, 3–18.
21. Constable, P.A.; Ring, M.; Gaigg, S.B.; Bowler, D.M. Problem-solving styles in autism spectrum disorder and the development of higher cognitive functions. *Autism* **2017**, *22*, 597–608. [CrossRef]
22. Molinero, C.; Bonete, S.; Gómez-Pérez, M.M.; Calero, M.D. Estudio normativo del "Test de 60 caras de Ekman" para adolescentes españoles. *Psicol. Conduct.* **2015**, *23*, 361.
23. Bonete, S.; Calero, M.D.; Fernández-Parra, A. Group training in interpersonal problem-solving skills for workplace adaptation of adolescents and adults with Asperger syndrome: A preliminary study. *Autism* **2014**, *19*, 409–420. [CrossRef]
24. White, S.; Scarpa, A.; Conner, C.M.; Maddox, B.B.; Bonete, S. Evaluating Change in Social Skills in High-Functioning Adults With Autism Spectrum Disorder Using a Laboratory-Based Observational Measure. *Focus Autism Other Dev. Disabil.* **2014**, *30*, 3–12. [CrossRef]
25. Buon, M.; Dupoux, E.; Jacob, P.; Chaste, P.; Leboyer, M.; Zalla, T. The Role of Causal and Intentional Judgments in Moral Reasoning in Individuals with High Functioning Autism. *J. Autism Dev. Disord.* **2012**, *43*, 458–470. [CrossRef] [PubMed]
26. Vanderborght, B.; Simut, R.; Saldien, J.; Pop, C.B.; Rusu, A.S.; Pintea, S.; Lefeber, D.; David, D.O. Using the social robot probo as a social story telling agent for children with ASD. *Interact. Stud.* **2012**, *13*, 348–372. [CrossRef]
27. Turner-Brown, L.M.; Perry, T.D.; Dichter, G.S.; Bodfish, J.W.; Penn, D.L. Brief report: Feasibility fo social cognition and interaction training for adults with high functioning autism. *J. Autism Dev. Disord.* **2008**, *38*, 1777–1784. [CrossRef] [PubMed]
28. Goddard, L.; Howlin, P.; Dritschel, B.; Patel, T. Autobiographical Memory and Social Problem-solving in Asperger Syndrome. *J. Autism Dev. Disord.* **2006**, *37*, 291–300. [CrossRef] [PubMed]
29. Channon, S.; Charman, T.; Heap, J.; Crawford, S.; Rios, P. Real-life-type problem-solving in Asperger's syndrome. *J. Autism Dev. Disord.* **2001**, *31*, 461–469. [CrossRef] [PubMed]
30. Schlosser, R.; Lee, D. Promoting generalization and maintenance in augmentative and alternative communication: A meta-analysis of 20 years of effectiveness research. *Augment. Altern. Commun.* **2000**, *16*, 208–226. [CrossRef]
31. Stokes, T.F.; Baer, D.M. An implicit technology of generalization1. *J. Appl. Behav. Anal.* **1977**, *10*, 349–367. [CrossRef]

32. Froehlich, A.; Anderson, J.; Bigler, E.; Miller, J.; Lange, N.; DuBray, M.; Cooperrider, J.; Cariello, A.; Nielsen, J.; Lainhart, J. Intact prototype formation but impaired generalization in autism. *Res. Autism Spectr. Disord.* **2012**, *6*, 921–930. [CrossRef]
33. Baron-Cohen, S.; Golan, O.; Wheelwright, S.; Hill, J.J. *Mind Reading: The Interactive Guide to Emotions*; London Jessica Kingsley Limited: London, UK, 2004.
34. Rao, P.A.; Beidel, D.C.; Murray, M.J. Social Skills Interventions for Children with Asperger's Syndrome or High-Functioning Autism: A Review and Recommendations. *J. Autism Dev. Disord.* **2007**, *38*, 353–361. [CrossRef]
35. Bonete, S.; Molinero, C. The interpersonal problem-solving process: Assessment and intervention. In *Newton, K. Problem-Solving: Strategies, Challenges and Outcomes*; Nova Science Publishers: New York, NY, USA, 2016; pp. 103–132.
36. Antshel, K.M.; Polacek, C.; McMahon, M.; Dygert, K.; Spenceley, L.; Dygert, L.; Miller, L.; Faisal, F. Comorbid ADHD and anxiety affect social skills group intervention treatment efficacy in children with autism spectrum disorders. *J. Dev. Behav. Pediatr.* **2011**, *32*, 439–446. [CrossRef]
37. Reynolds, C.R.; Kamphaus, R.W. *Reynolds Intelectual Assessment Scales (RIAS)*; PAR: Odessa, FL, USA, 2003.
38. Kim, S.H.; Hus, V.; Lord, C. Autism Diagnostic Interview-Revised. *Encycl. Clin. Neuropsychol.* **2013**, 345–349. [CrossRef]
39. Lord, C.; Risi, S.; Lambrecht, L.; Cook, E.H., Jr.; Leventhal, B.L.; DiLavore, P.C.; Pickles, A.; Rutter, M. The autism diagnostic observation schedule-generic: A standard measure of social and communication deficits associated with the spectrum of autism. *J. Autism Dev. Disord.* **2000**, *30*, 205–223. [CrossRef] [PubMed]
40. Paradiz, V. *The Integrated Self-Advocacy ISA Curriculum: A Program for Emerging Self-Advocates with Autism Spectrum and Other Conditions*; Autism Asperger Publishing Co.: Overland Park, KS, USA, 2009.
41. Neely, L.C.; Ganz, J.B.; Davis, J.L.; Boles, M.B.; Hong, E.R.; Ninci, J.; Gillliland, W.D. Generalization and maintenance of functional living skills for individuals with autism spectrum disorder: A Review and Meta-Analysis. *Rev. J. Autism Dev. Disord.* **2016**, *3*, 37–47. [CrossRef]
42. Siegel, J.M.; Spivack, G. Problem-solving therapy: The description of a new program for chronic psychiatric patients. *Psychother. Theory Res. Pract.* **1976**, *13*, 368. [CrossRef]
43. Shure, M.B.; Spivack, G. Interpersonal problem-solving in young children: A cognitive approach to prevention. *Am. J. Community Psychol.* **1982**, *10*, 341–356. [CrossRef]
44. Bauminger, N. The Facilitation of Social-Emotional Understanding and Social Interaction in High-Functioning Children with Autism: Intervention Outcomes. *J. Autism Dev. Disord.* **2002**, *32*, 283–298. [CrossRef]
45. Channon, S.; Crawford, S.; Orlowska, D.; Parikh, N.; Thoma, P. Mentalising and social problem solving in adults with Asperger's syndrome. *Cogn. Neuropsychiatry* **2013**, *19*, 149–163. [CrossRef]
46. Bauminger, N.; Shulman, C.; Agam, G. Peer interaction and loneliness in high-functioning children with autism. *J. Autism Dev. Disord.* **2003**, *33*, 489–507. [CrossRef]
47. Laugeson, E.A.; Frankel, F.; Gantman, A.; Dillon, A.R.; Mogil, C. Evidence-based social skills training for adolescents with autism spectrum disorders: The UCLA PEERS program. *J. Autism Dev. Disord.* **2012**, *42*, 1025–1036. [CrossRef]
48. Jacobson, N.S.; Truax, P. Clinical significance: A statistical approach to defining meaningful change in psychotherapy research. *J. Consult. Clin. Psychol.* **1991**, *59*, 12–19. [CrossRef]
49. Fletcher-Watson, S.; McConnell, F.; Manola, E.; McConachie, H. Interventions based on the Theory of Mind cognitive model for autism spectrum disorder (ASD). *Cochrane Database Syst. Rev.* **2014**, *2014*, CD008785. [CrossRef] [PubMed]
50. Baron-Cohen, S.; Jolliffe, T.; Mortimore, C.; Robertson, M. Another Advanced Test of Theory of Mind: Evidence from Very High Functioning Adults with Autism or Asperger Syndrome. *J. Child Psychol. Psychiatry* **1997**, *38*, 813–822. [CrossRef] [PubMed]
51. Estes, A.; Munson, J.; Rogers, S.J.; Greenson, J.; Winter, J.; Dawson, G. Long-Term Outcomes of Early Intervention in 6-Year-Old Children With Autism Spectrum Disorder. *J. Am. Acad. Child Adolesc. Psychiatry* **2015**, *54*, 580–587. [CrossRef] [PubMed]
52. Bottema-Beutel, K.; Park, H.; Kim, S.Y. Commentary on Social Skills Training Curricula for Individuals with ASD: Social Interaction, Authenticity, and Stigma. *J. Autism Dev. Disord.* **2017**, *48*, 953–964. [CrossRef]
53. Bottema-Beutel, K.; Turiel, E.; DeWitt, M.N.; Wolfberg, P.J. To include or not to include: Evaluations and reasoning about the failure to include peers with autism spectrum disorder in elementary students. *Autism* **2017**, *21*, 51–60. [CrossRef]
54. Bonete, S. Impacto del Entrenamiento de Habilidades Interpersonales Para la Adaptación Laboral en Jóvenes con Síndrome de Asperger. Doctoral Thesis, The University of Granada, Granada, Spain, 2013.

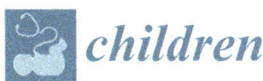

Article

Outcome Quality of Inpatient and Day-Clinic Treatment in Child and Adolescent Psychiatry—A Naturalistic Study

Leonhard Thun-Hohenstein [1,*], Franka Weltjen [1], Beatrix Kunas [1], Roman Winkler [2] and Corinna Fritz [1,3]

1. Paediatric and Adolescent Psychiatry, University Children's Hospital, Paracelsus Medical University (PMU), 5020 Salzburg, Austria; f.weltjen@gmail.com (F.W.); beatrix.kunas@stud.sbg.ac.at (B.K.); c.fritz@salk.at (C.F.)
2. Ludwig Boltzmann Institut for Health Technology Assessment, Ludwig Boltzmann Gesellschaft, 1090 Vienna, Austria; roman.winkler@goeg.at
3. Institute of Psychology, Paracelsus Private Medical University, 5020 Salzburg, Austria
* Correspondence: leonhard.thun@pmu.ac.at

Abstract: Background: Child and adolescent psychiatry has only recently been established as a separate specialty and is practiced in different settings. The epidemiology of psychological problems in childhood is high and varied, thus qualitative work is essential. Assessment of outcome as part of quality management is central to assure the service of psychiatric care to be effective. Method: Over a three-year period consecutively admitted patients from inpatient and day-clinic treatment were prospectively evaluated. A total of 200 from 442 patients (m = 80, f = 120; age 15.1 ± 2.8 y) agreed to participate. Patients, caregivers, and therapists answered a range of questionnaires to provide a multi-personnel rating. Questionnaires used for outcome assessment were Child Behavior Checklist (CBCL) and Youth-Self-Report (YSR) (at admission, discharge, and 6 weeks after discharge) and the problem score of the Inventory of Quality of Life for children (ILK), treatment satisfaction, and process quality by the Questionnaire for Treatment Satisfaction (FBB, at discharge) and as real-life outcome control assessment of quality of life (ILK) was added (admission, discharge, and 6 wks after discharge). Results: There was a significant reduction in psychopathologicalsymptoms (CBCL, YSR) and in the problem score. Furthermore, there was a significant increase in quality of life. QoL score and YSR/CBCL scores returned to normal levels. Treatment satisfaction was high and so was satisfaction with process quality. Factors significantly influencing outcome were severity of disease and the relationship to the therapist. No differences were found for gender and setting. Conclusion: The quality management analysis revealed significant improvements of symptom load, a significant increase in QoL and a high treatment satisfaction. Furthermore, process quality was scored highly by parents and therapists.

Keywords: child and adolescent psychiatry; inpatient; day-clinic; outcome quality; treatment satisfaction; quality of life

Citation: Thun-Hohenstein, L.; Weltjen, F.; Kunas, B.; Winkler, R.; Fritz, C. Outcome Quality of Inpatient and Day-Clinic Treatment in Child and Adolescent Psychiatry—A Naturalistic Study. *Children* **2021**, *8*, 1175. https://doi.org/10.3390/children8121175

Academic Editor: Matteo Alessio Chiappedi

Received: 3 November 2021
Accepted: 30 November 2021
Published: 11 December 2021

Publisher's Note: MDPI stays neutral with regard to jurisdictional claims in published maps and institutional affiliations.

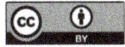

Copyright: © 2021 by the authors. Licensee MDPI, Basel, Switzerland. This article is an open access article distributed under the terms and conditions of the Creative Commons Attribution (CC BY) license (https://creativecommons.org/licenses/by/4.0/).

1. Introduction

In Austria, child and adolescent psychiatry (CAP) has only recently become a separate medical specialty by Austrian federal law. Up to 2007, when law was passed [1], it used to be an additive special medical education, only accessible for pediatricians, neurologists, and psychiatrists. The prevalence of psychological impairment among children and adolescents affects over 13.0% of the age group worldwide, 17.0% in Germany, and up to 35.0% in Austria [2]. Both late creation of the specialty and the epidemiology necessitate an increased need for intervention and prevention [3]. Diagnostic and therapeutic services are provided in private and public practice, day-clinics, outpatient clinics, and hospitals of different levels. During the last ten years, CAP services in Austria have grown significantly, but not sufficiently to meet the need for treatment [4].

Thus, the topic of quality management in the treatment of those affected is of particular importance. Quality management generally refers to—as defined by Austrian federal definition (ÖNORM EN ISO 9000:2000)—coordinated activities for the management and direction of an organisation, which aim to improve the quality of the products produced or the service offered. Theoretically, hospitals in Austria are obliged to systematically implement quality management, but until now there has been very little progress, as there are no officially defined benchmarks for CAP implementation. Bickman et al. [5] recommend the following topics to be included in quality strategies in child mental health: the severity and acuity of the child's symptoms; the child's functional impairment; the child's functional strengths; family functioning; the quality of family life; consumer satisfaction; the goals of treatment; the modality, strategy, and tactics of treatment; readiness for change; the quality of the therapeutic alliance and adherence to treatment. Usually, three areas are distinguished in quality management: structural quality, process quality and outcome quality [6].

Between 2004 and 2009 a new university department for child and adolescent psychiatry was developed in Salzburg. As part of a year-long organisational development process, a new departmental structure was developed as well as a basic treatment concept for inpatients and day-clinic patients [7]. For this, the structure of service and various working processes was defined, and the results were documented in an organisational manual. This is available to all employees via an online platform (Medikit https://medikit.net/de/).

The treatment concept is based on a systemic psychotherapeutic concept and aims to establish optimal cooperation conditions between the multiprofessional team, the patients and their families or guardians [8–10]. The systemic understanding of treatment places the patient in relationship to his network of relationships and understands psychological impairments as interactional disorders in the system [11]. The embedding of patients in relationship systems has a significant influence on the success of treatment [12]. Therapists and other support structures such as the care offered at the clinic act as new actors in the system and can activate resources [9].

All processes were designed according to the topics of the above-mentioned quality aspects, especially participation [13], solution orientation and resource orientation [8] and help for self-help. A distinction is made between different types of stay, each of which includes a specific and standardized procedure: acute stay (risis intervention), orientation stay (multimodal diagnostics and clearing) and project stay (psychotherapeutic treatment stay). These forms also differ in terms of motivation: in contrast to acute and orientation stays, project stays are planned electively and voluntarily with generally high motivation. In addition, depending on the diagnosis, disease-specific concepts (e.g., eating disorder treatment, etc.) are applied at the department—relying on the systemic concept.

After the development of the conceptual part and its implementation, an external assessment of employee rating (1–5; $n = 43/55$) concerning communication/cooperation, information/participation and organisation showed a high level of satisfaction (communication mean 1.85 ± 0.77, information 1.68 ± 0.68 and organisation 1.97 ± 0.7; personal data); additionally, the clinical impression of the implementation was of a very high standard. This gave rise to the idea of also investigating the outcome quality of the new therapeutic structures and processes.

Evaluation of outcome quality under most naturalistic conditions is described to be the possibly best case to ensure practical generalizability of results [14]. Furthermore, since this is no biological or physiological study [15] and to maintain control of our organisational and conceptual implementations, we decided to follow the concept of a naturalistic study. There is a lack of such studies, especially in children and adolescent psychiatry. Solid evaluations following the underlying systemic theory should be "multi-perspective", i.e., the various health professionals, parents, or primary caregivers and the children and adolescents themselves, should be included in the evaluation.

Foundations in the field of evaluation of child and adolescent psychiatry have been laid by the works of Remschmidt and Mattejat [16,17]. These authors introduced the Marburg evaluation project (Marburger System zur Qualitätssicherung und Therapieevaluation, MARSYS; [17]) which systematically investigated the success of the treatment in a local child and adolescent psychiatry hospital under naturalistic conditions. This work was used as a basis for the present evaluation project's structure and intention. Although Remschmidt and Mattejat's study is one of the pioneering works in Germany, there are only two Austrian studies on inpatient treatment outcomes in Austrian CAP departments [18,19].

The primary focus of assessment of outcome quality lies on the success of treatment. The comparison of a pre–post measurement of the extent of symptoms provides the central measure for evaluating treatment success. Evaluative studies in child and adolescent psychiatry consistently show a positive change in symptoms regardless of the disorder [19–23] as well as in a disorder-specific context [16]. The quality of the relationship between the patients and the therapist contributes significantly to the success of the treatment [24].

In addition to this primary parameter, recent research has been increasingly focused on the analysis of additional factors affecting treatment conditions in evaluations [16,20]. Closely associated with the success of treatment is treatment satisfaction within all participants in the treatment process. In the literature, the two parameters are regarded as the same construct (i.e., treatment success is determined by the treatment satisfaction; [22]) and as parallel constructs that correlate positively with each other [16,21]. In general, at least a moderate treatment satisfaction is achieved at the end of a successful treatment [17,25].

Treatment success and treatment satisfaction do not predict whether the children are going to do well in real life. It is important to look at the clinical significance of the results and, thus, the aspect of quality of life of patients has recently gained importance in medical evaluation research [26]. This is crucial, since, simply considering the change in clinical symptoms does not suffice to make valid statements on the improvement of function for the patients [27]. The additional recording of quality of life as a separate construct can, therefore, provide valuable additional information [28]. Reduced quality of life turns out to be a systematic feature of mentally impaired children and adolescents [29,30]. Consequently, this is increasingly regarded as a recommendation for therapeutic practice [31,32].

It has been shown that successful treatment is accompanied by an increase in the quality of life [16,28,33,34], as well as an increased accordance between the perspectives of all participants in the treatment process. [18,19,30]. Different perspectives can also provide exclusive information about the quality of life of patients [35].

Thus, for evaluating the results of the organisational project and the therapeutic concept a naturalistic study was designed, investigating treatment success, treatment satisfaction, and quality of life. It was assumed that the therapeutic concept provides significant reduction of symptoms with clinical relevance, accompanied by high treatment satisfaction and significant improvement of the quality of life.

In addition, the influences of gender and age on treatment success and treatment satisfaction were examined as various framework conditions of treatment: these included differences in the form of stay and the influence on the therapeutic relationship.

2. Materials and Methods

The study period lasted from April 2011 to January 2014 and was approved by the Salzburg Ethics Commission under E-1195 (28 April 2010). Within this period, at the time of admission, all patients were asked if they were willing to participate in the study. In the event of consent, participants and custodial providers were asked to sign a written declaration of consent (EVE). In the event of rejection, there were no disadvantages for the patients at any time during treatment. The sample also included the primary caregivers of the children and adolescents, as well as the treating physicians, psychologists or psychotherapists, educators, and social workers. Patients under the age of six years and patients displaying acute suicidality, psychosis, or cognitive impairment were excluded from the study. In the case of insufficient knowledge of German, interpreters were consulted. In the primary data collection, a total of four measurement time points were chosen: admission to the clinic (T1), discharge (T2), catamnesis six weeks after discharge (T3) and another catamnestic survey 18 months after discharge from the clinic (T4). The survey took place in a specially provided room, accompanied by study assistants. In the present work the measurement at timepoint T4 is not considered.

2.1. Measures

The data were collected using quantitative questionnaires. Treatment success, treatment satisfaction, and quality of life were measured multi-perspectively with different instruments at three time points: admission, discharge, and 6 weeks after discharge. Questionnaires were filled out digitally; patients were accompanied by a psychologist.

2.2. Instruments

Treatment success—as defined by a significant reduction of symptoms i.e., psychopathology, between T1, T2, and T3—was measured by Youth Self-Report (YSR) and Child Behavior Checklist (CBCL), using the Total Problem Scale, Internalizing and Externalizing scale [36].

Treatment satisfaction was measured by the Questionnaire for Treatment Satisfaction (FBB; Mattejat & Remschmidt, [37]), providing rating of treatment satisfaction by patients, parents/caregivers, and therapists. Statements are rated using a 5-point Likert scale, ranging from 0 (don't agree at all) to 4 (agree completely). This questionnaire also can be used as a quality assessment instrument, dividing the results into outcome (items 1,3,18,20 and 6) and process quality (all other items). Subscores for caregivers and patients were calculated for outcome quality: personal success and family success and for process quality: relationship to therapist and framework conditions. The latter were only rated by caregivers, as suggested by the manual. Internal consistency (Cronbach's alpha) is reported to be 0.88.

Quality of life (QoL) was measured by the Inventory for quality of life (ILK; Mattejat & Remschmidt, [38]) in children and adolescents and parents/caregivers. For analysis, the total score for quality of life and the problem score, assessing load of the disease and the treatment, were employed. Internal consistency (Cronbach´s alpha) for the total score is reported to be 0.55–0.76. Normative data are provided for healthy and mentally ill children and adolescents.

2.3. Statistical Analysis

Both correlation and difference hypotheses were formulated and evaluated with the program IBM SPSS Statistics 24 (IBM, Armonk, NY, USA) and R (version 4.0.1, R Core Team, Vienna, Austria) for Windows. If the requirements for the use of parametric methods were not met, their non-parametric equivalents were used. For the difference hypotheses in independent design, the Mann–Whitney U test was used for the comparison of two groups and the Kruskal–Wallis test for the comparison of more groups. Pairwise comparisons were performed in the Kruskal–Wallis test using the non-parametric post hoc test according to Dunn (Bonferroni correction). For the difference hypotheses in the dependent design, the t-test for dependent samples or the Wilcoxon signed-rank test was chosen for two samples, as well as the Friedman test for more than two groups. The correlation hypotheses were analyzed using spearman's rank correlation coefficient. For statistical description, absolute and relative frequency data, mean values, and standard deviations were used. If possible, 95% confidence intervals and effect sizes were specified. For the description of the effect sizes, the measure of Cohen's d was chosen for the mean value differences, and the correlation coefficient r was employed to evaluate the differences between medians and in the correlation calculations. The hypothesis tests were subject to two-sided calculations with a significance level p of $p = 0.05$ (*), $p = 0.01$ (**) and $p = 0.001$ (***). For the analysis of the hypotheses, in the case of missing data, the list-by-list case exclusion was chosen.

Sample Characteristics

The analyses included data from 442 patients treated during the aforementioned study period. Of this total, 328 were hospitalized once and 114 multiple times throughout the study period. Only the first hospitalization was included in the calculations. The consent for participation was given by $n = 200$, 148 of which were admitted once and 52 of which were admitted several times. Figure 1 illustrates the sampling process graphically. The sample size varies depending on the questionnaire and time of testing. At test time T1, data from 170 patients (85.0%) were available, while 163 data sets (81.5%) were available for T2 and 158 data sets (79.0%) for T3.

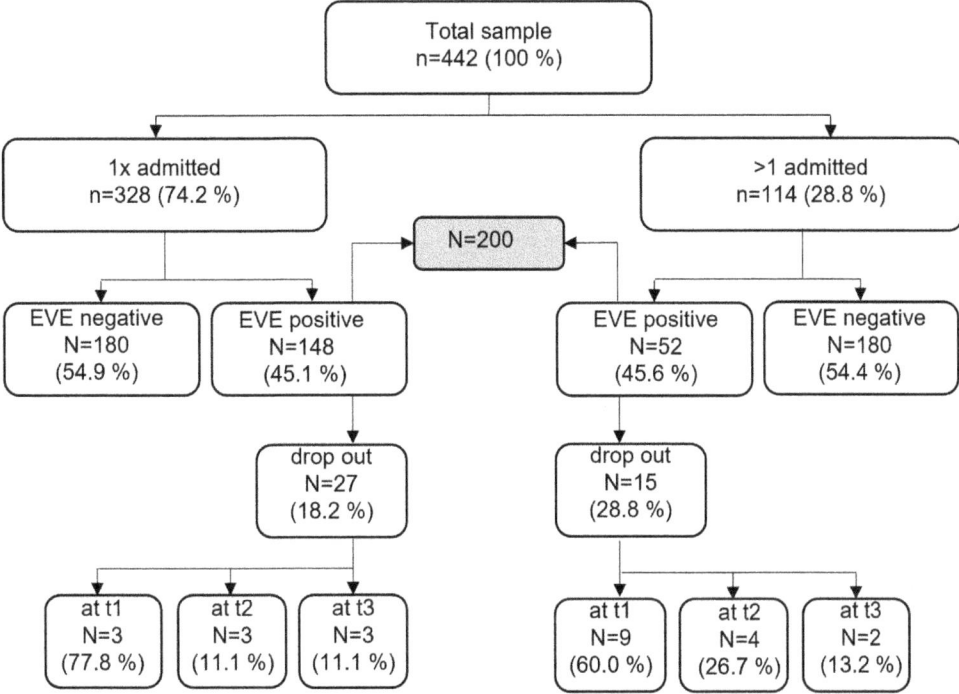

Figure 1. Consort diagram of study sample; EVE acceptance signature.

In the sample with positive consent ($n = 200$), there were 80 male (40.0%) and 120 female (60.0%) patients. The average age of patients was 15.14 years (SD = 2.83, [5,21]; female: M = 15.45, SD = 2.08, [7,21]; male: M = 13.49, SD = 3.42, [5,17]), with most patients in the age group between 14 and 17 years ($n = 135$, 67.5%). Diagnosis was classified at the end of hospitalization in 197 patients: anxiety disorders (F4; $n = 74$, 37.0%), eating disorders (F5; $n = 33$, 16.5%) and behavioral and emotional disorders (F9; $n = 50.0$, 25.0%). The average duration of treatment was 57.34 days (SD = 58.16, [1, 305]), with most patients ($n = 94$; 47.0%) being treated for more than 41 days. As a form of stay, 114 patients were in crisis stay (57.0%), while 67 patients were in orientation stay (33.5%) and 19 patients were in project stay (9.5%).

Patients with positive and negative EVE differed significantly regarding form of stay and form of admission (planned or unplanned). Patients with positive EVE were more likely to be admitted on a planned basis (U = 15,842, $p < 0.001$) and patients with negative EVE were more likely to be in crisis stay (U = 17,043, $p < .001$). Further descriptive information on the sample and a comparison of the characteristics of the subjects included as opposed to the not included are given in the Appendix A.

3. Results

Overview of all results is summarised in Table 1.

Table 1. Overview of sample sizes, means, and SD for all scales and participants.

	T1	T2	T3
FBB			
Therapists n (%)		131 (68.23)	
Therapists total score M (SD)		2.79 (0.51)	
Patients n (%)		128 (66.67)	
Patients total score M (SD)		2.98 (0.65)	
Main caregivers n (%)		99 (51.6)	
Main caregivers total score M (SD)		3.28 (0.57)	
CBCL n (%)	113 (54.5)	105 (52.5)	96 (48)
Externalizing problems M (SD)	61.89 (10.67)	58.08 (9.74)	57.13 (10.51)
Internalizing problems M (SD)	69.73 (8.92)	64.50 (9.27)	61.68 (11.44)
Total problems M (SD)	69.67 (8.13)	64.23 (8.45)	61.72 (10.83)
YSR n (%)	164 (82)	122 (61)	104 (52)
Externalizing problems M (SD)	58.05 (9.86)	54.12 (9.89)	53.02 (9.87)
Internalizing problems M (SD)	65.98 (9.88)	60.24 (11.26)	57.47 (11.15)
Total problems M (SD)	65.48 (9.06)	59.41 (10.89)	57.31 (10.26)
ILK			
Main caregivers n (%)	116 (58)	105 (52.5)	96 (48)
Problem score PR_{0-7} M (SD)	3.73 (1.67)	2.47 (1.86)	2.55 (2.07)
Quality-of-life score LQ_{0-28} M (SD)	16.41 (4.16)	19.36 (3.90)	19.47 (4.50)
Adolescents n (%)	148 (74)	111 (55.5)	94 (47)
Problem score PR_{0-7} M (SD)	3.34 (1.59)	2.08 (1.97)	1.96 (1.86)
Quality-of-life score LQ_{0-28} M (SD)	17.55 (4.01)	20.69 (4.48)	21.01 (4.25)
Children n (%)	28 (14)	26 (13)	23 (11.5)
Problem score PR_{0-7} M (SD)	2.75 (1.69)	2.15 (1.49)	2.3 (2.12)
Quality-of-life score LQ_{0-28} M (SD)	19.18 (4.36)	21.58 (3.84)	21.00 (5.55)

Abbr. FBB for Treatment Satisfaction; CBCL Child behavior Check List, YSR Youth self report; ILK Inventory for Quality of Life.

3.1. Treatment Success—Reduction of Psychopathology

The clinical symptoms rated by the children and adolescents showed a highly significant decrease between the times T1, T2, and T3 ($\chi^2 = 84.8$, $p < 0.001$) indicating treatment success. There was no difference between boys and girls ($U = 3512.5$, $z = 0.57$, $p = 0.571$, $r = 0.04$). Comparison of age groups (≤ 6; 6.1–14; 14–18; >18) showed no significant differences (2708; df = 3; $p = 0.439$).

The effect sizes are in the high range (T1–T2: $r = 0.66$; T1–T3: $r = 0.88$), while the effect size between T2 and T3 lies in the middle range ($r = 0.21$). This decrease also applies to the reported internalizing and externalizing symptoms (internalizing: $\chi^2 = 76.85$, $p < 0.001$; externalizing: $\chi^2 = 36.14$, $p < 0.001$): here, too, the effect sizes can be found in a similar spectrum (internalizing, T1–T2: $r = 0.64$; T1–T3: $r = 0.81$; T2–T3: $r = 0.17$; externalizing, T1–T2: $r = 0.37$; T1–T3: $r = 0.57$; T2–T3: $r = 0.21$). Assessment of the symptom change rated by the main caregivers showed a comparable picture of a significant decrease in clinical symptoms ($\chi^2 = 80.07$, $p < .001$). This effect applies also to both the internalizing and externalizing symptoms (internalizing: $\chi^2 = 57.91$, $p < 0.001$; externalizing: $\chi^2 = 56.38$, $p < 0.001$). The results are summarised in Table 2.

3.2. Treatment Satisfaction

On average patients showed positive treatment satisfaction (M = 2.94, SD = 0.63), a result that is significantly different from zero (t = 60.19, $p < 0.001$) and lies above the normative data (clinical sample mean 2.57 ± 1.31). There were no significant differences between treatment satisfaction of male and female patients (U = 3301.50, z = −0.12, $p = 0.903$). Treatment satisfaction also turned out to be equivalent in the different age groups ($\chi^2 = 4.34$, $p = 0.227$).

Table 2. Treatment success and quality of life over time and results of significance tests.

Measuring Instrument	Perspective	T1 Median	T2 Median	T3 Median	χ^2 Test Statistics
YSR	Patients' self-report				
	YSR-INT ($n = 99$)	21	13	10	76.85 ***
	YSR-EXT ($n = 99$)	13	10	9	36.14 ***
	YSR-GES ($n = 99$)	58	40	35	84.80 ***
CBCL	Main caregivers' rating				
	CBCL-INT ($n = 87$)	20	13	11.5	57.91 ***
	CBCL-EXT ($n = 86$)	13.5	10	8.5	56.38 ***
	CBCL-GES ($n = 86$)	57.5	37	34	80.07 ***
ILK	Children's self-report ($n = 24$)				
	ILK-PR$_{0-7}$	3.00	2.00	2.00	2.03
	ILK-LQ$_{0-28}$	19.00	21.00	22.00	10.17 **
	Adolescents' self-report ($n = 112$)				
	ILK-PR$_{0-7}$	4.00	2.00	2.00	78.42 ***
	ILK-LQ$_{0-28}$	18.00	21.00	21.00	85.19 ***
	Main caregivers' rating ($n = 97$)				
	ILK-PR$_{0-7}$	4.00	3.00	2.00	48.47 ***
	ILK-LQ$_{0-28}$	16.00	20.00	20.00	63.46 ***

Note. n = quantity. The table refers to the initial admissions of patients admitted to UK-KJP with positive informed consent. Means (M) and standard deviations (SD) of the CBCL, YSR, and FBB procedures were calculated using T values. The scales of the ILK have specific limits, see indices.

With regard to the form of hospitalization, there was no significant effect (H(15) = 5.64, $p = 0.060$, $\eta^2 = 0.02$, $d = 0.39$). A significant association was found between the severity of clinical symptoms at T1 and treatment satisfaction at T2. This effect applies equally to the age groups of children and adolescents, i.e., the higher the clinical symptoms were, the lower the treatment satisfaction of both children and adolescents was (children: rS = −0.56, 95% BCa CI [−0.78, −0.23], $p < 0.01$; Adolescents: rS = −0.27, 95% BCa CI [−0.42, −0.11], $p < 0.01$).

In relation to the quality assessment, the results of the FBB analysis at T2 are shown in Table 3, showing a high satisfaction of caregivers and patients concerning the different quality measures. Framework quality correlates significantly with outcome quality rated by patients (rS = 0.56, 95% BCa CI [0.43, 0.67], $p < 0.001$) and caregivers (rS = 0.25, 95% BCa CI [0.06, 0.43], $p < 0.05$.), i.e., the better the framework the higher the satisfaction with treatment.

3.3. Quality of Life

At T1 quality-of-life score was lower as the norm sample and significant improvements in quality of life were observed over the treatment period (see Table 2). At T3 the mean QoL score was above the norm population (19.25) for parents (19.47 ± 4.5), children (21.0 ± 5.6) and adolescents (21.0 ± 4.25). Large effects (Cohen's d ≥ 0.8) were found in terms of the overall assessment of quality of life (adolescents: z = 5.51, $p < 0.001$, d = 1.22; Main caregivers: z = 6.61, $p < 0.001$, d = 1.81) and mental health assessment (adolescents: z = 6.91, $p < 0.001$, d = 1.71; main reference persons: z = 5.71, $p < 0.001$, d = 1.42). Additionally, a significant reduction in the problem score (adolescents: z = 6.88,

$p < 0.001$, d = 1.71; Main caregivers: z = 5.09, $p = < 0.001$, d = 1.21) and a significant increase in the quality-of-life score 0–28 (adolescents: z = −7.72, $p < 0.001$, d = −2.13; Main reference persons: z = −6.43, $p < 0.001$, d = −1.72) illustrates an improvement in quality of life from the time T1 to T3. Furthermore, there was no significant difference between boys and girls (U = 1275.5; $p = 0.775$).

Table 3. Quality measures according FBB: percentage of categories 3 (mainly correct) and 4 (precisely correct) as well as the mean of the means of all ratings of patients (n = 111) and caregivers (n = 118).

Quality Measure	Submeasure	Caregivers		Patients	
		Mean %	Mean * Mean	Mean %	Mean * Mean
Outcome Quality	personal success	73.3 ± 13.7	3.2 ± 0.4	74.9 ± 5.0	3.0 ± 0.2
	family success	92.1	3.6 ± 0.7	53.3	2.6 ± 1.3
Process Quality	relation to therapist	83.8 ± 14.2	3.3 ± 0.4	85.4 ± 5.6	3.3 ± 0.1
	framework conditions	81.5 ± 5.8	3.1 ± 0.2		

FBB Questionnaire for treatment satisfaction. * Scale: 0 no success, 1 rather successless, 2 partially successful 3 mainly successful, 4 fully successful; shaded areas were not included in questionnaire for patients.

In the sample of children admitted to the UK-KJP (n = 24), a significant improvement in quality of life was found as well. The quality-of-life score at T2 is reported significantly higher than at T1 (z = −2.96, $p = 0.009$, d = −1.52), although this increase in quality of life is no longer detectable at T3 (z = −1.80, $p = 0.214$, d = −0.79); a result which may occur due to the small sample size.

4. Discussion

This study measures outcome quality within a naturalistic design at a department for child and adolescent psychiatry. Results show a significant reduction of psychopathology from admission to discharge and until six weeks after discharge. Effect sizes are high during the time of treatment and smaller, yet still significant, after discharge with high effect sizes also for general psychopathology as well as internalizing and externalizing symptoms. This means, the therapeutic setting provided leads to a significant symptom reduction. Symptom reduction is the first and main goal of treatment and, thus, the main outcome criteria for quality assessment [39]. In comparison to the two other Austrian studies [18,19] our results are aligned with previous findings. One of the departments evaluated by the older Austrian studies is also grounded on systemic therapy theory, the second is grounded on psychoanalytical theory. All three studies are naturalistic studies without a control group, without randomization and crossover, thus, mirroring the reality of daily treatment (treatment as usual) all over the world. It would be interesting to analyze the similarities of those departments in treatment provision, structure, and processes, to gain causal information about what "really helps". One principle of evidence-based medicine is to reach informed consent or shared decision-making, which this treatment process provides on a high level [13]. The other reason to perform a naturalistic study was the reality of treatment provision to kids of different ages, sex, with various different diseases and at different stages of disease, criteria which no known EBM protocol could provide. The therapeutic concept used in this study was developed to create a basic treatment situation, which is the grounding basis for an individual's recovery.

In all three Austrian studies treatment is successful in the sense of symptom reduction and clinical relevance, thus, arguably reaching at least a partial recovery—a results which has been documented by comparable international studies as well [20–23]. Recovery is defined as a "profound personal ... process to change attitudes, values, feelings, abilities, and roles to achieve a satisfactory, hopeful and productive way of life with the possible limitations of illness" [40]. Certainly, our study can only demonstrate recovery in the sense of symptom reduction and increased quality of life, but any recovery is important for lifelong prognosis of mental disorders. As a longer duration of mental health problems in adolescence is the main prognostic factor, it is essential to reduce symptom load and increase self-efficacy and quality of life [41]. Therefore, it is crucial to achieve a clinically relevant reduction. In our study, this is exemplified by reaching the normative symptom level of the CBCL scales and by the significant increase of the QoL score. Furthermore, the problem score of the QoL questionnaire also decreased significantly, providing even more information about the clinical relevance of the reported outcome quality.

From a quality management perspective treatment success—defined as satisfaction with treatment and with process—is the most important parameter. In our study, treatment satisfaction is high for caregivers, less but also very positive for patients and high for therapists. Looking at the subscores outcome quality is also in the high range and so are framework conditions and relationship to therapist. Both factors of process quality proved to be significantly associated with high satisfaction with treatment. In a recent qualitative survey Schneidtinger and Haslinger-Baumann [42] describe a model of recovery with 3 main facilitating factors. The basic level consists of supporting therapies, help with daily structures and the ward as a safe place. The next level is provided by peers´ understanding, community, and friendship, the third level by family factors as connectedness and parental support. As parents and patients rate the framework conditions satisfying the concept of department delivers the basic level of the recovery model. As parents are rating the improvement in family function equally positively as their children, effects on the third level can be assumed.

For future quality management in child and adolescent psychiatry there are several conclusions to draw. First, outcome measurement as performed in this study is useful and should be used in a continuous quality improvement concept [5,43] and performed as a measurement feedback system [44]. Reduction of symptoms and treatment satisfaction could be used as benchmarks, quality-of-life measures, and reduction of problem scores added for control of clinical relevance. However, as "recovery" would be the central goal of a profound quality management the quantitative assessment should be enriched by detailed analysis of, e.g., the severity and acuity of the child's symptoms; the child's functional impairment; the child's functional strengths; family functioning. Furthermore, assessment of the goals of treatment; the modality, strategy, and tactics of treatment; readiness for change; the quality of the therapeutic alliance and adherence to treatment should be added to the quantitative assessment of "recovery" [43].

Kelly [44] recommends multidimensional monitoring in three modules: a baseline follow-up module which assesses the child's and family's mental health status starting the entry to the system and lasting throughout treatment; a concurrent module which obtains information throughout the course of treatment; and a background module which assesses factors in the child's and family's background that moderates the course of treatment.

Furthermore, regular assessments of the employees' view of the structures and processes as well as their implementation—together with the measures described above—would give a 360-degree view of the therapeutic process a team provides. The results should be regularly assessed and reported back to the providing team for control, reflection, and supervision.

Limitations

In the sense of the strict rules of evidence-based medicine with the necessity of double blinded, randomized crossover studies the naturalistic design is the main limitation of this study. Nevertheless, critics of this strict interpretation of evidence-based research suggest also using alternative methods for gaining evidence [15]. The naturalistic approach is thought to evaluate concepts in the real situation, closely monitoring the real processes of the applied treatment service.

Moreover, participation of patients and caregivers was not complete, thus this may have caused a bias, although we checked the anamnestic details and found no difference between the participants and the non-participants concerning age, gender and several psychosocial items (see also Table A1).

5. Conclusions

Our study demonstrates strong therapeutic effects of a stringently organised and reflected multiprofessional treatment approach. Systemic theory gave rise to the values, vision, and mission of the project; it provided the basis for developing the respective structures and processes. Symptom reduction and treatment satisfaction is shown to be high, effect sizes are strong, and the clinical relevance—as measured by quality of life at discharge—is comparable to healthy children and adolescents.

Author Contributions: Conceptualization, C.F. and L.T.-H.; methodology, R.W., C.F.; formal analysis, C.F., B.K., F.W.; writing—original draft preparation, L.T.-H., F.W.; writing—review and editing, L.T.-H.; project administration, L.T.-H., C.F.; funding acquisition, L.T.-H. All authors have read and agreed to the published version of the manuscript.

Funding: Funding was partially provided by Ludwig-Boltzmann Institute for Health Technology Assessment (LBI-HTA), Vienna, and funds raised by charity events.

Institutional Review Board Statement: The entire study project was approved by the Ethics Committee of the Federal State of Salzburg (Austria; vote of 28.04.2010, E-No. 1195).

Informed Consent Statement: Informed consent was obtained from all subjects involved in the study.

Data Availability Statement: The data generated and analysed during the present study are not publicly available due to ethical restrictions but are available from the corresponding author upon reasonable request.

Acknowledgments: We thank all the patients, their caregivers, and all our employees, who are responsible for the application of the treatment process and supported the study.

Conflicts of Interest: The authors declare no conflict of interest. Furthermore, the funders had no role in the design of the study; in the collection, analyses, or interpretation of data; in the writing of the manuscript, or in the decision to publish the results.

Appendix A

Table A1. Sample characteristics and comparison of participants and non-participants.

Sample Characteristics	Total Sample n (%)	Sample with Positive EVE n (%)	Sample with Negative EVE n (%)
(Total)	442 (100)	200 (100)	242 (100)
Age			
≤6 years (Children [2])	5 (1.1)	4 (2)	1 (0.4)
≥7 to ≤13 years (underage minors [2])	105 (23.8)	45 (22.5)	60 (24.8)
≥14 to ≤17 years (minors of age [3])	311 (70.4)	135 (67.5)	176 (72.7)
≥18 years (Adults [3])	21 (4.8)	16 (8)	5 (2.1)
Sex			
female	250 (56.6)	120 (60)	130 (53.7)
male	192 (43.4)	80 (40)	112 (46.3)
Diagnosis [1] at T2	-	197 (98.5)	0 (0)
F3		23 (11.5)	
F4		74 (37.0)	
F5		33 (16.5)	
F9		50 (25.0)	
Other (F1, F2, F6, F8)		17 (8.5)	

Table A1. *Cont.*

Sample Characteristics		Total Sample n (%)	Sample with Positive EVE n (%)	Sample with Negative EVE n (%)
Missing			3 (1.5)	
Hospitalization form				
planned		133 (30.1)	98 (49)	35 (14.5)
unplanned		309 (69.9)	102 (51)	207 (85.5)
Type of stay				
Crisis stay		322 (72.9)	114 (57)	208 (86)
Orientation stay		97 (21.9)	67 (33.5)	30 (12.4)
Project stay		23 (5.2)	19 (9.5)	4 (1.7)
Department				
Day-clinical stay		63 (14.3)	46 (23)	17 (7)
In-patient stay		379 (85.7)	154 (77)	225 (93)
Duration of stay				
≤1 day		96 (21.7)	5 (2.5)	91 (37.6)
≥2 to ≤7 days		132 (29.9)	33 (16.5)	99 (40.9)
≥8 to ≤41 days		105 (23.8)	68 (34)	37 (15.3)
≥42 days		109 (24.7)	94 (47)	15 (6.2)
Legal basis of inpatient admission [1]		-	192 (100)	0 (0)
voluntary			152 (79.2)	
according to § 8 UBG			25 (13)	
according to § 9 UBG			1 (0.5)	
by court order			1 (0.5)	
other			13 (6.8)	
Legal duty of custody [1]		-	192 (100)	0 (0)
father			9 (4.7)	
mother			69 (35.9)	
both parents			97 (50.5)	
youth welfare			7 (3.6)	
other			10 (5.2)	
Parents' school-leaving qualification [1]		-	368 (100)	0 (0)
No school-leaving qualification	Mother		2 (0.5)	
	Father		0 (0)	
Special education school	Mother		1 (0.3)	
	Father		2 (0.5)	
Secondary school	Mother		41 (11.1)	
	Father		19 (5.2)	
Apprenticeship	Mother		63 (17.1)	
	Father		71 (19.3)	
Abitur/A-Level/vocational baccalaureate diploma	Mother		38 (10.3)	
	Father		26 (7.1)	
University degree	Mother		22 (6)	
	Father		26 (7.1)	
Unknown	Mother		17 (4.6)	
	Father		40 (10.9)	

Note: n = quantity. [1] Data were taken from baseline documentation (BADO). Therefore, no data are available for the sample with negative EVE. [2] Designated as children in the present study. [3] Designated as adolescents in the present study.

References

1. Ärzteausbildungsordnung (Medical Doctors' Education Regulation). Regulation of the Federal Minister of Health on Training as a General Practitioner and as a Specialist; 2015,) StF: BGBl. II Nr. 147/2015 §15(1)13. Available online: https://www.ris.bka.gv.at/GeltendeFassung.wxe?Abfrage=Bundesnormen&Gesetzesnummer=20009186 (accessed on 10 October 2021).
2. Philipp, J.; Zeiler, M.; Waldherr, K.; Nitsch, M.; Dür, W.; Karwautz, A.; Wagner, G. The Mental Health in Austrian Teenagers (MHAT)-Study: Preliminary results from a pilot study. *Neuropsychiatrie* **2014**, *28*, 198–207. [CrossRef]
3. Beck, N.; Warnke, A. Youth welfare needs after inpatient child and adolescent psychiatric treatment. *Zschr. Kinder Und Jugen Psychiatr. Psychother.* **2009**, *37*, 57–67. [CrossRef]
4. Fliedl, R.; Ecker, B.; Karwautz, A. Child and adolescent psychiatric care 2019 in Austria—Steps of care, current state and lookout. *Neuropsychiatrie* **2020**, *34*, 179–188. [CrossRef]

5. Bickman, L.; Noser, K. Meeting the challenges in the delivery of child and adolescent mental health services in the next millennium: The continuous quality improvement approach. *Appl. Prev. Psychol.* **1999**, *8*, 247–255. [CrossRef]
6. Kunkel, S.; Rosenquist, U.; Westerling, R. The structure of quality systems is important to the process and outcome, an empirical study of 386 hospital departments in Sweden. *BMC Health Serv. Res.* **2007**, *7*, 104. [CrossRef]
7. Thun-Hohenstein, L. Care situation of psychologically conspicuous and sick children and adolescents. In *Kindermedizin–Werte Versus Ökonomie*; Kerbl, R., Thun-Hohenstein, L., Vavrik, K., Waldhauser, F., Eds.; Springer: Berlin/Heidelberg, Germany, 2008; pp. 163–175.
8. de Shazer, S.; Berg, I.K.; Lipchik, E.; Nunnally, E.; Molnar, A.; Gingerich, W.; Weiner-Davis, M. Brief Therapy: Focused Solution Development. *Fam. Process.* **1986**, *25*, 207–221. [CrossRef] [PubMed]
9. Schweitzer, J.; Beher, S.; Sydow, K.; Retzlaff, R. Systemic therapy / family therapy. *Psychotherapeutenjournal* **2007**, *1*, 4–19.
10. Walter, G. Inpatient treatment as transition. *Systeme* **1998**, *12*, 52–62.
11. Working Group Systemic Therapy. Statement on the Theory and Practice of Systemic Therapy. 2009. Available online: https://www.dgsf.org/themen/berufspolitik/berufspolitik-bis2005/agst_stellungn_wiss_beirat.html (accessed on 25 June 2020).
12. Rotthaus, W. Systemic child and adolescent psychiatry and psychotherapy. In *Paar-Und Familientherapie*; Wirsching, M., Scheib, P., Eds.; Springer: Berlin/Heidelberg, Germany, 2002; pp. 525–535.
13. Thun-Hohenstein, L. Participation of children and adolescents in child and adolescent psychiatry. *Paediatr. Paedol.* **2014**, *49*, 42–47. [CrossRef]
14. Heekerens, H.P. From the laboratory to the field. *Psychotherapeut* **2005**, *50*, 357–366. [CrossRef]
15. Falissard, B. How should we evaluate non-pharmacological treatments in child and adolescent psychiatry. *Eur. Child Adolesc. Psychiatry* **2015**, *24*, 1011–1013. [CrossRef]
16. Mattejat, F.; Trosse, M.; John, K.; Bachmann, M.; Remschmidt, H. *Model Research Project on the Quality of Outpatient Child and Adolescent Psychiatric Treatments, Final Report*; Görich & Weiershäuser: Marburg, Germany, 2006.
17. Mattejat, F.; Remschmidt, H. The assessment of therapy outcome in child and adolescent psychiatry under naturalistic conditions—Conception and implementation of the Marburg System of Quality Assurance and Therapy Evaluation. *Z. Kinder Jugendpsychiatr Psychother.* **2006**, *34*, 445–454. [CrossRef]
18. Katzenschläger, P.; Fliedl, R.; Popow, C.; Kundi, M. Quality of life and satisfaction with inpatient treatment in adolescents with psychiatric disorders. *Neuropsychiatrie* **2018**, *32*, 75–83. [CrossRef]
19. Reinelt, P.D. Treatment Assessment and Quality of Life in Child and Adolescent Psychiatry Inventories, Progress and Correlation Analyses. Bachelor' Thesis, University of Klagenfurt, Klagenfurt, Austria, 2010. Available online: https://netlibrary.aau.at/obvuklhs/content/titleinfo/2413418 (accessed on 25 June 2021).
20. Bachmann, M.; Bachmann, C.J.; John, K.; Heinzel-Gutenbrunner, M.; Remschmidt, H.; Mattejat, F. The effectiveness of child and adolescent psychiatric treatments in a naturalistic outpatient setting. *World Psychiatry* **2010**, *9*, 111–117. [CrossRef]
21. Bredel, S.; Brunner, R.; Haffner, J.; Resch, F. Treatment success, treatment experience and treatment satisfaction from the point of view of patients, parents and therapists—results of an evaluative study from inpatient child and adolescent psychiatry. *Prax. Kinder Jugendpsychiatrie Psychol.* **2004**, *53*, 256–276.
22. Fleischhaker, C.; Bock, K.; Hennighausen, K.; Horwath, D.; Kuhn-Hennighausen, C.; Rauh, R.; Wewetzer, G.; Drömann, S.; Schulz, E. 20-year catamnesis of the child and adolescent psychiatric and psychosomatic clinic Haus Vogt. *Z. Kinder Jugendpsychiatrie Psychother.* **2008**, *36*, 191–203. [CrossRef] [PubMed]
23. Gutknecht, H. Patients' evaluation of day-to-day clinical treatment–aspects of treatment experiences and changes experienced. *Psychiatr. Prax.* **2005**, *32*, 342–348. [CrossRef]
24. Cropp, C.; Streeck-Fischer, A.; Jaeger, U.; Masuhr, O.; Schröder, A.; Leichsenring, F. The relationship between treatment experience and treatment success in inpatient psychotherapy with children and adolescents. *Z. Kinder Jugendpsychiatrie Psychother.* **2008**, *36*, 205–213. [CrossRef] [PubMed]
25. Kaplan, S.; Busner, J.; Chibnall, J.; Kang, G. Consumer satisfaction at a child and adolescent state psychiatric hospital. *Psychiatr. Serv.* **2001**, *52*, 202–206. [CrossRef] [PubMed]
26. Renneberg, B.; Lippke, S. Quality of life. In *Gesundheitspsychologie*; Renneberg, B., Hammelstein, P., Eds.; Springer: Berlin/Heidelberg, Germany, 2006; pp. 29–33.
27. Reinecke, M.A.; Shirk, S.R. Psychotherapy with adolescents. In *Oxford Textbook of Psychotherapy*; Gabbard, G.O., Beck, J.S., Holmes, J., Eds.; University Press Oxford: Oxford, UK, 2005; pp. 353–366.
28. Jozefiak, T.; Larsson, B.; Wichstrøm, L.; Wallander, J.; Mattejat, F. Quality of Life as reported by children and parents: A comparison between students and child psychiatric outpatients. *Health Qual. Life Outcomes* **2010**, *8*, 136. [CrossRef]
29. Balazs, J.; Miklosi, M.; Halasz, J.; Horváth, L.O.; Szentiványi, D.; Vida, P. Suicidal Risk, Psychopathology, and Quality of Life in a Clinical Population of Adolescents. *Front. Psychiatry* **2018**, *9*, 17. [CrossRef] [PubMed]
30. Bastiaansen, D.; Koot, H.M.; Ferdinand, R.F. Determinants of quality of life in children with psychiatric disorders. *Qual. Life Res.* **2005**, *14*, 1599–1612. [CrossRef]
31. Baumgarten, F.; Cohrdes, C.; Schienkiewitz, A.; Thamm, R.; Meyrose, A.K.; Ravens-Sieberer, U. Health-related quality of life and its relation to chronic diseases and mental health problems among children and adolescents: Results from KiGGS Wave 2. *Bundesgesundheitsblatt Gesundh. Gesundh.* **2019**, *62*, 1205–1214. [CrossRef] [PubMed]

32. Mattejat, F.; Simon, B.; König, U.; Quaschner, K.; Barchewitz, C.; Felbel DKatzenski, B. Quality of life in mentally ill children and adolescents: Results of the first multicenter study with the inventory for recording the quality of life in children and adolescents (ILK). *J. Child Adolesc. Psychiatry Psychother.* **2003**, *31*, 293–303. [CrossRef]
33. Flechtner, H.; Möller, K.; Kranendonk, S.; Luther, S.; Lehmkuhl, G. On the subjective quality of life of children and adolescents with mental disorders: Development and validation of a new survey instrument. *Prax. Kinderpsychol. Kinderpsychiatr.* **2002**, *51*, 77–91.
34. Ravens-Sieberer, U.; Erhart, M.; Wille, N.; Bullinger, M.; BELLA Study Group. Health-related quality of life in children and adolescents in Germany: Results of the BELLA study. *Europ. Child Adolesc. Psychiatr.* **2008**, *17*, 148–156. [CrossRef] [PubMed]
35. Kamp-Becker, I.; Schröder, J.; Muehlan, H.; Remschmidt, H.; Becker, K.; Bachmann, C.J. Health-related quality of life in children and adolescents with autism spectrum disorder. *Z. Kinder Jugendpsychiatr Psychoth.* **2011**, *39*, 123–131. [CrossRef]
36. Döpfner, M.; Plück, J.; Kinnen, C. *German School-Age Forms of the Child Behavior Checklist by Thomas, M. Achenbach: Parent Questionnaire on Child and Adolescent Behavior (CBCL/6-18R), Teacher Questionnaire on Child and Adolescent Behavior (TRF/6-18R), Questionnaire for Adolescents (YSR/11-18R)*; Hogrefe: Göttingen, Germany, 2014.
37. Mattejat, F.; Remschmidt, H. *Questionnaires for Treatment Satisfaction*; Hogrefe: Göttingen, Germany, 1998.
38. Mattejat, F.; Remschmidt, H. *Inventory for Quality of Life in Children and Adolescents*; Huber Bern: Edison, NJ, USA, 2006.
39. Becker, K.D.; Chorpita, B.F.; Daleiden, E.L. Improvement in Symptoms Versus Functioning: How do our best treatments measure up? *Adm. Policy Ment. Health* **2011**, *38*, 440–458. [CrossRef]
40. Ballesteros-Urpi, A.; Slade, M.; Manley, D.; Pardo-Hernandez, H. Conceptual framework for personal recovery in mental health among children and adolescents: A systematic review and narrative synthesis protocol. *BMJ Open* **2019**, *9*, e029300. [CrossRef]
41. Patton, G.C.; Coffey, C.; Romaniuk, H.; Mackinnon, A.; Carlin, J.B.; Degenhardt, L.; Olsson, C.A.; Moran, P. The prognosis of common mental disorders ion adolescents: A 14-year prospective study. *Lancet* **2014**, *383*, 1404–1411. [CrossRef]
42. Schneidtinger, C.; Haslinger-Baumann, E. The lived experience of adolescent user of mental health services in Vienna, Austria: A qualitative study of personal recovery. *J. Adolesc. Psychiatr. Nurs.* **2019**, *32*, 112–121. [CrossRef] [PubMed]
43. Bickman, L.; Nurcombe, B.; Townsend, C.; Belle, M.; Schut, J.; Karver, M. *Consumer Measurement Systems in Child and Adolescent Mental Health*; ACT: Canberra, Australia, 1998.
44. Kelly, S.D.; Bickman, L. Beyond outcomes monitoring: Measurement feedback systems in child and adolescent practice. *Curr. Opin. Psychiatry* **2009**, *22*, 363–368. [CrossRef] [PubMed]

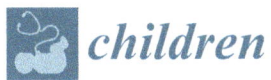

Article

Mental Imagery and Social Pain in Adolescents—Analysis of Imagery Characteristics and Perspective—A Pilot Study

Susan Muriel Schwarz *, Mersiha Feike and Ulrich Stangier

Department of Clinical Psychology and Psychotherapy, Goethe University, Varrentrappstraße 40-42, 60486 Frankfurt am Main, Germany; mersi.feike@stud.uni-frankfurt.de (M.F.); stangier@psych.uni-frankfurt.de (U.S.)
* Correspondence: s.schwarz@psych.uni-frankfurt.de; Fax: +49-69-798-28110

Abstract: Background: Mental imagery (MI) may play a key role in the development of various mental disorders in adolescents. Adolescence is known to be a fragile life period, in which acceptance by one's favored peer group is extremely important, and social rejection is particularly painful. This is the first pilot study investigating MI and its relationship to social pain (SP). Method: A sample of 80 adolescents (14–20 years; 75.3% female) completed a web-based quasi-experimental design about the contents and characteristics of their spontaneous positive and negative MI and associated emotions, and were asked to complete the Social Pain Questionnaire, the Becks Depression Inventory and the Social Phobia Inventory. Results: A higher score of SP was significantly associated with increased fear, sadness, and feelings of guilt, and less control over negative MI. Characteristics of negative MI were more precisely predicted by SP scores than depression- and social anxiety scores. Adolescents with higher SP-scores more often reported negative images including social situations and were more likely to perceive negative images in a combination of field-and observer perspectives than adolescents with lower SP scores. Conclusion: SP-sensitivity seems to be linked to unique characteristics of negative MI, which reveals the strong emotional impact of social exclusion in youths. The results do not allow causal conclusions to be drawn, but raise questions about previous studies comparing each imagery perspective individually.

Keywords: mental imagery; social pain; depression; anxiety; children; adolescents

1. Introduction

Adolescence is known to be a fragile life period in which acceptance by one's preferred peer group is more important than in other phases, and therefore, social rejection is especially painful [1,2]. The experience of pain as a consequence of interpersonal exclusion or ostracism, such as rejection by a peer group and bullying, or the loss of a loved one, is defined as social pain [3]. Social pain is one of the social emotions and can be triggered by actual or imagined situations with other people. Social emotions are emotions which a person has towards another person and they help acting communally and caring. Among these social emotions, a distinction is made between social-evaluative and social-relational emotions (in addition to positive and negative emotions). Social-evaluative emotions are sensations that a person feels towards other persons. These include, for example, hate or love. Social pain, like sadness, guilt, or shame, belongs to the social-relational emotions. These result from the perceived emotions of other persons toward oneself [4].

Social rejection by one's preferred peer group, for instance, has negative consequences for our wellbeing and health [5,6]. In adults, the experience of rejection seems to affect pain processing [7] and might be involved in the development of depression, borderline personality disorder, and anxiety disorders [8,9]. Previous studies have primarily investigated SP in adults, using the cyberball paradigm (which provides the most applied experimental induction possibilities for SP). Results have shown that there is a large overlap between

Citation: Schwarz, S.M.; Feike, M.; Stangier, U. Mental Imagery and Social Pain in Adolescents—Analysis of Imagery Characteristics and Perspective—A Pilot Study. Children 2021, 8, 1160. https://doi.org/10.3390/children8121160

Academic Editors: Matteo Alessio Chiappedi and Margarida Gaspar de Matos

Received: 15 September 2021
Accepted: 7 December 2021
Published: 8 December 2021

Publisher's Note: MDPI stays neutral with regard to jurisdictional claims in published maps and institutional affiliations.

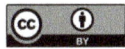

Copyright: © 2021 by the authors. Licensee MDPI, Basel, Switzerland. This article is an open access article distributed under the terms and conditions of the Creative Commons Attribution (CC BY) license (https://creativecommons.org/licenses/by/4.0/).

the processing of physical and social pain and therefore, researchers have postulated a common pain network of physical and social pain [10].

2. Mental Imagery

Many mental health problems have their onset in adolescence [11]. To treat these disorders, it is important to understand the processes leading to such emotional dysfunctions. For adults, studies indicate that mental imagery (MI) plays a key role in the development and maintenance of psychological disorders [12]. These mental images not only occur visually but can appear in any sensory form like auditory, gustatory and olfactory, physical sensations, and tactile impressions [13] and might be associated with emotions like joy, sadness, anger, disgust, and fear (e.g., [12,14]). Mental images can contain parts of memories and maybe comparable to flashbacks (as in post-traumatic stress disorders, PTSD). But MI can also contain an image of a future event. These "flash-forwards" can trigger positive emotions (such as when one thinks with joy of a future event concerning a favorite hobby) or, as found in adult patients with depression, an image of one's own suicide is linked to both distress *and* comfort [15,16]. Mental images are distressing and are linked to psychopathological symptoms when negative MI are frequent, associated with intense negative emotions and if they are experienced as intrusive and not controllable.

3. Mental Imagery in Psychopathology

There is also evidence that depression (in adolescents: [17–21]) and social anxiety disorder (SAD; adolescents: [22–27]) are linked to specific attributes of MI in adolescents (for a detailed review of the relevance of MI in psychopathology in children and adolescents, see [28]).

Adolescents with depression were more likely to perceive negative mental images as more vivid and more often from an observer perspective, than adolescents without depression [17,19–21]. Concerning SAD, they discovered that negative self-images were a result, rather than a significant causal factor of SAD, and therefore may play a different role in the disorder among adolescents. Furthermore, neither valence nor content of self-images, but simply *having* self-images was a substantial factor in SAD during adolescence [22]. This finding contrasts with studies with adults, indicating that self-imagery does indeed play a causal role in SAD [29]. Further studies investigating MI in adolescents with SAD or social anxiety symptoms showed more frequent and more vivid self-images [25], that these images were associated with greater distress and that negative self-imagery was more often perceived with an observer perspective in patients with SAD [26]. These results are in accordance with [23,24]. In both studies, adolescents with high anxiety levels had more images in an observer perspective (experience the image from a third-person-perspective) than adolescents with low anxiety levels. The observer perspective might be part of a cognitive avoidance tendency, as in adult patients with PTSD as the observer perspective is linked to decreased emotions and might be less anxiety-provoking than a field perspective (experience the image in a first-person perspective) and therefore, might be an important maintaining factor [30].

4. Social Pain and Mental Imagery

As there is an overlapping of the construct of social anxiety and SP as well as depression *and* SP, SP might also be associated with different characteristics of MI. Accordingly, patients suffering from SAD reported a fear of rejection and recovered more slowly from a current social rejection than patients without a SAD. Sensitivity to SP might also mediate the development of SAD [31,32]. Accordingly, sensitivity to social pain could be moderated by social anxiety symptoms as socially anxious individuals tend to perceive themselves and their social experiences more negatively [33].

The constructs of depression and SP are associated with one another since patients with depression also report a higher sensitivity to social rejection. The higher sensitivity to social rejection may lead to a key symptom of depression, namely social withdrawal.

Girls reported a stronger internalizing reaction, such as withdrawal, as a response to social rejection than boys, whereas boys tended to display stronger externalizing reactions and expressed more anger and aggression [34,35].

Thus, the present pilot study aimed to explore the association between characteristics of MI and SP scores, as well as to determine the content of MI in adolescents with high SP scores.

5. Hypotheses

Based on the literature search relating to adults and adolescents, we first hypothesized in negative images that higher SP-scores are linked to a higher frequency and vividness of negative images, as well as higher levels of reported emotions and distress. We also postulated that adolescents with a high-SP-sensitivity report images with social themes more often.

Concerning positive images, we assumed that higher SP scores would be significantly associated with a lower frequency and vividness of positive images, as well as lower levels of associated joy. Concerning the use of perspective, we hypothesized that adolescents in a group with high SP scores would report more frequent use of observer perspective. Given that so far, no study has investigated the controllability of MI, we exploratively investigated whether or not the experienced controllability is linked to SP scores. Furthermore, we explored whether the vividness and several specific characteristics of MI would predict SP-sensitivity over and above the predictive power of depression and social anxiety.

6. Method

We present data from an anonymous web-based study examining $N = 80$ adolescents, aged 14 to 20 years. The assessment was conducted using unipark (QuestBack GmbH, Berlin, Germany), an online survey software program. Participants were asked to generate two self-selected spontaneous images, a positive and a negative one. Questions were asked about the sensory qualities (visual, auditory, gustatory, and olfactory properties, physical sensations, and tactile impressions), the intensity of emotions (joy, fear, anger, sadness, disgust, shame, guilt), as well as the perspective of the two images. Additionally, the participants were requested to complete questionnaires about their experience of SP, depressive symptoms, and social anxiety symptoms. Participants specified whether or not their parents had agreed to the participation and data without parental consent was deleted. Permission from the ethics committee was obtained prior to the start of the study.

7. Procedure and Recruitment

The study was approved by the local ethics committee. Before starting the online survey, pilot data were collected for four adolescents (14 to 20 years old) to test the comprehensibility of the MI-questionnaire and the SP-questionnaire, neither of which had yet been used in an adolescent group. The time needed to complete the questionnaire was also stipulated. Participants were recruited using social media websites, e-mail distribution lists, online forums of soccer clubs, and local bulletin boards in Frankfurt, Heidelberg, and Ulm (Germany). In addition, flyers were distributed containing the goals of the study, as well as a QR-Code and hyperlink to the home page of the online survey. The survey started with a description of the study goals and participants were requested to provide informed consent. Participants specified whether or not their parents had agreed to the participation. Adolescents without parental consent were not allowed to complete the survey. Socio-demographic variables including age, gender, type of school, grade level, mother tongue, and existing mental diagnoses were requested. The online survey was conducted between January 2019 and July 2019. To increase motivation for participation, an iPad and cinema tickets were raffled. The email addresses (to contact the winners) of this raffle were saved completely independently of the questionnaire responses, to ensure anonymity.

8. Participants

The first page of the online assessment was opened $n = 436$ times. Informed consent was provided by $n = 149$, and of the starters, $n = 80$ (54%) participants completed the full survey. Participants were excluded if they had indicated that they were visiting a special school or were currently experiencing an acute suicidal crisis. The required time for completing the assessments varied from 35 to 60 min. The mean age of patients was $M = 17.66$ years ($SD = 1.76$; range: 14–20; 75.3% girls, $n = 61$). Forty-six adolescents stated attending a high school, 26 declared attending university, seven participants were undertaking some form of training, and one adolescent was already working. Furthermore, 18 adolescents stated to have an immigration background.

9. Measures

Mental Imagery Questionnaire for Youths (MIQ-Y, adapted by [36]; based on [37]). The MIQ-Y general structure was based on the items used in the *Imagery Interview* from [37]. In many studies with adults, the Imagery Interview has been shown to be a valid measure to assess mental imagery (e.g., [38]). As there are no validated tools for adolescents, we modified the *Imagery Interview*. A validation of the instrument could not be done due to the small sample size.

A general description of a mental image was provided (e.g., Mental images are pictures which we can see with our "inner eye" like a photo or a film in our heads. They are sometimes based on real memories. The contents of these images can also seem very funny to you and do not necessarily have to be real, they can also be more like fantasy images. These mental images can refer to past events, the present, or the future. They can be pleasant or uncomfortable. The images sometimes appear although you do not want them to. Many people have such inner mental images some have them often, some seldom. Afterward, participants were asked to imagine and describe two self-selected spontaneous mental images, first a positive one and then a negative one. After each specific image, they described what they experienced in each sensory impression (including visual, auditory, gustatory, and olfactory properties, physical, and tactile sensations) and rated the clarity on a five-step scale (from 1 = no image at all to 5 = as vivid as real life) and also the strength of the associated emotions (joy, anger, fear, sadness, disgust, shame, guilt), controllability (the control over the mental image itself) on a scale from 0 (no associated emotions, no distress, no control) to 10 (very strong emotions, high distress, full control). Respondents are also asked for the perspective (field, observer, combination of field and observer, not specified). Furthermore, participants report the frequency of occurrence in the last six months (from 1 = almost never, only if I'm asked to think about it to 5 = always, at least once a day).

The different descriptions of the participants were divided into categories according to [39], based on an inductive procedure. The two superordinate categories for positive images are social reward and physical reward. For negative images, the two superordinate categories are physical threat and interpersonal threat. Five categories for positive images (social reward: *enjoying time with family or friends, romantic situations*; physical reward: *enjoying nature, pursuing a sport*) and seven categories for negative images (interpersonal threat: *conflicts with friends/family, death of a close relative, loneliness, failure in a performance situation, social embarrassment*; physical threat: *unintended/accidental physical injury to oneself; physical harm of another person*) were identified.

Social Pain Questionnaire (SPQ; [40]). The *Social Pain Questionnaire* consists of 18 items, each involving a statement about the perception of SP (e.g., if I am excluded by a group, it offends me a lot; if someone ignores me, it hurts me a lot). Participants rate these statements on a 5-point scale (ranging from *not applicable* to *fully applicable*). Internal consistency of the questionnaire has been established as high (Cronbach's $\alpha = 0.95$). Past research has also confirmed highly significant, positive correlations and good convergent validity between the sensitivity to SP and depression ($r = 0.55$, $p < 0.01$), social anxiety ($r = 0.64$, $p < 0.01$), and an anxious ($r = 0.34$, $p < 0.01$) and avoiding attachment style ($r = 0.49$, $p < 0.01$) in an adult-sample ($M = 32.61$ years, $SD = 11.13$). This questionnaire has not yet been validated for youths [40]. The contents of the questionnaire were adjusted (changing words from "valid" to "important", "colleagues" to "classmates", providing examples of somatic syndromes like headache or nausea) to ensure age-appropriateness. Based on a factor analysis, we were able to identify that in our sample, the SPQ is based on a one-dimensional construct, and the internal consistency of the total scale in our sample is high (Cronbach's $\alpha = 0.938$).

Beck Depression Inventory (BDI-II; [41]). The BDI-II assesses depressive symptoms such as changes in appetite, sleeping problems, and bad moods. Twenty-one items have to be rated on a four-point scale. The BDI-II is a reliable instrument for assessing depressive symptoms in clinical and non-clinical populations (from 13 years old). The BDI-II was found to have a Cronbach's $\alpha \geq 0.84$ for non-depressed and acutely depressed samples, as well as adequate content validity and sufficient retest reliability in non-clinical samples [42].

Social Phobia Inventory (SPIN); originally developed by [43]; German version by [44]. The German version of the SPIN consists of 17 items that assess social anxiety symptoms. Participants rate these items on a 5-point Likert scale ranging from 1 (not stressful) to 5 (extremely stressful). The measure displays high internal consistency (Cronbach's $\alpha = 0.89$ and $\alpha = 0.95$) and good retest reliability $r_{tt} = 0.85$ in populations aged 14 to 93 years [44].

10. Statistical Analyses

Prior to the data analysis, participants were screened based on previously outlined exclusion criteria (no participant had to be excluded), and the data set was checked for completeness and correctness, as well as the fit between the distributions and the assumptions of multivariate analysis, according to [45]. Because all of the responses were 'forced-choice', no missing data was generated. We also checked and can confirm that our data meet the requirements (homogeneous variability and normal distributions) for the parametric analysis.

To examine the degree of association between SP scores and MI characteristics, we used correlation analyses. The following variables were included in the correlation analysis: imagery frequency, imagery vividness, controllability, emotional distress, as well as the strength of associated emotions (joy, fear, anger, sadness, disgust, shame, guilt). We conducted two correlation analyses, one for positive imagery and one for negative. To explore the influence of the covariates *social anxiety-* and *depression scores*, as well as *gender*, we used partial correlation analysis. For each analysis, we included all individuals ($n = 80$).

To compare students with different levels of SP concerning the occurrence of MI and the use of perspective in positive and negative imagery, the sample was split into quartiles, in line with [46]. The *high symptom* group (high-SP group) was based on the top 25% of the scores in the social pain measure (SPQ) and the *low symptom* group (low-SP group) consisted of the participants scoring in the lowest 25% on the measure. The limit for the lowest 25% was a sum of 39 points, and for the highest 25%, the sum was 61. After splitting the sample into quartiles, the high- and low-symptom groups each consisted of 20 individuals. The groups were compared demographic variables such as age and sex, using an independent sample *t*-test and *Fisher–Yates* tests. To examine differences in *imagery perspective* (options: observer-, field perspective, the combination of both perspectives, not specified) and *occurrence* between the high-SP group and low-SP group, we used χ^2-tests for positive and negative MI. To investigate the differences in the content of negative and positive MI between SP groups, χ^2-test and *Fisher–Yates* tests were conducted. With a coefficient of determination of $R^2 = 0.18$, statistical power of 0.9, $\alpha = 0.05$, a sample size of $n = 76$ would be needed for a significant overall model for the comparison of contents between SP-groups.

Two sequential linear regression analyses, one for negative MI and one for positive MI, were computed to examine whether SP-, depression- or social anxiety scores significantly predict MI characteristics (frequency, vividness, controllability, associated emotions).

11. Results

11.1. Correlation Analysis of Characteristics of Negative Imagery and Social Pain-Scores

To explore the link between SP-scores and the variables imagery frequency, imagery vividness, controllability, emotional distress and emotions (joy, fear, anger, sadness, disgust, shame, guilt) in negative imagery, a correlation analysis was conducted. Even after including social anxiety- and depression-scores in a partial analysis, significant correlations were found. As significant differences between high- and low-SP groups appeared, *gender* was also included as a covariate. Table 1 displays significant correlations of every partial analysis.

Table 1. Significant correlations between SP-scores and characteristics of negative MI.

	Correlations with SPQ-Scores		SPIN-Scores Partialled Out		BDI-Scores Partialled Out		Gender Partialled Out	
	r	p	r	p	r	p	r	p
Frequency	0.367	0.001			0.268	0.017	0.312	0.005
Vividness	0.307	0.006					0.231	0.040
Controllability	−0.379	0.001 **	−0.253	0.024	−0.313	0.005	−0.325	0.003
Emotional Distress	0.344	0.002			0.261	0.020	0.284	0.011
Emotions								
fear	0.365	0.001	0.304	0.006	0.315	0.005	0.315	0.005
guilt	0.433	0.001 **	0.331	0.003	0.327	0.003	0.434	0.001 **
shame	0.337	0.002			0.322	0.004	0.294	0.008
sadness	0.292	0.009	0.224	0.047	0.224	0.048	0.241	0.032
anger	0.229	0.041						

Note. SP = Social Pain; MI = Mental imagery; SPQ = Social-Pain-Questionnaire. BDI-II = Becks-Depression-Inventory. SPIN = Social Phobia Inventory. Correlations that sustained are in bold. ** $p \leq 0.001$.

11.2. Correlation Analysis of Characteristics of Positive Imagery and Social Pain-Scores

To explore the link between SP-scores and the variables imagery frequency, imagery vividness, controllability, emotional distress, and *emotions* (joy, fear, anger, sadness, disgust, shame, guilt) in positive imagery, a correlation analysis was conducted. No significant correlations ($p \geq 0.05$) were found for SP scores and characteristics of positive images.

11.3. Prediction of Characteristics of Positive and Negative MI by Clinical Measures

Using all individuals, ($n = 80$), a sequential linear regression analysis was used to examine whether SP-, depression-, or social anxiety-scores predict negative MI characteristics in the most suitable manner. One more sequential analysis was computed to explore whether SP-, depression-, or social anxiety scores predict positive MI characteristics.

In negative images, SP scores made the largest contribution to the prediction of the *imagery vividness* ($\beta = 0.31$, $p = 0.006$), *emotional distress* ($\beta = 0.34$, $p = 0.002$) as well as *anxiety* ($\beta = 0.37$, $p = 0.001$), *shame* ($\beta = 0.34$, $p = 0.002$), *sadness* ($\beta = 0.29$, $p = 0.01$), and *anger* ($\beta = 0.23$, $p = 0.04$). *Imagery frequency* ($\beta = 0.43$, $p \leq 0.001$) was most accurately predicted by social anxiety-scores. Feelings of *guilt* were also most accurately predicted by SP-scores ($\beta = 0.43$, $p \leq 0.001$) and depression-scores ($\beta = 0.25$, $p = 0.02$). For *controllability*, *joy*, and *disgust*, no clinical measure was found to predict these variables reliably.

For positive images, *emotional distress* ($\beta = 0.26$, $p = 0.02$), *controllability* ($\beta = -0.33$, $p = 0.003$), and *joy* ($\beta = -0.24$, $p = 0.03$), were most accurately predicted by depression-scores. For *imagery vividness* and *frequency*, *anxiety*, *disgust*, and *shame*, no clinical measure was found to predict these variables accurately.

11.4. Group Differences among SP-Groups

To compare students with different levels of SP concerning the occurrence of positive and negative imagery and the use of perspective, the sample was split into quartiles. A Fisher–Yates test showed a significant difference in *gender* ($p = 0.01$) and *education* ($p = 0.02$) between the SP-groups. The high-SP group includes more females and fewer high school students than in the low-SP group. No significant differences in *age* emerged between the groups ($p = 0.74$). Individuals in the high-SP group show not only significantly higher scores for the SP questionnaire, but also for the depression ($p \leq 0.001$) and social anxiety questionnaires ($p \leq 0.001$). Table 2 shows the demographic characteristics and clinical measures of the two groups.

Table 2. Demographic characteristics and clinical measures.

	Low-SP n (%) or Mean (SD)	High-SP n (%) or Mean (SD)	Statistic
Age	17.50 (1.91)	17.50 (1.81)	$t_{(38)} = -0.34; p = 0.74$
Gender (%)	10 Female (50%) 9 Male (45%) 1 not specified (5%)	18 (90%) 1 Male (5%) 1 not specified (5%)	$\chi^2_{(2,38)} = 8.99; p = 0.01$ *
Education			
Basic School	1 (5%)	3 (15%)	
Advanced School	15 (75%)	7 (35%)	
University	2 (10%)	9 (45%)	
Training	1 (5%)	1 (5%)	
Working	1 (5%)	0	$\chi^2_{(2,38)} = 9.35; p = 0.02$ *
Clinical measures			
SPQ	32.10 (5.05)	70.10 (7.57)	$t_{(38)} = -18.69; p \leq 0.001$ **
BDI-II	7.70 (6.95)	18.50 (10.42)	$t_{(38)} = -3.86; p \leq 0.001$ **
SPIN	9.55 (6.84)	23.70 (13.21)	$t_{(38)} = -4.25; p \leq 0.001$ **

Note. SP = Social Pain; Low-SP = Group of adolescents with a low score on a social pain measure; High-SP = Group of adolescents with a high score on a social pain measure. SPQ = Social-Pain-Questionnaire. BDI-II = Becks-Depression-Inventory. SPIN = Social Phobia Inventory. ** $p \leq 0.001$. * $p < 0.05$.

Differences in occurrence and content of MI between high- and low-SP groups. The results showed significant differences in the occurrence of negative mental images between the high- and low-SP groups ($\chi^2_{(1,39)} = 5.63$ $p = 0.02$). Of 20 individuals in the high-SP group, 19 reported having negative images, in the low-SP group 13 adolescents reported experiencing negative images, seven adolescents in the low-SP group did not report negative imagery.

Concerning the superordinate content of negative images, differences were significant in a χ^2-test ($\chi^2_{(1,38)} = 5.78$ $p = 0.029$). Adolescents in the high-SP group were more likely to report images about *interpersonal threat*. A *Fisher–Yates* test investigating the difference in subcategories showed no significant group differences ($\chi^2_{(6,32)} = 13.77; p = 0.055$). Table 3 shows the frequency distribution of the different contents for negative images.

Table 3. Frequency distribution of contents in negative mental imagery for social pain.

Content of Negative Images	Low-SP n (%)	High-SP n (%)
Interpersonal threat	5 (25%)	14 (70%)
Conflicts with friends/family (e.g., "crying at my desk, reading an awful message from my boyfriend")	1	3
Loneliness (e.g., "being alone, not being able to speak")	1	2
Social embarrassment (e.g., "pupils making fun of me, insulting me, laughing at me")	1	6
Failure in a performance situation (e.g., "sitting in my final exams, forgot everything I've learned")	2	3
Physical threat	9 (45%)	4 (20%)
Physical harm to another person (e.g., "a friend of mine falls down the stairs at school, hearing his crying and falling sounds")	1	3
Death of someone I care about (e.g., "seeing my grandpa lying in a coffin")	5	1
Accidental/unintended physical injury of oneself (e.g., "getting a door slammed into my face, feel blood running down my face")	3	0
No image	6 (30%)	2 (10%)

Note. Content of negative mental images in an adolescent sample aged 14–20 years. SP = Social Pain; Low-SP = Group of individuals with a low score on social pain measure; High-SP = Group of individuals with a high score on a social pain measure.

Concerning the experience of positive images, a χ^2-test showed no significant difference in the occurrence of positive mental images between the high- and low-SP groups ($\chi^2_{(1,39)} = 1.026\ p = 1.00$). All 20 individuals in the low-SP group reported having positive images, in the high-SP group, 19 of the 20 adolescents reported experiencing positive images.

Concerning the contents of positive images, there were no significant differences either in the χ^2 -test (for superordinate categories: $\chi^2_{(1,38)} = 0.1.48; p = 0.224$) or in the Fisher–Yates tests (for subcategories: $\chi^2_{(4,39)} = 3.69\ p = 0.450$) between the two SP-groups. Table 4 shows the frequency distribution of the different contents for positive images.

Table 4. Frequency distribution of contents in positive mental imagery for social pain.

Content of Positive Images	Low-SP n (%)	High-SP n (%)
Social reward	10 (50%)	14 (70%)
Enjoying time with family or friends (e.g., "it's Christmas eve and I'm playing ball with my grandpa")	7	11
Romantic situation (e.g., "kissing my girlfriend, smelling her perfume and feeling her lips")	3	3
Physical reward	10 (50%)	5 (25%)
Enjoying nature (e.g., "walking through the forest in good weather and enjoying the fresh air")	7	3
Pursuing a sport (e.g., "being on a horse farm and taking care of my favorite pony")	3	2
No image	0 (0%)	1 (5%)

Note. Content of positive mental images in an adolescent sample aged 14–20 years. Note: SP = Social Pain; Low-SP = Group of individuals with a low score on the social pain measure; High-SP = Group of individuals with a high score on the social pain measure.

Differences in adopted imagery perspective between high- and low-SP groups. To examine differences between the high- and low-SP groups in the use of the perspective options (observer-, field perspective, the combination of both perspectives, not specified), we used a *Fisher–Yates* test. The test showed a significant difference in the use of perspective in negative images between the high- and low-SP groups ($\chi^2_{(3,39)} = 10.41; p = 0.01$). Table 5 shows the frequency distribution of the different perspective options.

Table 5. Frequency distribution of perspective options in negative mental imagery for social pain.

Perspective Options	Low-SP n (%)	High-SP n (%)
Field perspective	10 (50%)	8 (40%)
Observer Perspective	3 (15%)	2 (10%)
Combination of both	1 (5%)	9 (45%)
Not specified	6 (30%)	1 (5%)

Note: SP = Social Pain; Low-SP = Group of individuals with a low score on the social pain measure; High-SP = Group of individuals with a high score on a social pain measure.

Most of the individuals in the low-SP-group reported perceiving the image in a field-perspective (50%), whereas one person reported perceiving it in a combination of both perspectives. Thirty percent could not specify in which perspective they perceived the image. In the high-SP group, adolescents reported observing the negative images in a field-perspective (40%) and a combination of both perspectives (45%). Differences in positive images were not found.

12. Discussion

The study aimed to investigate the link between social pain (SP) and mental imagery (MI). This is the first study to investigate imagery characteristics and the sensitivity to SP.

12.1. Social Pain and Negative Mental Imagery

It emerged that higher SP scores in adolescents were associated with a significantly higher imagery frequency, imagery vividness, associated emotional distress, fear, anger, sadness, shame, and especially feelings of guilt. Furthermore, higher SP scores were associated with less control over the negative image. Statistical analysis showed moderate correlations between the variables. Even after including social anxiety-, depression scores, and gender as covariates in a partial analysis, the significant correlations were sustained between SP-scores and associated fear, sadness, and guilt. Especially guilt, as a social emotion was associated in this context. This suggests that individuals with a high sensitivity to SP might have not reachable and very high internal moral standards [47]. The adjustment of these extreme standards could be a suitable goal in psychotherapy with patients with high-SP sensitivity. The result that higher SP scores were associated with less control over the negative image was also persistent. Therefore, SP sensitivity might play an important role in explaining variances in these characteristics. Furthermore, most characteristics of negative imagery were predicted most accurately by SP scores. Only imagery frequency was most accurately predicted by social anxiety scores. Therefore, SP sensitivity seems to be an important factor when investigating and dealing with MI in youths. Using methods that aim to reduce SP-sensitivity (like behavioral experiments, cognitive methods) might also have a beneficial effect on MI. Alternatively, techniques in therapy focusing on changing negative MI (like imagery rescripting) might also help to reduce SP-sensitivity. Looking at the results concerning controllability, it might also be appropriate to consider techniques in therapy to increase controllability over negative imagery in patients with higher sensitivity to SP. Our results also support the assumption that adolescence is a fragile life period in which social exclusion hurt particularly. The link between MI and SP reveals the strong emotional impact of social exclusion in adolescents, endorsing the use of methods reducing SP and gaining control over MI in therapy. The implementation of training to improve social skills, as these training might help to reinterpret difficult and ambiguous social situations in a more functionally and less painfully way.

12.2. Social Pain and Positive Mental Imagery

For positive images, characteristics were most accurately predicted by depression scores. Higher depression scores were associated with less controllability and joy, and more distress in fact due to positive images. This is in accordance with previous research exploring depression and MI, as depression seems to affect positive imagery and not only on negative imagery [15,20,48]. Thus, positive MI characteristics were linked most of all to depressive symptoms. However, causal attributions cannot be made, as the results only reveal associations between MI and SP.

The results also indicate a significantly increased frequency of negative images in adolescents with high-SP-sensitivity. There were no significant differences between SP groups in the frequency of positive images. Interestingly, the content of negative images involved close others more frequently in the high-SP- than in the low-SP group. A negative or positive image of an unpleasant or pleasant social situation could therefore be particularly hurtful or enjoyable for people with a high sensitivity for SP compared to positive images without a social theme. This needs to be investigated in an experimental design.

12.3. Social Pain and Attachment Styles

Since different attachment styles appear to be associated with different levels of sensitivity to social pain [49] and since the present study shows a relationship between the characteristics of mental images and sensitivity to SP, attachment styles may also influence the appearance and characteristics of mental images. For example, an insecure attachment style is strongly related to a high sensitivity to SP and could thus also be associated with particularly distressing and/or more frequent negative images. This hypothesis also needs further investigation.

12.4. Social Pain and Perspective of Mental Imagery

The results also showed significant differences in the use of perspective in negative MI between adolescents with high- and low SP-sensitivity. Remarkably, there was a more frequent use of the combination of both perspectives in the high-SP group. This raises questions about previous research comparing only field and observer perspectives, but not the combination of both. In previous studies, patients with different disorders reported having either field- or observer perspectives (e.g., SAD: [23,24,26]; depression: [17]; PTSD: [50]). In our sample, the combination of both perspectives was associated with a higher level of psychopathological symptoms (as the high- and low-SP groups also differed significantly in depression- and social anxiety scores). Possibly, using the combination of both perspectives is already an indication of higher psychopathological symptoms in general.

12.5. Social Pain and Physical Pain

As previous studies in adults showed a large overlap in the processing of physical and social pain, it could be postulated that a stimulus might have a parallel effect on the sensitivity of one type of pain and the other [51]. Thus, the influence of social support on physical pain is conceivable, as is the influence of painkillers on SP and consequently on MI. For example, the intake of paracetamol was shown to have an inhibitory effect on the perceived SP after social rejection and reduced anterior cingulate cortex activity [52]. Treating negative MI could therefore also lead to a reduction of SP and physical pain which might support the use of helpful imaginations during physical procedures.

13. Limitations

The study has several limitations. As already mentioned, nothing can be said about the causality of the relationship between SP sensitivity and characteristics of mental images, as we used a cross-sectional design in this study. Given that we recruited an analog adolescent sample and there were no external clinical assessments and no detailed diagnostic face-to-face interviews (and therefore no diagnosis can be made), there is only limited applicability and generalizability of any conclusions drawn, to clinical samples. As we only used self-report measures there is a lack of verifiability of the objectivity. Because of its exploratory nature, this study could be a preliminary study to an experimental study where one could manipulate social exclusion (e.g., via the cyberball) and evaluate the effects on mental imagery.

Although we gathered pilot data and tested the comprehensibility and clarity of the questionnaires, we cannot ignore the fact that the questionnaires may have been understood differently in terms of language (e.g., unsuitable wording, [53]), lack of adequate reading ability [54], or native language [55] as this could be common in adolescents compared to adults. The use of questionnaires (and not face-to-face interviews) might not be suitable for measuring such a complicated and nonfigurative construct as MI. Youths might have more problems reporting emotions, cognitions, and other mental processes, compared to adults, as they might have a less pronounced self-awareness. As most participants dropped out after the MiQ-Y, the questions may have been too conceptual for some of the adolescents, explaining the high educational status of our final sample. The responses of the participants in this study, who completed the whole survey, did not indicate that they had trouble understanding any questions, although the MIQ-Y was developed based on a semi-structured interview (Hackmann et al., 2000) and not based on a questionnaire. Although the interview of [37] has been widely used in adults and has shown to be a valid instrument, the validity of our measure is questionable.

Furthermore, the sample size is rather small, especially for the comparison of the contents of MI, which especially limits the informative value of the results concerning contents. Furthermore, our sample has a relatively high social status and education, as more than half are attending advanced schools or universities. Additionally, there are several limitations because the data are from an online survey. Certain age and social groups as well as individuals are more likely to take part in online surveys. For example, participants with a lower level of education might not respond to such a survey, which might also explain the generally high educational status [56]. We also cannot ensure that the information given on age or gender, for example, is true. To guarantee that a participant only completed the survey only one time, every IP-address only could participate once. However, we still cannot definitely ensure that participants completed the survey a second time. Furthermore, we could not control current mood or any kind of environmental emotional priming effects such as actual experience of social pain (e.g., bullying).

14. Conclusions

Despite these limitations, the current investigation is among the first to examine MI and its link to SP. Higher scores of SP were significantly associated with a higher score for anxiety, sadness, and guilt and with less control over negative MI. SP-scores seem to predict differences in negative MI more appropriately than social anxiety- or depression scores indicating that differences in SP-sensitivity need to be controlled in studies investigating methods using MI for treatment of mental disorders as possible group differences may falsify outcome measures. The relationship between SP-sensitivity and MI characteristics may explain why negative mental imagery manifests in childhood and adolescence and may contribute to the development of a mental disorder. Furthermore, the link between MI and SP reveals the strong emotional impact of social exclusion in youths. Adolescents in the high-SP group reported using the combination of both perspectives in negative images more often. Using the combination of both perspectives in MI might indicate more severe psychopathological symptoms in general. As this is the first study dealing with the combination of perspectives, the results raise questions about previous results comparing each perspective individually. Consequently, replications with clinical adolescent samples are needed, as well as longitudinal assessments of the MI, to deal satisfactorily with causal issues. The present pilot study also constitutes a starting point for future investigations of the association between SP and characteristics of MI.

Author Contributions: Conceptualization, S.M.S. and U.S.; methodology, S.M.S. and U.S.; software: S.M.S. and U.S.; validation, S.M.S. and U.S.; formal analysis, S.M.S. and U.S.; investigation, S.M.S., U.S. and M.F.; resources, U.S.; data curation, S.M.S. and M.F.; writing—original draft preparation, S.M.S. and U.S.; writing—review and editing, S.M.S. and U.S.; visualization, S.M.S.; supervision, U.S.; project administration, S.M.S. and U.S. All authors have read and agreed to the published version of the manuscript.

Funding: The authors declare no external funding source.

Institutional Review Board Statement: The study was conducted according to the guidelines of the Declaration of Helsinki, and approved by the Ethics Committee of the Goethe University Frankfurt am Main (2018-64; 07.12.2018).

Informed Consent Statement: Informed consent was obtained from all subjects involved in the study.

Data Availability Statement: The data presented in this study are available on request from the corresponding author. The data are not publicly available due to ethical reasons.

Acknowledgments: We thank Brian Bloch for his comprehensive editing of the manuscript.

Conflicts of Interest: The authors have no current or potential conflict of interest to declare that may have a direct bearing on the subject matter of the article.

References

1. Blakemore, S.-J.; Choudhury, S. Development of the adolescent brain: Implications for executive function and social cognition. *J. Child Psychol. Psychiatry* **2006**, *47*, 296–312. [CrossRef] [PubMed]
2. Sebastian, C.L.; Tan, G.C.; Roiser, J.P.; Viding, E.; Dumontheil, I.; Blakemore, S.-J. Developmental influences on the neural bases of responses to social rejection: Implications of social neuroscience for education. *NeuroImage* **2011**, *57*, 686–694. [CrossRef] [PubMed]

3. Dalgleish, T.; Walsh, N.D.; Mobbs, D.; Schweizer, S.; van Harmelen, A.-L.; Dunn, B.; Dunn, V.; Goodyer, I.; Stretton, J. Social pain and social gain in the adolescent brain: A common neural circuitry underlying both positive and negative social evaluation. *Sci. Rep.* **2017**, *7*, 42010. [CrossRef]
4. Leary, M.R. Affect, cognition, and the social emotions. In *Feeling and Thinking: The Role of Affect in Social Cognition*; Forgas, J.P., Ed.; Cambridge University Press: Cambridge, UK, 2000; pp. 331–356.
5. Baumeister, R.F.; Leary, M.R. The need to belong: Desire for interpersonal attachments as a fundamental human motivation. *Psychol. Bull.* **1995**, *117*, 497–529. [CrossRef] [PubMed]
6. Williams, K.D. Ostracism. *Annu. Rev. Psychol.* **2007**, *58*, 425–452. [CrossRef] [PubMed]
7. Bernstein, M.J.; Claypool, H.M. Social Exclusion and Pain Sensitivity. *Pers. Soc. Psychol. Bull.* **2011**, *38*, 185–196. [CrossRef] [PubMed]
8. Hawthorne, G. Perceived social isolation in a community sample: Its prevalence and correlates with aspects of peoples' lives. *Soc. Psychiatry Psychiatr. Epidemiol.* **2007**, *43*, 140–150. [CrossRef]
9. Stanley, B.; Siever, L.J. The Interpersonal Dimension of Borderline Personality Disorder: Toward a Neuropeptide Model. *Am. J. Psychiatry* **2010**, *167*, 24–39. [CrossRef]
10. Williams, K.D.; Cheung, C.K.T.; Choi, W. Cyberostracism: Effects of being ignored over the Internet. *J. Pers. Soc. Psychol.* **2000**, *79*, 748–762. [CrossRef] [PubMed]
11. Paus, T.; Keshavan, M.; Giedd, J.N. Why do many psychiatric disorders emerge during adolescence? *Nat. Rev. Neurosci.* **2008**, *9*, 947–957. [CrossRef]
12. Holmes, E.A.; Mathews, A. Mental imagery in emotion and emotional disorders. *Clin. Psychol. Rev.* **2010**, *30*, 349–362. [CrossRef]
13. Andrade, J.; May, J.; Deeprose, C.; Baugh, S.-J.; Ganis, G. Assessing vividness of mental imagery: The Plymouth Sensory Imagery Questionnaire. *Br. J. Psychol.* **2013**, *105*, 547–563. [CrossRef] [PubMed]
14. Blackwell, S.E. Mental imagery: From basic research to clinical practice. *J. Psychother. Integr.* **2019**, *29*, 235–247. [CrossRef]
15. Holmes, E.A.; Crane, C.; Fennell, M.J.; Williams, J.M.G. Imagery about suicide in depression—"Flash-forwards"? *J. Behav. Ther. Exp. Psychiatry* **2007**, *38*, 423–434. [CrossRef] [PubMed]
16. Moritz, S.; Hörmann, C.C.; Schröder, J.; Berger, T.; Jacob, G.A.; Meyer, B.; Holmes, E.A.; Späth, C.; Hautzinger, M.; Lutz, W.; et al. Beyond words: Sensory properties of depressive thoughts. *Cogn. Emot.* **2013**, *28*, 1047–1056. [CrossRef] [PubMed]
17. Kuyken, W.; Howell, R. Facets of autobiographical memory in adolescents with major depressive disorder and never-depressed controls. *Cogn. Emot.* **2006**, *20*, 466–487. [CrossRef] [PubMed]
18. McKinnon, A.C.; Nixon, R.D.; Brewer, N. The influence of data-driven processing on perceptions of memory quality and intrusive symptoms in children following traumatic events. *Behav. Res. Ther.* **2008**, *46*, 766–775. [CrossRef] [PubMed]
19. Meiser-Stedman, R.; Dalgleish, T.; Yule, W.; Smith, P. Intrusive memories and depression following recent non-traumatic negative life events in adolescents. *J. Affect. Disord.* **2012**, *137*, 70–78. [CrossRef] [PubMed]
20. Pile, V.; Lau, J.Y. Looking forward to the future: Impoverished vividness for positive prospective events characterises low mood in adolescence. *J. Affect. Disord.* **2018**, *238*, 269–276. [CrossRef]
21. Pile, V.; Lau, J.Y. Intrusive images of a distressing future: Links between prospective mental imagery, generalized anxiety and a tendency to suppress emotional experience in youth. *Behav. Res. Ther.* **2020**, *124*, 103508. [CrossRef] [PubMed]
22. Alfano, C.A.; Beidel, D.C.; Turner, S.M. Negative Self-Imagery Among Adolescents with Social Phobia: A Test of an Adult Model of the Disorder. *J. Clin. Child Adolesc. Psychol.* **2008**, *37*, 327–336. [CrossRef]
23. Hignett, E.; Cartwright-Hatton, S. Observer Perspective in Adolescence: The Relationship with Social Anxiety and Age. *Behav. Cogn. Psychother.* **2008**, *36*, 437–447. [CrossRef]
24. Ranta, K.; Tuomisto, M.T.; Kaltiala-Heino, R.; Rantanen, P.; Marttunen, M. Cognition, Imagery and Coping among Adolescents with Social Anxiety and Phobia: Testing the Clark and Wells Model in the Population. *Clin. Psychol. Psychother.* **2013**, *21*, 252–263. [CrossRef] [PubMed]
25. Schreiber, F.; Höfling, V.; Stangier, U.; Bohn, C.; Steil, R. A Cognitive Model of Social Phobia: Applicability in a Large Adolescent Sample. *Int. J. Cogn. Ther.* **2012**, *5*, 341–358. [CrossRef]
26. Schreiber, F.; Steil, R. Haunting self-images? The role of negative self-images in adolescent social anxiety disorder. *J. Behav. Ther. Exp. Psychiatry* **2012**, *44*, 158–164. [CrossRef]
27. Vassilopoulos, S.P.; Moberly, N.J.; Douratsou, K.-M. Social Anxiety and the Interaction of Imagery and Interpretations in Children: An Experimental Test of the Combined Cognitive Biases Hypothesis. *Cogn. Ther. Res.* **2011**, *36*, 548–559. [CrossRef]
28. Schwarz, S.; Grasmann, D.; Schreiber, F.; Stangier, U. Mental Imagery and its Relevance for Psychopathology and Psychological Treatment in Children and Adolescents: A Systematic Review. *Int. J. Cogn. Ther.* **2020**, *13*, 303–327. [CrossRef]
29. Hirsch, C.R.; Mathews, A.; Clark, D.M.; Williams, R.; Morrison, J.A. The causal role of negative imagery in social anxiety: A test in confident public speakers. *J. Behav. Ther. Exp. Psychiatry* **2006**, *37*, 159–170. [CrossRef] [PubMed]
30. Kenny, L.M.; Bryant, R.A. Keeping memories at an arm's length: Vantage point of trauma memories. *Behav. Res. Ther.* **2007**, *45*, 1915–1920. [CrossRef] [PubMed]
31. Fung, K.; Alden, L.E. Once Hurt, Twice Shy: Social Pain Contributes to Social Anxiety. *Emotion* **2017**, *17*, 231–239. [CrossRef]
32. Zadro, L.; Boland, C.; Richardson, R. How long does it last? The persistence of the effects of ostracism in the socially anxious. *J. Exp. Soc. Psychol.* **2006**, *42*, 692–697. [CrossRef]

33. Moscovitch, D.A.; Orr, E.; Rowa, K.; Reimer, S.G.; Antony, M.M. In the absence of rose-colored glasses: Ratings of self-attributes and their differential certainty and importance across multiple dimensions in social phobia. *Behav. Res. Ther.* **2009**, *47*, 66–70. [CrossRef]
34. DeRosier, M.E.; Kupersmidt, J.B.; Patterson, C.J. Children's Academic and Behavioral Adjustment as a Function of the Chronicity and Proximity of Peer Rejection. *Child Dev.* **1994**, *65*, 1799–1813. [CrossRef]
35. London, B.; Downey, G.; Bonica, C.; Paltin, I. Social Causes and Consequences of Rejection Sensitivity. *J. Res. Adolesc.* **2007**, *17*, 481–506. [CrossRef]
36. Schwarz, S.; Schreiber, F. *Fragebogen zur Erfassung mentaler Bilder bei Jugendlichen (FEMB-J)*; Goethe-University: Frankfurt am Main, Germany, 2016; Unpublished Manuscript.
37. Hackmann, A.; Clark, D.; McManus, F. Recurrent images and early memories in social phobia. *Behav. Res. Ther.* **2000**, *38*, 601–610. [CrossRef]
38. Day, S.; Holmes, E.; Hackmann, A. Occurrence of imagery and its link with early memories in agoraphobia. *Memory* **2004**, *12*, 416–427. [CrossRef]
39. Mayring, P. *Einführung in Die Qualitative Sozialforschung*; Beltz: Weinheim, Germany, 2002.
40. Stangier, U.; Schüller, J.; Brähler, E. Development and validation of a new instrument to measure social pain. *Sci. Rep.* **2021**, *11*, 8283. [CrossRef] [PubMed]
41. Beck, A.T.; Steer, R.A.; Brown, G.K. *Manual for the Beck Depression Inventory-II*; Psychological Corporation: San Antonio, TX, USA, 1992.
42. Kühner, C.; Bürger, C.; Keller, F.; Hautzinger, M. Reliabilität und Validität des revidierten Beck-Depressionsinventars (BDI-II). *Der Nervenarzt* **2007**, *78*, 651–656. [CrossRef] [PubMed]
43. Connor, K.M.; Davidson, J.R.T.; Churchill, E.; Sherwood, A.; Foa, E.; Weisler, R.H. Psychometric properties of the Social Phobia Inventory (SPIN). *Br. J. Psychiatry* **2000**, *176*, 379–386. [CrossRef] [PubMed]
44. Consbruch, K.; Stangier, U.; Heidenreich, T. *SOZAS: Skalen zur Sozialen Angststörung: Soziale-Phobie-Inventar (SPIN), Soziale-Interaktions-Angst-Skala (SIAS), Soziale-Phobie-Skala (SPS), Liebowitz-Soziale-Angst-Skala (LSAS): Manual, 1. Auflage*; Hogrefe: Oxford, UK, 2016.
45. Tabachnick, B.G.; Fidell, L.S. *Using Multivariate Statistics*, 5th ed.; Allyn & Bacon/Pearson Education: Boston, MA, USA, 2007.
46. Hodson, K.J.; McManus, F.V.; Clark, D.M.; Doll, H. Can Clark and Wells' (1995) cognitive model of social phobia be applied to young people. *Behav. Cogn. Psychother.* **2008**, *36*, 449–461. [CrossRef]
47. Ferguson, T.J.; Stegge, H.; Miller, E.R.; Olsen, M.E. Guilt, shame, and symptoms in children. *Dev. Psychol.* **1999**, *35*, 347–357. [CrossRef]
48. Morina, N.; Deeprose, C.; Pusowski, C.; Schmid, M.; Holmes, E.A. Prospective mental imagery in patients with major depressive disorder or anxiety disorders. *J. Anxiety Disord.* **2011**, *25*, 1032–1037. [CrossRef]
49. Chester, D.S.; Pond, R.S.J.; Richman, S.B.; DeWall, C.N. The optimal calibration hypothesis: How life history modulates the brain's social pain network. *Front. Evol. Neurosci.* **2012**, *4*, 10. [CrossRef]
50. McIsaac, H.K.; Eich, E. Vantage Point in Traumatic Memory. *Psychol. Sci.* **2004**, *15*, 248–253. [CrossRef]
51. Macdonald, G.; Leary, M.R. Why Does Social Exclusion Hurt? The Relationship Between Social and Physical Pain. *Psychol. Bull.* **2005**, *131*, 202–223. [CrossRef] [PubMed]
52. DeWall, C.N.; MacDonald, G.; Webster, G.D.; Masten, C.L.; Baumeister, R.F.; Powell, C.; Combs, D.; Schurtz, D.R.; Stillman, T.F.; Tice, D.M.; et al. Acetaminophen Reduces Social Pain. *Psychol. Sci.* **2010**, *21*, 931–937. [CrossRef]
53. Campbell, M.A.; Rapee, R.M. Current Issues in the Assessment of Anxiety in Children and Adolescents: A Developmental Perspective. *Behav. Chang.* **1996**, *13*, 185–193. [CrossRef]
54. Vasey, M.W.; Dalgleish, T.; Silverman, W.K. Research on information-processing factors in child and adolescent psychopathology: A critical commentary. *J. Clin. Child Adolesc. Psychol.* **2003**, *32*, 81–93. [CrossRef]
55. Alfano, C.; Beidel, D.C.; Turner, S.M. Cognition in childhood anxiety: Conceptual, methodological, and developmental issues. *Clin. Psychol. Rev.* **2002**, *22*, 1209–1238. [CrossRef]
56. Blasius, J.; Brandt, M. Repräsentativität in online-befragungen. In *Umfrageforschung*; VS Verlag für Sozialwissenschaften: Wiesbaden, Germany, 2009; pp. 157–177. [CrossRef]

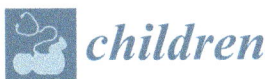

Case Report

Stimulus Control Procedure for Reducing Vocal Stereotypies in an Autistic Child

Marco Esposito [1,*], Laura Pignotti [2], Federica Mondani [3], Martina D'Errico [4], Orlando Ricciardi [3], Paolo Mirizzi [5], Monica Mazza [1] and Marco Valenti [6]

1. Department of Applied Clinical Sciences and Biotechnology, University of L'Aquila, 67100 L'Aquila, Italy; monica.mazza@univaq.it
2. Department of Psychology, University of Rome La Sapienza, 00185 Roma, Italy; la.pignotti@gmail.com
3. Autism Research and Treatment Centre, Una Breccia nel Muro, 00168 Roma, Italy; federica.mondani@unabreccianelmuro.org (F.M.); orlandoricciardi1989@gmail.com (O.R.)
4. Modern Cultures and Literatures, University of Rome La Sapienza, 00185 Roma, Italy; derrico.1797479@studenti.uniroma1.it
5. Department of Psychology, University of Bari, 70121 Bari, Italy; paolomirizzi@yahoo.it
6. Regional Centre for Autism, Abruzzo Region Health System, 67100 L'Aquila, Italy; marco.valenti@univaq.it
* Correspondence: marco.esposito@unabreccianelmuro.org

Abstract: Stereotyped vocal behavior exhibited by a seven-year-old child diagnosed with autism spectrum disorder and maintained by automatic reinforcement was placed under stimulus control through discrimination training. The training consisted of matching a green card (SD) with free access to vocal stereotypy and a red card (SD-absent) with interruption of stereotypy and vocal redirection. At the same time, appropriate behaviors were reinforced. After discrimination training, the child rarely engaged in vocal stereotypy in the red card condition and, to a greater extent, in the green card condition, demonstrating the ability to discriminate between the two different situations. After the training, the intervention began. Once they reached the latency criterion in the red stimulus condition, the child could have free access to vocal stereotypy (green card condition). The latency criterion for engaging in stereotypy was gradually increased during the red card condition and progressively decreased during the green card condition. The intervention follows a changing criterion design. This study indicates that stimulus discrimination training is a useful intervention to reduce vocal stereotypy in an autistic child.

Keywords: vocal stereotypies; autism spectrum disorder; automatic reinforcement; stimulus control; changing criterion design

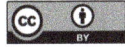

1. Introduction

Children diagnosed with autism spectrum disorders (ASD) are characterized by social communication deficit and a tendency to engage in a pattern of restricted and repetitive behavior [1]. Moreover, autistic children can present impairments in a large variety of developmental abilities, from social–cognitive to behavioral challenges. Although cases of autism have been increasing, currently effective educational interventions for these children are widely diffused, and progress has been demonstrated in intellectual, language, behavior, social, and adaptive skills [2]. Stereotypies are included in core symptoms and they are defined as topographically invariant and repetitious behaviors [3], representing a diagnostic feature of autism spectrum disorder (ASD) according to the current diagnostic criteria of the Diagnostic and Statistical Manual of Mental Disorders. Vocalizing, echolalia, and a-contextual speech are examples of stereotypies maintained by automatic positive reinforcement [3,4]. Stereotypies can become a barrier to learning if their reinforcing value exceeds other stimuli in the environment, and the behavior absorbs too many daily activities of children. Indeed, stereotyped behaviors may compete with other activities and develop control of the stimulus and instruction interfering with learning [5]. In addition, stereotypies can be socially stigmatizing and limit opportunities for socialization and learning in daily life, such as engagement in leisure, vocational, self-care, and may interfere with skill acquisition in academic settings [3,6–8]. Regarding academic settings, Cook and Rapp [9] guide teachers and clinicians through different considerations prior to the implementation of behavior interventions. In sum, the extent to which direct treatment of vocal stereotypy is required for academic tasks varies on an individual basis; essentially, an assessment concerning some conditions including the impact of standard teaching on stereotypies or access of music and others aspects could evoke more or less the stereotypies in children. The mentioned model can also guide practitioners in selecting the least intrusive and most efficient intervention during the academic curriculum. For example, an individual may require multiple preferred items to compete with stereotypy during conditions with low ambient stimulation and adult interaction, but may require either a different or no intervention during academic instruction since only instructions and praises can limit challenging behaviors. At same time, consider the individual without his environment as school context can shed light only on the part of the current issue. Also, treating stereotypies could decrease the stigma that others perceive when children with ASD displays the behavior, impeding social interactions. A recent study [10] has administered a questionnaire to college students after having watched a child engaging in the motor and vocal stereotypy evaluating their perception. Results indicated that observers negatively rated the child when he displayed motor stereotypy, the additional vocal stereotypy yielded more negative judgements than motor stereotypy alone. Stereotyped behaviors exhibit several topographies, including echolalia [11], repetitions of meaningless sounds [12], instances of non-contextual or non-functional speech [13]. Echolalia behavior may be immediate or delayed. Fay [14] defined immediate echolalia as "meaningless repetition of a word or word group just spoken by another person" (p. 39). Differently, delayed echolalia requires longer durations, including repeats of expressions heard even several days earlier. There seems to be a lack of understanding of the sound being repeated and of communicative intent in both cases.

1.1. Function Analysis of Stereotypies

Several studies have reported that reinforcement contingencies could maintain vocal and motor stereotypy behavior for access to attention [15–18] and by reinforcement contingencies for access to the tangible [15]. However, according to Rapp and Vollmer [3], more than 90% of the published functional analyses of stereotypies show that they are maintained by automatic positive reinforcement, a stimulus produced independently of the social environment. Results indicate that the repetitive behaviors (motor and vocal) observed on different individuals with various developmental disabilities are reinforced by the stimulation that was directly generated by the behavior [19], on the other hand, it is maintained by the sensory consequences it produces. Additionally, although repetitive vocalizations may be maintained by social consequences, a recent review [20] focused report behaviors maintained by nonsocial consequences since: (a) stereotypy generally persists in the absence of social reinforcement; (b) interventions for socially reinforced vocalizations considerably differ and would require a separate review; and (c) repetitive vocalizations maintained by social consequences would be more accurately labeled using the verbal operants described and defined by Skinner. Therefore, the current study uses the term vocal stereotypy to refer to any repetitive sounds or words produced by an individual's vocal apparatus that are maintained by nonsocial reinforcement.

1.2. Behavioral Interventions

Vocal and motor stereotypies maintained by automatic reinforcement are difficult to treat due to the challenging control of access to and retention of the sensory consequence it produces [21]. Some studies have used mild punishment to treat automatic reinforcement in vocal stereotypies in individuals diagnosed with autism. For example, Ahearn, Clark, MacDonald and Chung [22] found that target response interruption and redirection to appropriate vocalizations (RIRD; response interruption and redirection) positively reduced vocal stereotypy in at least four interventions with autistic children. The findings were later confirmed by Athens and Vollmer [23] and Cassella, Sidener, Sidener and Progar [24]. Interventions based on RIRD [25] involve interrupting vocal or motor stereotypy and replacing it with response exercises to simple questions concerning social rules or how to request an object [22]. This procedure conforms to ethical requirements that behavior analysts do not use aversive methods or punishment procedures until all reinforcement options have been exhausted [26]. In RIRD, the response blocking of the stereotypies is associated with the social reinforcement provided by therapist in contingency of the appropriate vocal responses of the child [24]. Rapp, Patel, Ghezzi, O'Flaherty, and Titterington [27] have highlighted how antecedent—and consequence—based interventions reduce vocal stereotypy in children with ASD [12,13,22,28]. Research has highlighted how effective discrimination training is on problem behavior maintained by automatic reinforcement. Discrimination training is a procedure that reinforces a target behavior in the presence of certain antecedent stimuli, indicates that the reinforcer will not be available in that contingency, and prevents reinforcement of the same target behavior in the presence of other antecedent stimuli [29]. The outcome of such training involves the subject producing appropriate responses in the presence of predictive reinforcing stimuli and appropriate behaviors (the non-emission of stereotyped behavior) in the presence of predictive extinction or punishment stimuli. This stimulus control procedure has been used in some research to teach adaptive responses to individuals diagnosed with autism, including communication, social, academic, vocational, and self-care skills [30,31]. Several recent studies document the effects of decreasing maladaptive behavior by making use of discrimination training [27,32–35]. Rapp et al. [27] and O'Connor, Prieto, Hoffmann, DeQuinzio, and Taylor [36], referring to previous studies, confirmed and demonstrated that environmental stimuli can exert an inhibitory control on behavior automatically reinforced after discrimination training. Specifically, they combined a red card using a verbal reprimand (positive punishment) or toys removal (negative punishment) to interrupt vocal stereotypy. In contrast, no programmed consequences were applied when the occurrence of stereotypy was paired with a green card. Their research suggests that stereotypy passed under the card's control occurring less in the presence of the red card and more when paired with the green card. The basic principle of this procedure is that the green card stimulus assumes the function of conditional positive reinforcement when applied contingently to the absence of stereotypy in the red card condition [32]. During the intervention, when the subject met the criterion in the red card condition, he had access to the green card condition (access to stereotypy). The criterion consisted in the non-emission of stereotypy for a progressively longer time. At the same time, the duration of access to the green stimulus was systematically decreased. The red and green stimuli were scaled down from posters to 10 cm colored cards, and stimulus control was generalized to the participant's classroom and community environment (public library). Results were discussed in terms of discrimination training as a useful intervention for reducing motor and vocal stereotypy. Also, a more recent study [37] reported the effects of a stimulus control procedure involving contingent reprimands on stereotypies of five children with ASD. A brief functional analysis indicated that motor and vocal stereotypy persisted in the absence of social consequences. Subsequently, results indicated that contingent verbal reprimands decreased the targeted stereotypy of the children. The present study describes and evaluates the effectiveness of the application of discrimination training using a RIRD procedure. The main objective was to reduce stereotyped vocal behaviors and implement contextually appropriate alternative behaviors during solitary play in a seven-year-old child diagnosed with autism.

2. Method

2.1. Participant

The participant, Robert, was a seven-year-old boy diagnosed with ASD according to the criteria of the DSM–5 [1]. The child attended the first year of primary school. Robert followed an applied behavior analysis (ABA) treatment at a center and home for 8-h a week (divided in 4 h at clinical center and 4 h at home). Please, note that we refer to the child using disability-first language against the use of first-person one, since the disability is part of a person's identity [38]. Robert engaged in vocal stereotypy for much of his play time and at school. His parents and school teachers reported that this behavior interfered with his learning distressing his classmates. At school, the main difficulties of the child were reported in sustained attention to academic activities, including play time with peers. The family required to clinical staff a specific intervention for the reduction of the vocal stereotypies and provided informed consent in order to participate to the training. The child profile concerning abilities was assessed using the revised Assessment of Basic Language and Learning Skills [39]. Robert was able to give attention to an adult and materials. He described a short story with flashcards, simple comments with respect to an object or activities, and answered questions regarding objects, details, function, categories, and personal characteristics. Robert utilized adjectives and some verbs in phrases. Likewise, his request level was formed by common verbs, nouns, and adjectives (generally, three or four words every request). At the time of the current study, he was learning the past simple tense to describe events along with reading-writing letters and syllables. Concerning social interaction, Robert preferred to play alone; some social initiatives were supported by therapists. Nevertheless, the child played in turn with other peers but he didn't engage in symbolic plays. Finally, preschooler autonomies and imitations were preserved, and no physical impediments were observed. Concerning his challenging behaviours about stereotypies, Robert frequently repeated entire strings of cartoons that he had previously watched on television or YouTube channels (e.g., "Like a little bird from my nest I will now fly"). The behavior was defined as delayed echolalia, since it occurred hours or days after the first contact with the stimulus. In order to understand the recurrent function of the above-mentioned behavior, we applied a descriptive functional assessment (Antecedent-Behavior-Consequence, ABC) which suggested us that the vocal stereotypy of Robert occurred in different environments, especially while he was playing alone in his room. The behavior appeared to be maintained by automatic reinforcement. Although the clinical staff well-identified the function of the behavior, we suggest the use of ABC narrative recordings and open-ended functional assessment interviews along with traditional functional analysis (FA), since they have reported limited empirical support (47% and 71% of cases, respectively, matched with FA) concerning hypotheses on the functions of challenging behavior [40].

2.2. Setting and Materials

Experimental sessions were held in the clinical room at the center and at home of the child with two therapists, two sessions a week. The rooms were furnished with a desk and chairs, a large rug, and various toys and books. Throughout the discrimination training, the child alternated play sessions either at the desk or on the carpet. The intervention started at home while the last three sessions were held at the clinical center. It was not possible to conduct the intervention at school due to restrictions related to the COVID-19 emergency. The discrimination training consisted of presenting two discriminative stimuli during the child played on the carpet or table with high preference available toys. The plays most selected were the marble race truck and a book with pictures and written words. Two 10 cm × 10 cm red and green cards were used as stimuli for discrimination training, such as in the study of Rapp et al. [27] and O'Connor et al. [36]. The green card was faded by resizing to 5 cm × 5 cm during the training until its gradual removal with no card condition, whereas a red elastic bracelet replaced the red card for a major portability (this arrangement could guarantee a more efficacy training during transitions in different places).

2.3. Data Collection and Dependent Variable

For all conditions of the experiment, the dependent variable was the occurrence of stereotyped vocal behavior defined as vocalizing: (a) non-communicative and not appropriate to the context (e.g., repeating movie phrases or words while playing with the track) or (b) repetitive (more than three repetitions of phrases or words within 15 s). Appropriate behavior was defined as playing without vocal stereotypy. Therefore, the dependent variable was the latency between the verbal instruction, "You can play now", given by the therapist and the first exhibition of the vocal stereotypy (the therapist measured the latency time with a digital stopwatch); this data collection based on latency was applied only during the baseline and intervention phase. Conversely, during discrimination training, stereotypy was scored on a partial interval time recording (PIR) into a 5-min session divided into twenty 15-s intervals when the child remained alone. Consequently, the intervals were scored as positive if the participant engaged in stereotypy at any point during the 15-s. The dependent measure in the discrimination phase was, hence, the percentage of 15-s intervals engaged in stereotypy during playing. On the contrary, when the participant did not engage in stereotypy for the entirety of the 15-s interval (whole interval), it was scored as negative. The measurement was converted to the percentage of time when the child was engaged in stereotyped vocal behavior (number of positive intervals divided number of totals intervals $\times$ 100). Inter-observer agreement (IOA) was calculated by two therapists only for discrimination training by dividing the number of agreements by the number of agreements plus disagreements and multiplying by 100. Treatment integrity data were collected for 30% of sessions at a mean score of 100% accuracy.

2.4. Experimental Design

Three conditions were implemented in this study. Firstly, a baseline assessment was conducted, followed by discrimination training and an intervention phase. The purpose of the discrimination training was to control vocal stereotypy by matching programmed consequences with red and green stimuli. At the same time, the child played alone with building blocks, marble tracks, or books of his choice. During the intervention phase, the experimental design used was the changing-criterion design to evaluate the effectiveness of the intervention on increasing the latency time in which the child engages in vocal stereotypy.

2.5. Procedure: Baseline, Discrimination Training and Intervention

In the baseline condition, Robert was in his room, sitting or standing and having free access to various familiar plays. The child was alone while the therapists could observe him from another room via the video camera. In baseline condition, the stereotyped vocal behavior was not interrupted, and no reinforcement or suggestions were provided during appropriate play. Similarly, red and green cards were not present. The eight sessions lasted one minute and successively the discrimination training started. In order to bring the behavior of the child under the stimulus control, discriminating the color of the cards, we have delivered a positive punishment in the presence of the red color (reducing stereotypies) and positive reinforcement in the presence of the green color (free access for stereotypies). In the red card condition Robert was sitting at the table and was allowed to access his toys. The therapist was behind the child and pointed to him the red card saying "Red card, you play without talking". As a result, when the child emitted vocal stereotypies, the contingency included a mild reprimand ("Red card, you play without talking"), the interruption of the game, and vocal redirection (e.g., "How many balls are missing?", "I see a dog with..."). Therefore, when the behavior was appropriate (contextual commentary on the play activities), the contingency included reinforcement with tangibles (e.g., access to the game and more pieces of a toy) and a praise with encouragement (descriptive reinforcement such as "Good, you are playing well, yes the balls are yellow"). The green card condition followed the red card condition. In this condition, the child was seated at the small table and had free access to his games, while on the table was a green card that the therapists pointed to by saying, "Green card, you can play", leaving him alone in the room. There were no contingencies in this condition, so Robert could continue to play emitting stereotypies. The discrimination training was divided into five phases (every phase comprised a different number of the sessions lasted five minutes), each representing a different schedule of reinforcement. Reinforcements (tangible and praise) were identified through a preference assessment, and they were delivered based on a variable interval (IV) reinforcement schedule, contingently the appropriate behavior. Once the child reached zero rates of stereotypy, the reinforcement schedule was thinned. Reinforcements were provided on average every 15 s (I and II phase), every 20 s (III phase), and every 25 s (IV phase). In the second phase, the red bracelet placed on the child's wrist replacing the red card. The fifth phase did not include any reinforcement or prompt.

The intervention began after the discrimination training. The intervention included 32 sessions, each lasted five minutes. A changing criterion design was applied to assess the effectiveness of the green stimulus (or simply red card removal) as an access to automatic reinforcer, in order to increase the latency to engage in stereotypy during red conditions (since green stimulus occurred after the removal of red one, the free access to stereotypy could become a motivation for Robert engaging less with vocal stereotypies in order to have the access to automatic behaviour). Hence, reaching criterion in one condition, the child was required not to emit stereotypy for a longer time to access the automatic reinforcer. Anyhow, the sessions took place in his bedroom and in living room/kitchen. The child was sitting at the table or on the carpet and had access to his toys. The child played alone while his mother was busy with daily activities. The last three sessions were held in the centre with different therapists. During the intervention, the red card condition was called red bracelet and the green card condition (from session 35 onwards) no card (gradually we faded the green stimulus). During the red condition, the therapist put on child's wrist the red bracelet saying, "now you can play". After the instruction, he started the stopwatch monitoring the child from a video connected to the video camera. Contrary to discrimination training, the therapist did not give instructions such as "Red card, you play without talking" and did not use any prompts or additional reinforcement to the contextual comments. When Robert did not engage in the stereotyped vocalizations, he was allowed access to the green card/no card condition for the residual time of the 5-min session (since the sessions lasted 5 min, when the child reached the predefined latency criterion starting by 30 to 300 s during the sessions as showed in Table 1, if he respected the latency criterion could access or not to stereotypy consuming the residual time of each single session). On the other hand, if he showed stereotypies before the end of the predefined criterion, Robert wouldn't have access to the green card condition, and the session ended. During the green card/no card condition, the child did not wear the red bracelet and could emit the target behaviour without intervention. In the red bracelet condition, the latency criterion in order to access to automatic reinforcement (access to the green card/no card condition) was progressively greater during each session:

Table 1. Sessions of the intervention with related changing criterion time.

Sessions (Range)	Criterion Time (Seconds)
1–8	baseline
9–11	30
12–14	60
15–17	90
18–19	120
20–22	180
23–24	120 (>stereotypies)
25–25	180
26–28	210
29–31	240
32–34	270 (fading green card)
35–40	300 (no card)

Note. The sessions lasted 5 min, the latency criterion (30 to 300 s) to access to stereotypy gradually increased. During sessions 23–24 the child needed a backstep since he reported a problem to maintain functional behaviors for a longer time. From session 39 we faded green card since the only removal of red card could evoke the automatic behaviors.

2.6. Generalization of the Intervention

Generalization was assessed conducting the last three sessions of the intervention in the clinical room with different toys and activities, likewise different operators, and interacting with a peer. Robert was sitting at the table with another child sharing a construction game (sessions 38–39). The child was wearing only the red bracelet. However, he was not reminded of the condition. After having reached the predefined criterion (5 min), the bracelet placed on the wrist was removed, leaving free access to the stereotypies. During session 40, Robert was on the carpet alone, wearing the red bracelet. He was watching a book labelling pictures and reading the written words. Having completed the first book, he chose flashcards with pictures and letters continuing to play through related comments. Likewise, when Robert reached the predetermined criterion of 5 min, his bracelet was removed.

3. Results

The related graphs show the results for the conditions examined in this study.

Concerning the discrimination training, at the beginning of phase 1, the child did not discriminate between the red and green stimuli. During the second session of phase 1, Robert engaged in stereotypy for the 55% of the intervals in the red bracelet condition and 80% in the green card condition. In session three, he demonstrated a clear discrimination between the two conditions (percentage of the stereotypies in red/green condition correspondingly 0/100%). Furthermore, in the other phases, discrimination between stimuli was observed. Finally, in the last phase, Robert did not emit any stereotypy in the red condition and engaged in stereotyped behaviour approximately 75% the green condition. In order to gather more information, please see Figure 1.

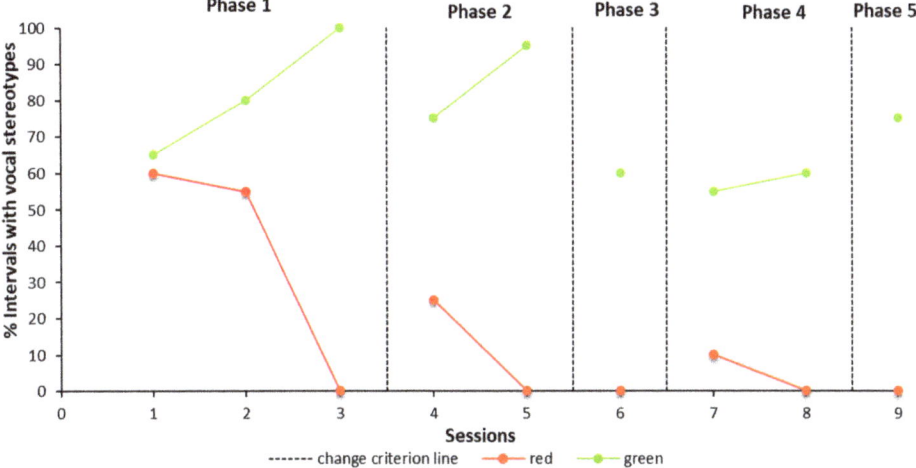

Figure 1. Discrimination Training, vocal stereotypies showed for both of the conditions (red card/green card) during five phases. Note: Percentage of 15-s intervals in which the child emitted the stereotyped vocal behavior. During phase 2 the red card was replaced with a red bracelet. The red lines represent the red card condition and the green lines the green card. The dotted lines (change criterion) represent the different phases where reinforcements (tangible and praise) were delivered through a variable interval schedule.

Regarding the baseline and intervention, the sessions of the baseline lasted one minute. Latency in engaging in stereotyped behaviour was of 11.7 s (average). On the other hand, the intervention was divided into sub-phases, each of which corresponds to a different reinforcement criterion. Each phase gradually approached to the final behavioural goal; the latency gradually increased. In sessions 23 and 24, a bi-directional change was observed, a return back to a previous criterion was implemented since the latency to engage in stereotypy was 2 min (as previous sessions 18–19), a useful return to a previous criterion concurred to evaluate the functional relationship between the variables, as can be seen in the Figure 2. The arrows on the graph indicate the fading steps of the green card stimulus. In sessions 32–34, the green card was faded in colour. Then, from session 35, the green card was eliminated (no card). Sessions 38–40 refer to the generalization of the intervention. In the generalization phase, sessions took place in the clinical room and the child shared play with a peer. In this phase even after the red bracelet condition, the child continued to play commenting the pictures appropriately without vocal stereotypies.

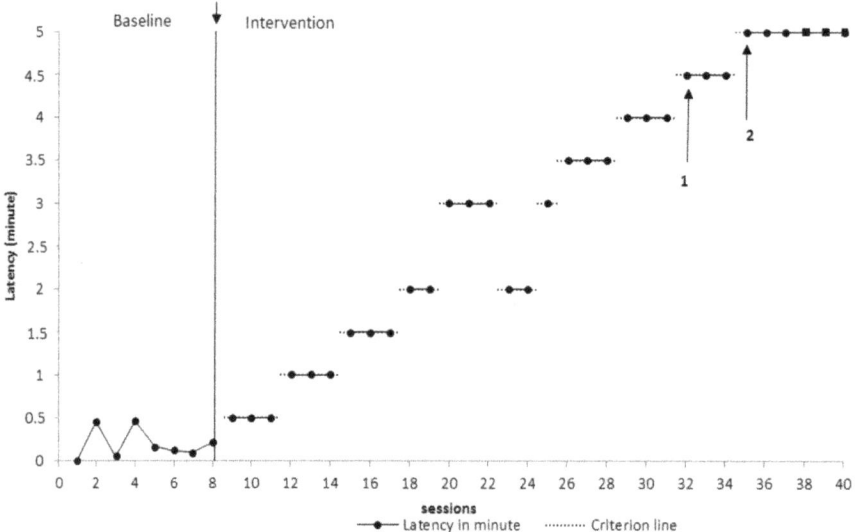

Figure 2. Latency in minutes to engage in stereotyped vocal behaviour during baseline sessions and interventions. Note: Arrows with numbers 1 and 2 indicate fading steps of the green card stimulus (Arrow #1 = fading sessions 32–34; Arrow #2 = no-card sessions 35–40). The arrow between the BL and intervention indicates discrimination training between the baseline and the intervention. Also, the dependent variable is the latency in minute, hence the time spent between the end of the given stimulus ("now you can play") and the beginning of the stereotypy. The horizontal dotted lines represent the pre-established criteria in order to provide the reinforcement (access to the green card condition). The predetermined criterion is gradually increasing.

4. Discussion

Children diagnosed with autism spectrum disorders can display impairments in a large variety of developmental abilities, including behavioural challenges. Stereotypes including core symptoms often become for people an obstacle to academic learning, incentivizing their social stigma and limiting social interactions. However, literature reviews suggest that behavioural interventions have demonstrated efficacy in decreasing and replacing vocal stereotypies [20,41]. Moreover, recent scientific literature concerning the function of these repetitive behaviours suggest that stereotypies are maintained by non-social consequences since they generally persist in the absence of social reinforcement [20]. Vocal stereotypies maintained by automatic reinforcement are difficult to treat [21]. Some studies have used mild punishment or response interruption and redirection [22]. According to Rapp et al. [27] and O'Connor et al. [36], the results of this study indicate that stimulus discrimination training is a helpful intervention for reducing vocal stereotypy in an autistic child. In this study, we find that vocal stereotypy is under the control of the red card/green card. Moreover, the stereotyped behaviour occurs less in the presence of the red card and more in the presence of the green card, due to the inhibitory stimulus control, inducing a decrease of the stereotypies during red card condition. Furthermore, during the intervention, the green card stimulus or simply the removal of the red card, becomes a stimulus evocating automatic reinforcement, applied contingently to the absence of stereotypy in the red card condition. Actually, the access to stereotyped vocal behaviour in the green card/no card condition becomes a reinforcement in the red card condition since the child engages to decrease the vocal stereotypies. It will be interesting to study the increment of functional vocalizations of children in order to understand if a RIRD procedure [42,43], where the therapist block the self-stimulation prompting the correct response is enough to address these challenging behaviours. Future research studies could investigate the efficacy of stimulus control, comparing it with behaviour redirections. On the other hand, we believe it essential to explore the predictors of functional language development. Note that Robert showed an intermediate educational curriculum regarding language, and as a result the personal characteristic could have influenced the outcomes. As a result, it is necessary to gather more information concerning stimulus control and RIRD applications with children with different linguistic levels, especially about children following base curriculum and poor expressive language skills. Likewise, we suggest that one should conduct group analysis or multiple baselines across participants in order to address the mentioned methodology issues. Nevertheless, the current results encourage the research in this research field, demonstrating a clinical impact on autistic people and related disabilities. In fact, it has been observed that Robert, when he reached the predetermined criterion removing the red bracelet, he continued to play appropriately commenting contextually play activities. As a result, we suggest to gather more information about behaviours occurring during no card conditions and related functional comments of children.

However, the current study has other limitations. Firstly, we have noted a lack of observers' agreement during the baseline and the intervention. The educational plan of the child was divided between the centre and home providing a one-to-one therapy. Hence, it is no easy to enrol a second observer to collect data. Another important limitation is the no-extension of the intervention to the other contexts of the daily life. Nevertheless, the use of the bracelet should encourage a generalization of treatment to public places (e.g., school, gym). Additionally, we have provided a poor definition of appropriate behaviour. It was not directly measured as well. These limitations are all aspects to be considered for the future. Regarding future studies, in our opinion measurements regarding the description and the increment of appropriate behaviour could be added. In addition, validating the effectiveness of the procedure, this study confirms that it is possible to use a stereotype to reinforce, in fact, the absence of the stereotype itself. Also, following researches could evaluate whether the results are maintained for a long time (follow-ups) or whether it is necessary to revise the training adding or removing procedural components [44].

Despite these limitations, in part related to the COVID-19 emergency, this study demonstrates how automatic behaviour can be addressed through training in discrimination and stimulus control, and how the access to stereotypy can be used as reinforcement. Finally, we would like to show to students and behavioural therapists different evidence-based strategies to address challenging behaviour in children with neuropsychiatric disorders, comprising vocal and motor stereotypies [45]. Similarly, we would suggest that any behavioural interventions should be trained by a behaviour analyst and certified therapists (generally with Master in ABA). Generally, a certified training appropriate to implement these behavioural programs should respect predefined requirements. Internationally, people can accomplish the task list concerning registered behaviour technician in order to learn contents of ABA interventions and training with behavioural analysts (https://www.bacb.com/wp-content/uploads/2020/05/RBT-2nd-Edition-Task-List_181214.pdf, accessed on 15 October 2021), although in these cases affording persistent challenging behaviours a more high-level training could be necessary (as assistant analyst). Finally, the behavioural treatments should be always supervised by a Board-Certified Behaviour Analyst (BCBA). As reminded during the method section a functional analysis assessment a tailored educational program including evidence-based behavioural interventions is necessary to guarantee the efficacy of a training about dysfunctional behaviours.

Concerning parents there are various aspects to consider. Firstly, parents of children emitted stereotypies in more contexts should receive a specific training, overall, on the implemented procedure, planning their parent inclusion. Also, parents should provide planned activities to child in order to facilitate the generalization process. Concerning the current training including stimulus control, the parents could deliver red card conditions to reduce the stereotypy, in particular during daily activities in community (parties, restaurant, playgrounds, gym, and so on) without providing the access to vocal stereotypies as reinforcement (in the current procedure during green card/no card conditions). Generally, parents of children with ASD suffer perceived problem behaviours emitted by the child, and as a result they could be encouraged to provide only punitive consequences, avoiding to furnish self-stimulations as reinforcement. All of these aspects should be considered during parent training. On the other hand, there are various positive side effects of these interventions. Commonly, problem behaviours limit daily life of families and their social relationships. Consequently, when families start a well-organized educational program including an effective parent training, it permits them to meliorate their quality of life. Likewise, stereotypy could represent a limit in classrooms either limiting learning or social interaction, increasing social stigma [10] and learning opportunities [9]. Therefore, clinical staff should select an appropriate behavioural technique in order to reduce the motor and vocal stereotypies in school settings or generalizing effective procedures implemented in structured ones. Accordingly, behavioural procedures based on stimulus control, interruption and redirection should be considered. Conversely, these interventions generally need a private cost (50 USD/hour) and many families are not available to afford it. In these cases, it could be necessary a study of cost/benefit regarding the efforts involved in planned and supervised training.

5. Conclusions

Children diagnosed with autism spectrum disorders are also characterized by restricted and repetitive behaviours, vocalizing, echolalia, and a-contextual speech. These are examples of stereotypies maintained by automatic positive reinforcement becoming a barrier to learning if their reinforcing value exceeds other stimuli in the environment, absorbing too many daily activities of children and their families. Undeniably, stereotyped behaviours interfere with different aspects as learning in academic setting, social skills, leisure time, and vocational and self-care time. In order to address these challenging behaviours, some behavioural interventions have been proposed in the literature including mild punishment, response interruption and redirection to appropriate vocalizations, response blocking, antecedent based interventions, reinforcement schedules, and discrimination training. Likewise, the current research suggests that stereotypy can pass under the card's control occurring less in the presence of the red card and more when paired with the green card/no card. During the intervention, we trained a child to discriminate two conditions (red card and green card) evoking through RIRD procedure two opposed behaviours (respectively the absence and access of vocal stereotypies). Subsequently, after the discrimination training we furnished an intervention where the child watched a red card (or red bracelet) and without prompting had to maintain gradually a greater time without vocal stereotypies. In case the child respected the latency time requested, he could access to vocal stereotypies (green or no card) for the residual time of the session. Therefore, during the sessions the child increased the time passed without stereotypy, and as a result the current procedure indicates that stimulus discrimination training is a useful intervention to reduce vocal stereotypy in an autistic child. Likewise, these behavioural interventions applied by certified professionals could support therapists and families in different daily life settings as playgrounds, school, the home, and the community. Finally, a training to reduce stereotypy should be derived from individualized educational plans and appropriate functional analysis assessments combining manualized behavioural techniques in order to maximise the outcomes.

Author Contributions: Regarding literature, conceptualization, writing and methodology including data analysis (F.M., O.R., L.P. and M.D.), while concerning review and editing (M.E., M.M., P.M. and M.V.). All authors have read and agreed to the published version of the manuscript.

Funding: This research received no external funding, and the APC was funded by voluntary association una breccia nel muro, operating for autism services in Italy.

Institutional Review Board Statement: The study was conducted according to the guidelines of the Declaration of Helsinki and according to the code of behavior analysts (BACB).

Informed Consent Statement: Informed consent was obtained from parents of child involved in the study. The related documents were shared with editorial office.

Data Availability Statement: In order to receive the data, the user need to write at info@unabreccianelmuro.org.

Conflicts of Interest: The authors declare no conflict of interest.

References

1. APA—American Psychiatric Association. *Diagnostic and Statistical Manual of Mental Disorders—DSM 5*; APA: Washington, DC, USA, 2013.
2. Wong, C.; Odom, S.L.; Hume, K.A.; Cox, A.W.; Fettig, A.; Kucharczyk, S.; Brock, M.E.; Plavnick, J.B.; Fleury, V.P.; Schultz, T.R. Evidence-based practices for children, youth, and young adults with autism spectrum disorder: A comprehensive review. *J. Autism Dev. Disord.* **2015**, *45*, 1951–1966. [CrossRef] [PubMed]
3. Rapp, J.T.; Vollmer, T.R. Stereotypy I: A review of behavioral assessment and treatment. *Res. Dev. Disabil.* **2005**, *26*, 527–547. [CrossRef]
4. Lanovaz, M.J.; Sladeczek, I.E. Vocal stereotypy in children with autism: Structural characteristics, variability, and effects of auditory stimulation. *Res. Autism Spectr. Disord.* **2011**, *5*, 1159–1168. [CrossRef]
5. Sundberg, M.L. *Verbal Behavior Milestones Assessment and Placement Program: The VBMAPP*; AVB Press: Concord, CA, USA, 2008.
6. Koegel, R.L.; Covert, A. The relationship of self-stimulation to learning in autistic children. *J. Appl. Behav. Anal.* **1972**, *5*, 381–387. [CrossRef] [PubMed]
7. Koegel, R.L.; Firestone, P.B.; Kramme, K.W.; Dunlap, G. Increasing spontaneous play by suppressing self-stimulation in autistic children 1. *J. Appl. Behav. Anal.* **1974**, *7*, 521–528. [CrossRef]
8. Lanovaz, M.J.; Robertson, K.M.; Soerono, K.; Watkins, N. Effects of reducing stereotypy on other behaviors: A systematic review. *Res. Autism Spectr. Disord.* **2013**, *7*, 1234–1243. [CrossRef]
9. Cook, J.L.; Rapp, J.T. To what extent do practitioners need to treat stereotypy during academic tasks? *Behav. Modif.* **2020**, *44*, 228–264. [CrossRef]
10. Coon, J.C.; Rapp, J.T. Brief report: Evaluating college students' perceptions of a child displaying stereotypic behaviors: Do changes in stereotypy levels affect ratings? *J. Autism Dev. Disord.* **2020**, *50*, 1827–1833. [CrossRef]
11. Ahearn, W.H.; Clark, K.M.; DeBar, R.; Florentino, C. On the role of preference in response competition. *J. Appl. Behav. Anal.* **2005**, *38*, 247–250. [CrossRef]
12. Taylor, B.A.; Hoch, H.; Weissman, M. The analysis and treatment of vocal stereotypy in a child with autism. *Behav. Interv.* **2005**, *20*, 239–253. [CrossRef]
13. Falcomata, T.S.; Roane, H.S.; Hovanetz, A.N.; Kettering, T.L.; Keeney, K.M. An evaluation of response cost in the treatment of inappropriate vocalizations maintained by automatic reinforcement. *J. Appl. Behav. Anal.* **2004**, *37*, 83–87. [CrossRef]
14. Fay, W.H. On the basis of autistic echolalia. *J. Commun. Disord.* **1969**, *2*, 31–41. [CrossRef]
15. Ahearn, W.H.; Clark, K.M.; Gardener, N.C.; Chung, B.I.; Dube, W.V. Persistence of stereotypic behavior: Examining the effects of external reinforcers. *J. Appl. Behav. Anal.* **2003**, *36*, 439–448. [CrossRef] [PubMed]
16. Durand, V.M.; Carr, E.G. Social influences on "self-stimulatory" behavior: Analysis and treatment application. *J. Appl. Behav. Anal.* **1987**, *20*, 119–132. [CrossRef] [PubMed]
17. Kennedy, C.H.; Meyer, K.A.; Knowles, T.; Shukla, S. Analyzing the multiple functions of stereotypical behavior for students with autism: Implications for assessment and treatment. *J. Appl. Behav. Anal.* **2000**, *33*, 559–571. [CrossRef] [PubMed]
18. Repp, A.C.; Felce, D.; Barton, L.E. Basing the treatment of stereotypic and self-injurious behaviors on hypotheses of their causes. *J. Appl. Behav. Anal.* **1988**, *21*, 281–289. [CrossRef] [PubMed]
19. Lovaas, O.I.; Newsom, C.; Hickman, C. Self Stimulatory behavior and perceptual reinforcement. *J. Appl. Behav. Anal.* **1987**, *20*, 45–68. [CrossRef] [PubMed]
20. Lanovaz, M.J.; Sladeczek, I.E. Vocal stereotypy in individuals with autism spectrum disorders: A review of behavioral interventions. *Behav. Modif.* **2012**, *36*, 146–164. [CrossRef]

21. Vollmer, T.R. The concept of automatic reinforcement: Implications for behavioral research in developmental disabilities. *Res. Dev. Disabil.* **1994**, *15*, 187–207. [CrossRef]
22. Ahearn, W.H.; Clark, K.M.; MacDonald, R.P.F.; Chung, B.I. Assessing and treating vocal stereotypy in children with autism. *J. Appl. Behav. Anal.* **2007**, *40*, 263–275. [CrossRef]
23. Athens, E.S.; Vollmer, T.R. An analysis of vocal stereotypy and therapist fading. *J. Appl. Behav. Anal.* **2008**, *41*, 291–298. [CrossRef] [PubMed]
24. Cassella, M.D.; Sidener, T.M.; Sidener, D.W.; Progar, P.R. Response interruption and redirection for vocal stereotypy in children with autism: A systematic replication. *J. Appl. Behav. Anal.* **2011**, *44*, 169–173. [CrossRef] [PubMed]
25. Love, J.J.; Miguel, C.F.; Fernand, J.K.; LaBrie, J.K. The effects of matched stimulation and response interruption and redirection on vocal stereotypy. *J. Appl. Behav. Anal.* **2012**, *45*, 549–564. [CrossRef] [PubMed]
26. Behavior Analyst Certification Board. BACB Professional and Ethical Compliance Code for Behavior Analysts. 2017. Available online: https://www.bacb.com/wp-content/uploads/2020/05/BACB-Compliance-Code-english_190318.pdf (accessed on 25 October 2021).
27. Rapp, J.T.; Patel, M.R.; Ghezzi, P.M.; O'Flaherty, C.H.; Titterington, C.J. Establishing stimulus control of vocal stereotypy displayed by young children with autism. *Behav. Interv.* **2009**, *24*, 85–105. [CrossRef]
28. Rapp, J.T. Toward an empirical method for identifying matched stimulation for automatically reinforced behavior: A preliminary investigation. *J. Appl. Behav. Anal.* **2006**, *39*, 137–140. [CrossRef] [PubMed]
29. Cooper, J.O.; Heron, T.E.; Heward, W.L. *Applied Behavior Analysis*, 2nd ed.; Pearson Prentice Hall: Upper Saddle River, NJ, USA, 2007.
30. Green, G. Behavior analytic instruction for learners with autism: Advances in stimulus control technology. *Focus Autism Other Dev. Disabil.* **2001**, *16*, 72–85. [CrossRef]
31. Miller, T.L.; Lignugaris-Kraft, B. The effects of text structure discrimination training on the performance of students with learning disabilities. *J. Behav. Educ.* **2002**, *11*, 203–230. [CrossRef]
32. Brusa, E.; Richman, D. Developing stimulus control for occurrences of stereotypy exhibited by a child with autism. *Int. J. Behav. Consult. Ther.* **2008**, *4*, 264. [CrossRef]
33. Doughty, S.S.; Anderson, C.M.; Doughty, A.H.; Williams, D.C.; Saunders, K.J. Discriminative control of punished stereotyped behavior in humans. *J. Exp. Anal. Behav.* **2007**, *87*, 325–336. [CrossRef]
34. Haley, J.L.; Heick, P.F.; Luiselli, J.K. Use of an antecedent intervention to decrease vocal stereotypy of a student with autism in the general education classroom. *Child Fam. Behav. Ther.* **2010**, *32*, 311–321. [CrossRef]
35. McKenzie, S.D.; Smith, R.G.; Simmons, J.N.; Soderlund, M.J. Using a stimulus correlated with reprimands to suppress automatically maintained eye poking. *J. Appl. Behav. Anal.* **2008**, *41*, 255–259. [CrossRef] [PubMed]
36. O'Connor, A.S.; Prieto, J.; Hoffmann, B.; DeQuinzio, J.A.; Taylor, B.A. A stimulus control procedure to decrease motor and vocal stereotypy. *Behav. Interv.* **2011**, *26*, 231–242. [CrossRef]
37. Cook, J.L.; Rapp, J.T.; Gomes, L.A.; Frazer, T.J.; Lindblad, T.L. Effects of verbal reprimands on targeted and untargeted stereotypy. *Behav. Interv.* **2014**, *29*, 106–124. [CrossRef]
38. Kenny, L.; Hattersley, C.; Molins, B.; Buckley, C.; Povey, C.; Pellicano, E. Which terms should be used to describe autism? Perspectives from the UK autism community. *Autism* **2016**, *20*, 442–462. [CrossRef] [PubMed]
39. Partington, J.W. *The Assessment of Basic Language and Learning Skills—Revised (ABLLS–R)*; Behavior Analysts: Walnut Hill, CA, USA, 2006.
40. Gossou, K.M.; Lanovaz, M.J.; Giannakakos, A. Concurrent Validity of Functional Analysis, ABC Narrative Recordings, and Open-Ended Functional Assessment Interviews. *PsyArXiv* **2020**. [CrossRef]
41. Neely, L.; Gerow, S.; Rispoli, M.; Lang, R.; Pullen, N. Treatment of echolalia in individuals with autism spectrum disorder: A systematic review. *Rev. J. Autism Dev. Disord.* **2016**, *3*, 82–91. [CrossRef]
42. Dickman, S.E.; Bright, C.N.; Montgomery, D.H.; Miguel, C.F. The effects of response interruption and redirection (RIRD) and differential reinforcement on vocal stereotypy and appropriate vocalizations. *Behav. Interv.* **2012**, *27*, 185–192. [CrossRef]
43. Shawler, L.A.; Dianda, M.; Miguel, C.F. A comparison of response interruption and redirection and competing items on vocal stereotypy and appropriate vocalizations. *J. Appl. Behav. Anal.* **2020**, *53*, 355–365. [CrossRef]
44. Call, N.A.; Simmons, C.A.; Mevers, J.E.L.; Alvarez, J.P. Clinical outcomes of behavioral treatments for pica in children with developmental disabilities. *J. Autism Dev. Disord.* **2015**, *45*, 2105–2114. [CrossRef] [PubMed]
45. Fontani, S. Interventi educativi Evidence Based per la diminuzione delle stereotipie nei Disturbi dello Spettro Autistico. *Ital. J. Spec. Educ. Incl.* **2016**, *4*, 67–83. Available online: https://www.researchgate.net/publication/323074926 (accessed on 25 October 2021).

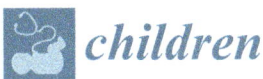

Case Report

Additional Evidence for Neuropsychiatric Manifestations in Mosaic Trisomy 20: A Case Report and Brief Review

Marco Colizzi [1,2,3,*], **Giulia Antolini** [1], **Laura Passarella** [1], **Valentina Rizzo** [1], **Elena Puttini** [1] **and Leonardo Zoccante** [1]

[1] Child and Adolescent Neuropsychiatry Unit, Maternal-Child Integrated Care Department, Integrated University Hospital of Verona, 37126 Verona, Italy; giuliaantolini11@gmail.com (G.A.); laura.passarella17@gmail.com (L.P.); valentinaannarizzo@gmail.com (V.R.); elena.puttini@aovr.veneto.it (E.P.); leonardo.zoccante@aovr.veneto.it (L.Z.)
[2] Section of Psychiatry, Department of Neurosciences, Biomedicine and Movement Sciences, University of Verona, 37134 Verona, Italy
[3] Department of Psychosis Studies, Institute of Psychiatry, Psychology and Neuroscience, King's College London, London SE5 8AF, UK
* Correspondence: marco.colizzi@univr.it; Tel.: +39-045-812-6832

Citation: Colizzi, M.; Antolini, G.; Passarella, L.; Rizzo, V.; Puttini, E.; Zoccante, L. Additional Evidence for Neuropsychiatric Manifestations in Mosaic Trisomy 20: A Case Report and Brief Review. *Children* **2021**, *8*, 1030. https://doi.org/10.3390/children8111030

Academic Editor: Matteo Alessio Chiappedi

Received: 21 September 2021
Accepted: 8 November 2021
Published: 10 November 2021

Publisher's Note: MDPI stays neutral with regard to jurisdictional claims in published maps and institutional affiliations.

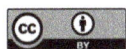

Copyright: © 2021 by the authors. Licensee MDPI, Basel, Switzerland. This article is an open access article distributed under the terms and conditions of the Creative Commons Attribution (CC BY) license (https://creativecommons.org/licenses/by/4.0/).

Abstract: Mosaic trisomy 20 is a genetic condition in which three chromosomes 20 are found in some cells. Its clinical phenotype seems to be highly variable, with most features not reported across all individuals and not considered pathognomonic of the condition. Limited and recent evidence indicates that neuropsychiatric manifestations may be more present in the context of trisomy 20 than was once thought. Here, we present a case of a 14-year-old female adolescent of White/Caucasian ethnicity with mosaic trisomy 20, who was admitted twice to an inpatient Child and Adolescent Neuropsychiatry Unit for persisting self-injury and suicidal ideation. A severe and complex neuropsychiatric presentation emerged at the cognitive, emotional, and behavioral levels, including mild neurodevelopmental issues, isolation, socio-relational difficulties, depressed mood, temper outbursts, irritability, low self-esteem, lack of interest, social anxiety, panic attacks, self-cutting, and low-average-range and heterogeneous intelligence quotient profile. Particularly, the patient was considered at high risk of causing harm, mainly to self, and appeared to be only partially responsive to medication, even when polypharmacy was attempted to improve clinical response. Except for school bullying, no other severe environmental risk factors were present in the patient's history. The patient received a diagnosis of disruptive mood dysregulation disorder.

Keywords: pediatric conditions; psychiatric genetics; anger; self-regulation; aneuploidy; autosomal trisomy

1. Introduction

Aneuploidy in natural conception is an estimated 0.3% [1], with 0.6 per 10,000 births presenting a rare mosaic trisomy [2] and trisomy 20 accounting for 16% of all mosaicisms [3]. Trisomy 20 is a genetic condition caused by an extra chromosome at position 20. While complete trisomy 20 is rare and suggested not to be compatible with life, a mosaic form of trisomy 20, where three chromosomes 20 are found only in some cells, may be possible, and thought to result in a grossly normal phenotype in most of the cases [4]. However, a recent review of the scientific literature revealed a paucity of studies reporting the phenotypic manifestations potentially associated with the condition [5]. To date, the clinical phenotype of trisomy 20 seems to be highly variable. In fact, most features are not reported across all individuals and are not considered pathognomonic of the condition, as they are also found in the general population, although at a lower rate [4]. More specifically, a number of craniofacial [4,6–13], cutaneous [11,14,15], cardiovascular-pulmonary [7,16–19], gastrointestinal [20], endocrinological [15], reproductive [10,15], locomotor [4,7,13,16,20–22], nervous [4,10,14,19,21,23], and cognitive and mental [4,7,13,15,18,20,22–25] features have been reported.

Recent evidence indicates that neuropsychiatric manifestations may be more present in the context of trisomy 20 than was once thought, with also potential forensic implications [5]. So far, it has been suggested that children with trisomy 20 may present with social [20], emotional [20], and learning [20,22] deficits, as per altered neurodevelopment [20,24]. Less clear is the persistence of psychiatric and behavioral features through adolescence and early adulthood.

Here, we report the case of a 14-year-old female adolescent of White/Caucasian ethnicity with mosaic trisomy 20, who was admitted twice to the inpatient Child and Adolescent Neuropsychiatry Unit of the Integrated University Hospital of Verona for persisting self-injury and suicidal ideation. Such admissions followed a neuropsychiatric assessment in the community and a presentation to the Accident & Emergency (A&E) Department, respectively. These were her first presentations to a neuropsychiatric ward. Her developmental history, neuropsychiatric presentation at admission, diagnosis, and clinical evolution are presented in detail in the following sections.

2. Case Report
2.1. Medical History

A detailed medical history was obtained from the patient and her parents. She was raised by her mother and father and currently lives at home with both her parents and her only sibling, an older sister. Her family history is positive for depressive disorder in her paternal grandmother, obsessive-compulsive disorder symptoms in her mother, self-injury in her sister, motor tics (self-limited childhood tics, including eye-winking movements as well as hand and finger twitching/stretching) in her mother and sister, and epileptic manifestations in her sister, maternal aunt, and paternal second cousin. A family history of joint laxity and hernias was also reported. As the patient's sister was not considered to have a clinically detectable mosaicism, formal genetic testing has never been performed, also considering the difficulties of ascertaining low-level mosaicism where most cell lineages are not affected. A full pedigree providing a graphic depiction of the patient's family structure and medical history is reported in Figure 1.

She was born to term out of her parents' third pregnancy (the first ended in a spontaneous abortion). The pregnancy was uncomplicated, but amniocentesis, performed due to advanced maternal age, showed a karyotype of 47,XX + 20/46,XX in 10 of 32 metaphases analyzed. Her Apgar score, birth weight, length, and head circumference were all within normal ranges. Successively performed abdominal ultrasound and transfontanelle ultrasonography turned out negative. Overall, her development milestones proceeded regularly and on time, except for a slight delay in gross and fine motor skills. Starting from the pediatric age, physical examination findings related to her genetic condition included a broad and depressed nasal bone, low-set ears, hypotonia, and joint laxity. Physiatric assessment also highlighted the presence of flatfoot, a slight degree of shoulders asymmetry, and left convex scoliosis. During the years of primary school, facial tics and compulsive repetitive behaviors made their first appearance, together with the findings of a slight degree of dysgraphia and astigmatism. In secondary school, following episodes of bullying and cyberbullying, a progressive decline in her school performance was observed, along with the tendency to isolate herself from others, with difficulties in building relationships with peers, resulting in a poor friendship network. Furthermore, a continuous depressed mood throughout the day, associated with temper outbursts and irritability (in the absence of clear mood swings), low self-esteem, a lack of interest in any activity, significant social anxiety, panic attacks, daily episodes of self-cutting (occurring both at school and at home), and suicidal ideation were reported. Such symptoms did not appear to negatively affect the sleep–wake cycle.

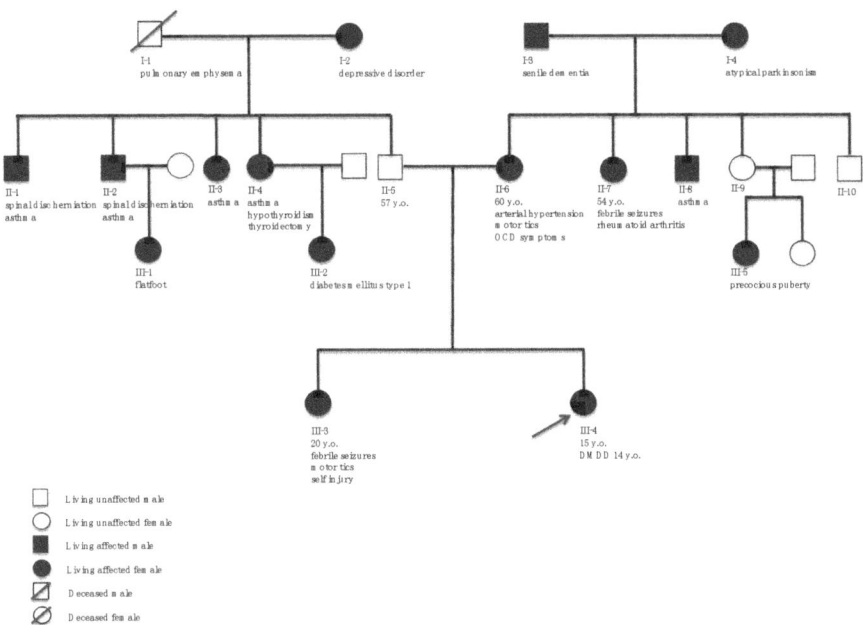

Figure 1. Pedigree of the patient. DMDD, disruptive mood dysregulation disorder.

Due to her neuropsychiatric distress, the patient was referred to the Childhood Neuropsychiatry Territorial Service, where a psychotherapeutic intervention was implemented, along with pharmacological treatment consisting of sertraline oral solution 20 mg/mL, at a dosage of 1.25 mL per day, and alprazolam 0.75 mg/mL oral concentrate, at a dosage of 0.125 mg per day (5 drops). Such therapy did not bring any benefit to the patient. Therefore, it was decided to admit her to the inpatient Child and Adolescent Neuropsychiatry Unit.

2.2. Clinical Course, Diagnostic Conclusions, and Outpatient Follow-Up

During hospitalization, she maintained overall good health and the following clinical evaluations were performed, aimed at monitoring her at both the clinical and the therapeutic level: COVID-19 nasal swab testing prior to admission, routine blood exams, urinalysis, and electrocardiogram; all of these turned out negative. Based on preexisting documentation and direct clinical observation, information was gathered with reference to her trisomy 20 manifestations. A detailed report of signs and symptoms, as contrasted to what is to be expected based on the current literature, is provided in Table 1.

Table 1. Trisomy 20 manifestations in the current case as compared to the previous literature.

Body Systems and Functions	Symptoms/Signs	Current Case + Present X Not Present
Craniofacial		
Korkontzelos (2017) [6], Velissariou et al. (2002) [7]	Underdeveloped nasal bone	+
Hsu et al. (1991) [4], Mavromatidis et al. (2010) [8], Myers and Prouty (1989) [9], Ensenauer et al. (2005) [10]	Ear morphology abnormalities	+
Velissariou et al. (2002) [7], Warren et al. (2001) [11]	Micrognathia and retrognathia	X
Stromme et al. (2005) [12]	Cleft lip and palate	X

Table 1. *Cont.*

Body Systems and Functions	Symptoms/Signs	Current Case + Present X Not Present
Hsu et al. (1991) [4], Velissariou et al. (2002) [7], Reish et al. (1998) [13]	Abnormal periorbital region morphology	X
Cutaneous		
Powis and Erickson (2009) [14]	Thin and brittle nails	X
Warren et al. (2001) [11], Powis and Erickson (2009) [14], Girard et al. (2005) [15]	Hypomelanosis of Ito	X
Hartmann et al. (2004) [18]	Linear and whorled nevoid hypermelanosis	X
Velissariou et al. (2002) [7]	Mongolian spots	X
Cardiovascular-Pulmonary		
Morales et al. (2010) [16]	Pulmonary isomerism	X
Velissariou et al. (2002) [7], Karaoguz et al. (2007) [17], Hartmann et al. (2004) [18], Hsieh et al. (1992) [19]	Congenital heart defects	X
Gastrointestinal		
Willis et al. (2008) [20]	Stipsis	+
Endocrinological		
Girard et al. (2005) [15]	Growth hormone deficiency	X
Reproductive		
Ensenauer et al. (2005) [10], Girard et al. (2005) [15]	Cryptorchidism	X
Locomotor		
Willis et al. (2008) [20], Stein et al. (2008) [21]	Sloped shoulders	+
Velissariou et al. (2002) [7], Willis et al. (2008) [20]	Abnormal spinal column morphology	+ (Scoliosis)
Velissariou et al. (2002) [7], Reish et al. (1998) [13], Willis et al. (2008) [20], Stein et al. (2008) [21], Holzgreve et al. (1986) [22]	Central and peripheral altered muscle tone	+ (Hypotonia)
Velissariou et al. (2002) [7]	Ligamentous laxity	+
Morales et al. (2010) [16]	Camptodactyly	X
Hsu et al. (1991) [4], Velissariou et al. (2002) [7]	Clinodactyly	X
Montplaisir (2019) [5]	Polydactyly	X
Stein et al. (2008) [21]	Rib anomalies	X
Nervous		
Powis and Erickson (2009) [14]	Epileptic manifestations	X
Ensenauer et al. (2005) [10]	Hearing impairment	X
Hsu et al. (1991) [4], Salafsky et al. (2001) [23]	Microcephaly	X
Hsieh et al. (1992) [19], Stein et al. (2008) [21]	Abnormal neuroimaging findings	X
Cognitive and Mental		
Willis et al. (2008) [20]	Preserved IQ and learning disabilities	+
	Repetitive behaviors	+
	Isolation	+
	Social and emotional difficulties	+
	Pragmatic/Social communication difficulties	+

Table 1. *Cont.*

Body Systems and Functions	Symptoms/Signs	Current Case + Present X Not Present
Wallerstein et al. (2005) [24]	Atypical neurodevelopment with attention deficit	X
	Impulsivity	+
	Atypical social reciprocity	+
Girard et al. (2005) [15]	Speech difficulties	X
Hsu et al. (1991) [4], Velissariou et al. (2002) [7], Girard et al. (2005) [15], Hartmann et al. (2004) [18], Salafsky et al. (2001) [23], Miny et al. (1989) [25]	Developmental psychomotor difficulties	+
Reish et al. (1998) [13]	Impaired fine and gross motor abilities	+
Holzgreve et al. (1986) [22]	Developmental language difficulties	X
Montplaisir (2019) [5]	Self-injury	+
Montplaisir (2019) [5]	Hallucinations	X

A psychological assessment was also carried out using the Child Behavior Checklist (CBCL) 6–18 [26] compiled by both the patient and her mother, who was with her throughout the hospitalization. CBCL subscales suggesting pathological symptoms (scores > 70) were "Anxious/Depressed", "Withdrawn/Depressed", "Social Problems", "Thought Problems", "Attention Problems", "Depressive Problems", "Anxiety Problems", "Sluggish Cognitive Tempo", and "Stress Problems". "Somatic Complaints" and "Obsessive-Compulsive Problems" were borderline symptoms according to her mother, while being rated as pathological by the patient (Table 2).

Throughout her hospital stay, the patient remained disheveled and unkempt. Self-cutting injuries were evident on her hands and neck, and upon further examination, they covered most of the forearms and thighs. The injuries were shallow and appeared to be in multiple stages of healing. She wore loose-fitting clothing, mostly in black. During interviews, she spoke reticently and only after requesting that her mother left the room. She appeared tense and had difficulty sustaining eye contact. Her speech was scarce, low in volume, and lacking modulation. She only answered questions when prodded, and her replies lacked articulation. She was coherent and oriented to person, place, and time. There were no signs of perceptual abnormalities. Hallucinations, depersonalization, derealization, and dissociative phenomena were denied. The patient did not show any loosening of association, flight of ideas, tangentiality, or circumstantiality. Her affect was flat but not inappropriate to the content of her speech, which was focused on the circumstances of her hospitalization, her emotional malaise, and her continued self-harm ideation. Some anxiety through repetitive wringing of her hands was observed. She reported that she had no appetite but had no trouble sleeping at night.

Considering the suboptimal symptom control, a change in pharmacological treatment was made. In particular, sertraline and alprazolam were discontinued, whereas pregabalin at a dosage of 150 mg, fluvoxamine at a dosage of 50 mg, and quetiapine extended release at a dosage of 50 mg were initiated. The patient received a diagnosis of disruptive mood dysregulation disorder (DMDD), according to the Diagnostic and Statistical Manual of Mental Disorders, -Fifth Edition DSM-5 [27], and was discharged 7 days later in good clinical condition, with the indication to continue the treatment with pregabalin, fluvoxamine, and quetiapine.

Table 2. Neurocognitive and psychological assessment.

Neurocognitive Assessment	
Wechsler Intelligence Scale for Children–Fourth Edition (WISC-IV)	Score (95% Confidence Interval; subtest raw score)
Full-Scale Intelligence Quotient	80 (75–87)
Verbal Comprehension	78 (72–86; Similarities: 7; Comprehension: 3; Vocabulary: 7; Information (supplemental subtest): 5)
Perceptual Reasoning	95 (87–103; Block Design: 11; Matrix Reasoning: 9; Picture Concepts: 8)
Working Memory	79 (72–90; Subtest: Digit Span: 7; Letter–Number Sequencing: 6; Arithmetic (supplemental subtest): 3)
Processing Speed	85 (77–97; Coding: 8; Symbol Search: 7)

Psychological Assessment			
Child Behavior Checklist (CBCL)	T-Scores (Patient)	T-Scores (Mother)	Clinical: T ≥ 70 Borderline: 65 ≥ T < 70 Non-clinical: T < 65
Syndrome Scale Scores			
Social Problems	70	70	Clinical
Thought Problems	73	73	Clinical
Attention Problems	83	70	Clinical
Internalizing Problems			
Withdrawn/Depressed	100	100	Clinical
Anxious/Depressed	100	74	Clinical
Somatic Complaints	70	65	Clinical/Borderline
Externalizing Problems			
Rule-Breaking Behavior	60	57	Non-clinical
Aggressive Behavior	58	58	Non-clinical
Total Problems			
Internalizing Score	86	77	Clinical
Externalizing Score	59	58	Non-clinical
Total Problems Score	74	70	Clinical
DSM-Oriented Scales			
Depressive Problems	88	79	Clinical
Anxiety Problems	94	73	Clinical
Somatic Problems	59	59	Non-clinical
Attention Deficit	69	60	Borderline/Non-clinical
Oppositional Defiant Problems	59	63	Non-clinical
Conduct Problems	61	55	Non-clinical
Other Scales			
Sluggish Cognitive Tempo	80	73	Clinical
Obsessive-Compulsive Problems	87	66	Clinical/Borderline
Stress Problems	86	78	Clinical

At a follow-up visit, planned 1 week later, the patient presented with symptoms of a potential relapse. Thus, the dosages of fluvoxamine and quetiapine extended release were increased to 75 mg and 150 mg, respectively. However, after 1 more week, she entered the A&E Department presenting with the same symptoms she had when she was admitted for the first time, namely remarkable social anxiety and panic attacks, significantly low mood, daily episodes of self-injury, and suicidal ideation. Using a pencil sharpener blade, she had cut her forearms, abdomen, and legs, to the point where she had carved the word "help" into the skin of her left thigh. The neuropsychiatrist assessment advised for another hospitalization, and she was hence admitted after a negative COVID-19 nasal swab. Besides multiple routine blood exams and electrocardiograms, all of which turned out negative, this time a plastic surgical evaluation and a cardiological assessment with color-Doppler ultrasound were also performed, which showed nothing pathological.

Despite the initial improvement, as the pharmacological treatment had not led to clinical stability, it was modified as follows: pregabalin and quetiapine were discontinued, whereas lithium prolonged release at a dosage of 166 mg per day and olanzapine at a dosage of 10 mg per day were introduced. Moreover, the fluvoxamine dosage was increased to 150 mg. The previous diagnosis of disruptive mood dysregulation disorder (DMDD), according to DSM-5, was confirmed, and she was discharged 13 days later in good overall clinical condition, with the indication to continue the treatment with lithium prolonged release, fluvoxamine, and olanzapine.

A post-discharge assessment performed 2 weeks later found the patient overall clinically stable but only partially responsive to treatment. Despite improvement, her mood was still oriented toward depression and socio-emotional difficulties were still reported, resulting in outbursts and irritability. An abdominal ultrasound was also performed, which turned out negative, with liver, hepatic ducts, portal vein, gallbladder, kidneys, spleen, pancreas, and bladder all normal in appearance and echotexture. Furthermore, after about 4 weeks of pharmacological treatment stability, a neurocognitive assessment was performed using the Wechsler Intelligence Scale for Children–Fourth Edition (WISC-IV) [28]. The patient's full-scale intelligence quotient (FSIQ) was in the low average range as for normative data (FSIQ = 80), and a heterogeneous profile emerged, with "Perceptual Reasoning" falling in the average range, "Processing Speed" in the low average range, and "Verbal Comprehension" and "Working Memory" in the very low range (Table 2).

3. Discussion

The past decades have witnessed an increasing interest in the role of genetics in shaping human behavior. Genome-wide association studies (GWASs) have helped detect the polygenic architecture of psychiatric disorders, with potential applications in clinical settings [29]. Disruptive mood dysregulation disorder (DMDD) is no exception. Since its introduction in the DSM-5 [27], studies have investigated the role of genetics in modulating emotional and behavioral functioning in youth suffering from the condition. Research interest has focused on genetic variation affecting the function of neurobiological systems, such as the opioid system, that are known to modulate cognitive, emotional, and social behaviors [30]. In addition, studies support developmentally dynamic genetic effects on core features of the disorder, such as irritability, with genetic influences being higher in the female gender and as compared to environmental features [31]. However, the environment is still believed to exert a modulatory effect [32]. Consistently, evidence from gene-by-environment-interaction studies suggests that genetic variation in the hypothalamic–pituitary–adrenal (HPA) axis may interact with the effect of chronic stress in increasing the risk of presenting with a negative affect [33]. The latter is considered one of the factors predicting later psychopathology [34] as well as stability of DMDD symptoms, such as an irritable–angry mood and temper outbursts, through adolescence and early adulthood.

The first linkage study of psychosis using empirically derived, clinically homogeneous phenotypes, defined by symptomatic profiles rather than operationalized diagnostic criteria, revealed an unexpected linkage to chromosome 20 for "Schizomania" and "Mania" latent classes of psychotic illness as well as the highest logarithm of the odds (LOD) score of any latent class in the genome for the "Deficit Syndrome" class [35]. That chromosome 20 may be involved in both manic/positive and depressive/negative symptoms of psychosis is supported by genome scan studies and meta-analyses finding evidence of linkage for bipolar disorder and schizophrenia [35–40], as well as a comprehensive gene-based association study of 327 genes on chromosome 20, identifying two loci, *R3HDML* and *C20orf39*, associated with depressive symptoms in psychotic illness [41]. Taken together, these studies are compelling in their support of chromosome 20 harboring genes relevant to the affective component of schizophrenia and conditions presenting with admixtures of mood and psychotic symptoms [42]. Further, chromosome 20 has been associated with affective psychoses characterized by suicidal attempts [40], and a recent genome-wide association study identified a number of single-nucleotide polymorphisms (SNPs), all on chromosome 20, supporting a genetic transmission of suicide attempts, not entirely accounted for by suffering from a mental disorder [43]. Interestingly, functional SNPs on chromosome 20 influencing gene expression and bipolar disorder susceptibility have been shown to modulate hippocampal volume and cognitive performance in healthy individuals [44].

Along with numerical chromosome anomalies, such as mosaicism, structural anomalies of the chromosome 20, including ring chromosome [45], deletion of the short arm [46], microduplication within the short arm [47], and microdeleletion of the long arm [48], have also been associated with alterations in several body systems and functions as well as neurocognitive difficulties and neuropsychiatric features. Commonly reported behavioral manifestations include developmental delay, intellectual disability, sensory processing disorder, poor motor coordination, impaired speech and executive abilities, apathy or hyperactivity, loss of social skills and poor emotional regulation, obsessive behavior, psychosis, and autistic features.

Of further interest, the activity-dependent neuroprotective protein (ADNP) syndrome, which was only discovered in 2014, is a neurodevelopmental genetic disorder caused by changes (mostly de novo mutations) in the *ADNP* gene, which is located on the long arm of chromosome 20. It is frequently associated with developmental delays, intellectual delays, motor planning delays, delayed or absent speech, and autism features of varying degrees [49]. A potential role in self-injurious behavior has also been suggested [50]. Multiple body systems may be affected, including the brain (e.g., developmental delay, intellectual disability), heart (e.g., atrial septal defect, patent ductus arteriosus), immune system (e.g., frequent infections), gastrointestinal system (e.g., gastroesophageal reflux, constipation), endocrine system (e.g., early puberty, thyroid hormone problems), and musculoskeletal system (e.g., joint hypermobility, scoliosis) [49]. Finally, several pathogenic and possibly pathogenic variants in the coding region of the prion protein gene (*PRNP*), which is also located on chromosome 20, have been associated with different clinical phenotypes of neurodegenerative diseases, including Creutzfeldt–Jakob disease, Gerstmann–Sträussler–Scheinker disease, fatal familial insomnia, and other types of dementia [51].

In summary, increasing evidence from studies of the numerical and structural variation of the genome at the chromosomal and subchromosomal levels supports a role of chromosome 20 in the manifestation of a wide range of neuropsychiatric features. A recent case report on a young adult male individual with trisomy 20 reported some novel neuropsychiatric symptoms that had never been associated with the condition, such as childhood-onset visual hallucinations and self-injury, including biting self and headbanging, hypothesizing an underestimation of the extent of mental disorders in the context of trisomy 20 [5]. In addition, authors suggested that several environmental risk factors encountered in their case, such as child abuse, family discord, and exposure to domestic violence, may have at least partially accounted for the unusually severe psychiatric presentation as compared to previously reported cases, where, instead, milder or subthreshold psychiatric symptoms may have been overlooked [5]. Noteworthy, in that case, trisomy 20 was successfully applied as a mitigating factor in a capital murder trial [5].

The current trisomy 20 case revealed a severe and complex neuropsychiatric presentation at the cognitive, emotional, and behavioral levels. In addition, the patient was considered at high risk of causing harm, mainly to self, and appeared to be only partially responsive to medication, even when polypharmacy was attempted to improve clinical response. To the best of our knowledge, except for school bullying and the potentially stressful impact of the sister's self-harm, no other severe environmental risk factors were present in the patient's history.

Due to mosaicism, a remarkable variability in clinical symptoms between cases is not surprising. It is plausible to hypothesize that depending on the degree of mosaicism, body systems may be differentially affected, with implications for the severity of the phenotypic expression. Further, the potential correlation between the level of trisomic cells and clinical outcome is currently unknown and deserves investigation, as for other chromosomal mosaicisms [52]. In fact, it is likely that patients with trisomy 20 presenting with more evident neuropsychiatric distress have a higher percentage of affected cells in the brain as well as systems other than the central nervous system (CNS), such as the immune, cardiometabolic, and hypothalamic–pituitary–adrenal (HPA) systems, which have been involved in the onset of major psychiatric disorders [53].

Author Contributions: Conceptualization, M.C., G.A., L.P., V.R., E.P. and L.Z.; methodology, M.C., G.A., L.P., V.R., E.P. and L.Z.; validation, M.C., G.A., L.P., V.R., E.P. and L.Z.; investigation, M.C., G.A., L.P., V.R., E.P. and L.Z.; resources, M.C., G.A., L.P., V.R., E.P. and L.Z.; data curation, M.C., G.A., L.P., V.R., E.P. and L.Z.; writing—original draft preparation, M.C., G.A., L.P., V.R. and E.P.; writing—review and editing, M.C., G.A., L.P., V.R., E.P. and L.Z.; visualization, M.C., G.A., L.P., V.R., E.P. and L.Z.; supervision, M.C. and L.Z. All authors have read and agreed to the published version of the manuscript.

Funding: This research received no external funding.

Institutional Review Board Statement: The study was conducted according to the guidelines of the Declaration of Helsinki, and ethical approval was not required.

Informed Consent Statement: The patient and her parents agreed to this publication by written consent.

Data Availability Statement: The data reported in this paper are available from the medical history of the patient.

Acknowledgments: The authors would like to acknowledge infrastructure from the Integrated University Hospital of Verona and the University of Verona.

Conflicts of Interest: M.C. has been a consultant/advisor to GW Pharma Limited and F. Hoffmann-La Roche Limited, outside of this work. All the other authors declare no conflict of interest.

References

1. Chuang, T.-H.; Chang, Y.-P.; Lee, M.-J.; Wang, H.-L.; Lai, H.-H.; Chen, S.-U. The Incidence of Mosaicism for Individual Chromosome in Human Blastocysts Is Correlated with Chromosome Length. *Front. Genet.* **2021**, *11*, 1677. [CrossRef]
2. Pertile, M.D. Genome-Wide Cell-Free DNA-Based Prenatal Testing for Rare Autosomal Trisomies and Subchromosomal Abnormalities. In *Noninvasive Prenatal Testing (NIPT)*; Page-Christiaens, L., Klein, H.-G., Eds.; Academic Press: Cambridge, MA, USA, 2018; pp. 97–123.
3. Hsu, L.Y.F.; Kaffe, S.; Perlis, T.E. Trisomy 20 mosaicism in prenatal diagnosis–a review and update. *Prenat. Diagn.* **1987**, *7*, 581–596. [CrossRef] [PubMed]
4. Hsu, L.Y.F.; Kaffe, S.; Perlis, T.E. A revisit of trisomy 20 mosaicism in prenatal diagnosis—An overview of 103 cases. *Prenat. Diagn.* **1991**, *11*, 7–15. [CrossRef] [PubMed]
5. Montplaisir, R.; Lee, E.; Moreno-De-Luca, D.; Myers, W.C. Mosaic trisomy 20 and mitigation in capital crimes sentencing: A review and case report. *Behav. Sci. Law* **2019**, *37*, 512–521. [CrossRef] [PubMed]
6. Korkontzelos, I. Prenatal diagnosis of trisomy 20 mosaicism associated with hypoplastic nasal bone as a single sonographic marker. *Eur. J. Obstet. Gynecol. Reprod. Biol.* **2017**, *213*, 140–141. [CrossRef]
7. Velissariou, V.; Antoniadi, T.; Gyftodimou, J.; Bakou, K.; Grigoriadou, M.; Christopoulou, S.; Hatzipouliou, A.; Donoghue, J.; Karatzis, P.; Katsarou, E.; et al. Maternal uniparental isodisomy 20 in a foetus with trisomy 20 mosaicism: Clinical, cytogenetic and molecular analysis. *Eur. J. Hum. Genet.* **2002**, *10*, 694–698. [CrossRef] [PubMed]
8. Mavromatidis, G.; Dinas, K.; Delkos, D.; Vosnakis, C.; Mamopoulos, A.; Rousso, D. Case of prenatally diagnosed non-mosaic trisomy 20 with minor abnormalities. *J. Obstet. Gynaecol. Res.* **2010**, *36*, 866–868. [CrossRef] [PubMed]
9. Myers, T.L.; Prouty, L.A. Non-mosaic trisomy 20 in amniotic fluid cultures with minor anomalies in the fetus. *Clin. Genet.* **2008**, *35*, 233–236. [CrossRef]
10. Ensenauer, R.E.; Shaughnessy, W.J.; Jalal, S.M.; Dawson, D.B.; Courteau, L.K.; Ellison, J.W. Trisomy 20 mosaicism caused by a maternal meiosis II error is associated with normal intellect but multiple congenital anomalies. *Am. J. Med. Genet. Part A* **2005**, *134A*, 202–206. [CrossRef]
11. Warren, N.; Soukup, S.; King, J.; Dignan, P. Prenatal diagnosis of trisomy 20 by chorionic villus sampling (CVS): A case report with long-term outcome. *Prenat. Diagn.* **2001**, *21*, 1111–1113. [CrossRef]

12. Strømme, P.; Van Der Hagen, C.B.; Haakonsen, M.; Risberg, K.; Hennekam, R. Follow-up of a girl with cleft lip and palate and multiple malformations: Trisomy 20 mosaicism. *Scand. J. Plast. Reconstr. Surg. Hand Surg.* **2005**, *39*, 178–179. [CrossRef] [PubMed]
13. Reish, O.; Wolach, B.; Amiel, A.; Kedar, I.; Dolfin, T.; Fejgin, M. Dilemma of trisomy 20 mosaicism detected prenatally: Is it an innocent finding? *Am. J. Med. Genet.* **1998**, *77*, 72–75. [CrossRef]
14. Powis, Z.; Erickson, R.P. Uniparental disomy and the phenotype of mosaic trisomy 20: A new case and review of the literature. *J. Appl. Genet.* **2009**, *50*, 293–296. [CrossRef] [PubMed]
15. Girard, C.; Guillot, B.; Rivier, F.; Vale, F.D.; Bessis, D. Mosaïcisme pigmentaire de type Ito révélant une trisomie 20 en mosaïque. *Ann. Dermatol. Venereol.* **2005**, *132*, 151–153. [CrossRef]
16. Morales, C.; Cuatrecasas, E.; Mademont-Soler, I.; Clusellas, N.; Peruga, E.; Català, V.; Garrido, C.; Milà, M.; Soler, A.; Sánchez, A. Non-mosaic trisomy 20 of paternal origin in chorionic villus and amniotic fluid also detected in fetal blood and other tissues. *Eur. J. Med. Genet.* **2010**, *53*, 197–200. [CrossRef] [PubMed]
17. Karaoguz, M.Y.; Pala, E.; Kula, S.; Karaer, K.; Kan, D.; Nas, T.; Tunaoglu, S. Transposition of great arteries in an infant born after prenatal diagnosis of trisomy 20 mosaicism. *Genet. Couns.* **2007**, *18*, 437–443.
18. Hartmann, A.; Hofmann, U.B.; Hoehn, H.; Broecker, E.B.; Hamm, H. Postnatal Confirmation of Prenatally Diagnosed Trisomy 20 Mosaicism in a Patient with Linear and Whorled Nevoid Hypermelanosis. *Pediatr. Dermatol.* **2004**, *21*, 636–641. [CrossRef] [PubMed]
19. Hsieh, C.C.; Hsu, J.J.; Lo, L.M.; Hsieh, T.T.; Soong, Y.K. Non-mosaic trisomy 20 in cultures of amniotic fluid from a fetus with serious congenital malformation. *J. Formos. Med. Assoc.* **1992**, *91*, 543–544.
20. Willis, M.J.; Bird, L.M.; Dell'Aquila, M.; Jones, M.C. Expanding the phenotype of mosaic trisomy 20. *Am. J. Med. Genet. Part A* **2008**, *146A*, 330–336. [CrossRef]
21. Stein, Q.P.; Boyle, J.G.; Crotwell, P.L.; Flanagan, J.D.; Johnson, K.J.; Davis-Keppen, L.; Van Eerden, P.; Woltanski, A.R.; Watson, W.J. Prenatally diagnosed trisomy 20 mosaicism associated with arachnoid cyst of basal cistern. *Prenat. Diagn.* **2008**, *28*, 1169–1170. [CrossRef]
22. Holzgreve, W.; Golabi, M.; Bradley, J. Multiple congenital anomalies in a child born after prenatal diagnosis of trisomy 20 mosaicism. *Clin. Genet.* **1986**, *29*, 342–344. [CrossRef]
23. Salafsky, I.S.; MacGregor, S.N.; Claussen, U.; Von Eggeling, F. Maternal UPD 20 in an infant from a pregnancy with mosaic trisomy 20. *Prenat. Diagn.* **2001**, *21*, 860–863. [CrossRef] [PubMed]
24. Wallerstein, R.; Twersky, S.; Layman, P.; Kernaghan, L.; Aviv, H.; Pedro, H.F.; Pletcher, B. Long term follow-up of developmental delay in a child with prenatally-diagnosed trisomy 20 mosaicism. *Am. J. Med. Genet. Part A* **2005**, *137A*, 94–97. [CrossRef] [PubMed]
25. Miny, P.; Karabacak, Z.; Hammer, P.; Schulte-Vallentin, M.; Holzgreve, W. Chromosome Analyses from Urinary Sediment: Postnatal Confirmation of a Prenatally Diagnosed Trisomy 20 Mosaicism. *N. Engl. J. Med.* **1989**, *320*, 809. [CrossRef] [PubMed]
26. Achenbach, T.M.; Rescorla, L.A. *Manual for the ASEBA School-Age Forms & Profiles*; University of Vermont Research Center for Children, Youth & Families: Burlington, VT, USA, 2001.
27. APA. *Diagnostic and Statistical Manual of Mental Disorders*, 5th ed.; American Psychiatric Publishing: Arlington, TX, USA, 2013.
28. Wechsler, D. *Wechsler Intelligence Scale for Children*, 4th ed.; APA PsycNet: Washington, DC, USA, 2003.
29. Ikeda, M.; Saito, T.; Kanazawa, T.; Iwata, N. Polygenic risk score as clinical utility in psychiatry: A clinical viewpoint. *J. Hum. Genet.* **2020**, *66*, 53–60. [CrossRef] [PubMed]
30. Cimino, S.; Carola, V.; Cerniglia, L.; Bussone, S.; Bevilacqua, A.; Tambelli, R. The μ-opioid receptor gene A118G polymorphism is associated with insecure attachment in children with disruptive mood regulation disorder and their mothers. *Brain Behav.* **2020**, *10*, e01659. [CrossRef]
31. Roberson-Nay, R.; Leibenluft, E.; Brotman, M.A.; Myers, J.; Larsson, H.; Lichtenstein, P.; Kendler, K.S. Longitudinal Stability of Genetic and Environmental Influences on Irritability: From Childhood to Young Adulthood. *Am. J. Psychiatry* **2015**, *172*, 657–664. [CrossRef]
32. Moore, A.A.; Lapato, D.M.; Brotman, M.A.; Leibenluft, E.; Aggen, S.H.; Hettema, J.M.; York, T.P.; Silberg, J.L.; Roberson-Nay, R. Heritability, stability, and prevalence of tonic and phasic irritability as indicators of disruptive mood dysregulation disorder. *J. Child Psychol. Psychiatry* **2019**, *60*, 1032–1041. [CrossRef]
33. Starr, L.R.; Dienes, K.; Li, Y.I.; Shaw, Z.A. Chronic stress exposure, diurnal cortisol slope, and implications for mood and fatigue: Moderation by multilocus HPA-Axis genetic variation. *Psychoneuroendocrinology* **2019**, *100*, 156–163. [CrossRef]
34. Dougherty, L.R.; Barrios, C.S.; Carlson, G.A.; Klein, D.N. Predictors of Later Psychopathology in Young Children with Disruptive Mood Dysregulation Disorder. *J. Child Adolesc. Psychopharmacol.* **2017**, *27*, 396–402. [CrossRef]
35. Arinami, T.; Ohtsuki, T.; Ishiguro, H.; Ujike, H.; Tanaka, Y.; Morita, Y.; Mineta, M.; Takeichi, M.; Yamada, S.; Imamura, A.; et al. Genomewide High-Density SNP Linkage Analysis of 236 Japanese Families Supports the Existence of Schizophrenia Susceptibility Loci on Chromosomes 1p, 14q, and 20p. *Am. J. Hum. Genet.* **2005**, *77*, 937–944. [CrossRef] [PubMed]
36. Detera-Wadleigh, S.D.; Badner, J.A.; Yoshikawa, T.; Sanders, A.R.; Goldin, L.R.; Turner, G.; Rollins, D.Y.; Moses, T.; Guroff, J.J.; Kazuba, D.; et al. Initial Genome Scan of the NIMH Genetics Initiative Bipolar Pedigrees: Chromosomes 4, 7, 9, 18, 19, 20, and 21q. *Am. J. Med. Genet.* **1997**, *74*, 254–262. [CrossRef]

37. Lewis, C.; Levinson, D.F.; Wise, L.H.; DeLisi, L.E.; Straub, R.E.; Hovatta, I.; Williams, N.M.; Schwab, S.G.; Pulver, A.E.; Faraone, S.; et al. Genome Scan Meta-Analysis of Schizophrenia and Bipolar Disorder, Part II: Schizophrenia. *Am. J. Hum. Genet.* **2003**, *73*, 34–48. [CrossRef] [PubMed]
38. Moises, H.; Yang, L.; Kristbjarnarson, H.; Wiese, C.; Byerley, W.; Macciardi, F.; Arolt, V.; Blackwood, D.; Liu, X.; Sjögren, B.; et al. An international two-stage genome–wide search for schizophrenia susceptibility genes. *Nat. Genet.* **1995**, *11*, 321–324. [CrossRef]
39. Ross, J.; Berrettini, W.; Coryell, W.; Gershon, E.S.; Badner, J.A.; Kelsoe, J.R.; McInnis, M.G.; McMahon, F.; Murphy, D.L.; Nurnberger, J.; et al. Genome-wide parametric linkage analyses of 644 bipolar pedigrees suggest susceptibility loci at chromosomes 16 and 20. *Psychiatr. Genet.* **2008**, *18*, 191–198. [CrossRef] [PubMed]
40. Radhakrishna, U.; Senol, S.; Herken, H.; Gücüyener, K.; Gehrig, C.; Blouin, J.-L.; Akarsu, N.; Antonarakis, S. An apparently dominant bipolar affective disorder (BPAD) locus on chromosome 20p11.2–q11.2 in a large Turkish pedigree. *Eur. J. Hum. Genet.* **2001**, *9*, 39–44. [CrossRef]
41. Bigdeli, T.B.; Maher, B.S.; Zhao, Z.; Oord, E.J.C.G.V.D.; Thiselton, D.L.; Sun, J.; Webb, B.T.; Amdur, R.L.; Wormley, B.; O'Neill, F.A.; et al. Comprehensive Gene-Based Association Study of a Chromosome 20 Linked Region Implicates Novel Risk Loci for Depressive Symptoms in Psychotic Illness. *PLoS ONE* **2011**, *6*, e21440. [CrossRef]
42. Hamshere, M.L.; Schulze, T.G.; Schumacher, J.; Corvin, A.; Owen, M.J.; Jamra, R.A.; Propping, P.; Maier, W.; Diaz, G.O.Y.; Mayoral, F.; et al. Mood-incongruent psychosis in bipolar disorder: Conditional linkage analysis shows genome-wide suggestive linkage at 1q32.3, 7p13 and 20q13.31. *Bipolar Disord.* **2009**, *11*, 610–620. [CrossRef]
43. Erlangsen, A.; Appadurai, V.; Wang, Y.; Turecki, G.; Mors, O.; Werge, T.; Mortensen, P.B.; Starnawska, A.; Børglum, A.; Schork, A.; et al. Genetics of suicide attempts in individuals with and without mental disorders: A population-based genome-wide association study. *Mol. Psychiatry* **2018**, *25*, 2410–2421. [CrossRef]
44. Li, M.; Luo, X.-J.; Landén, M.; Bergen, S.; Hultman, C.M.; Li, X.; Zhang, W.; Yao, Y.-G.; Zhang, C.; Liu, J.; et al. Impact of a cis-associated gene expression SNP on chromosome 20q11.22 on bipolar disorder susceptibility, hippocampal structure and cognitive performance. *Br. J. Psychiatry* **2016**, *208*, 128–137. [CrossRef]
45. Peron, A.; Catusi, I.; Recalcati, M.P.; Calzari, L.; Larizza, L.; Vignoli, A.; Canevini, M.P. Ring Chromosome 20 Syndrome: Genetics, Clinical Characteristics, and Overlapping Phenotypes. *Front. Neurol.* **2020**, *11*, 1617. [CrossRef] [PubMed]
46. Kamath, B.M.; Thiel, B.D.; Gai, X.; Conlin, L.K.; Munoz, P.S.; Glessner, J.; Clark, D.; Warthen, D.M.; Shaikh, T.H.; Mihci, E.; et al. SNP array mapping of chromosome 20p deletions: Genotypes, phenotypes, and copy number variation. *Hum. Mutat.* **2009**, *30*, 371–378. [CrossRef] [PubMed]
47. Khattak, S.; Jan, M.; Warsi, S.; Khattak, S. Chromosome 20p Partial De Novo Duplication Identified in a Female Paediatric Patient with Characteristic Facial Dysmorphism and Behavioural Anomalies. *Case Rep. Genet.* **2020**, *2020*, 7093409. [CrossRef] [PubMed]
48. Hanafusa, H.; Morisada, N.; Ishida, Y.; Sakata, R.; Morita, K.; Miura, S.; Ye, M.J.; Yamamoto, T.; Okamoto, N.; Nozu, K.; et al. The smallest de novo 20q11.2 microdeletion causing intellectual disability and dysmorphic features. *Hum. Genome Var.* **2017**, *4*, 17050. [CrossRef] [PubMed]
49. Van Dijck, A.; Silfhout, A.T.V.-V.; Cappuyns, E.; van der Werf, I.M.; Mancini, G.M.; Tzschach, A.; Bernier, R.; Gozes, I.; Eichler, E.E.; Romano, C.; et al. Clinical Presentation of a Complex Neurodevelopmental Disorder Caused by Mutations in ADNP. *Biol. Psychiatry* **2018**, *85*, 287–297. [CrossRef] [PubMed]
50. Breen, M.S.; Garg, P.; Tang, L.; Mendonca, D.; Levy, T.; Barbosa, M.; Arnett, A.B.; Kurtz-Nelson, E.; Agolini, E.; Battaglia, A.; et al. Episignatures Stratifying Helsmoortel-Van Der Aa Syndrome Show Modest Correlation with Phenotype. *Am. J. Hum. Genet.* **2020**, *107*, 555–563. [CrossRef]
51. Bagyinszky, E.; Van Giau, V.; Youn, Y.C.; An, S.S.A.; Kim, S. Characterization of mutations in *PRNP* (prion) gene and their possible roles in neurodegenerative diseases. *Neuropsychiatr. Dis. Treat.* **2018**, *14*, 2067–2085. [CrossRef]
52. Griffith, C.B.; Vance, G.H.; Weaver, D.D. Phenotypic variability in trisomy 13 mosaicism: Two new patients and literature review. *Am. J. Med. Genet. Part A* **2009**, *149A*, 1346–1358. [CrossRef] [PubMed]
53. Pillinger, T.; D'Ambrosio, E.; McCutcheon, R.; Howes, O.D. Is psychosis a multisystem disorder? A meta-review of central nervous system, immune, cardiometabolic, and endocrine alterations in first-episode psychosis and perspective on potential models. *Mol. Psychiatry* **2018**, *24*, 776–794. [CrossRef]

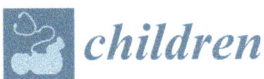

Article

Validation of the Proposed Specifiers for Conduct Disorder (PSCD) Scale in a Sample of Italian Students

Pietro Muratori [1], Carlo Buonanno [2], Anna Gallani [3], Giuseppe Grossi [2], Valentina Levantini [1], Annarita Milone [1], Simone Pisano [4], Randall T. Salekin [5], Gianluca Sesso [1], Gabriele Masi [1,*] and Annalaura Nocentini [6]

1. IRCCS Stella Maris, Scientific Institute of Child Neurology and Psychiatry, 56128 Pisa, Italy; pietro.muratori@fsm.unipi.it (P.M.); valentina.levantini@hotmail.it (V.L.); annarita.milone@fsm.unipi.it (A.M.); gianluca.sesso@fsm.unipi.it (G.S.)
2. Scuola Psicoterapia Cognitiva, 00185 Roma, Italy; buonanno@apc.it (C.B.); g.grossi@hotmail.it (G.G.)
3. Specialized Centre for Learning Disabilities, Uonpia Ausl, 40127 Ferrara, Italy; anna.gallani@gmail.com
4. Department of Translational Medical Sciences, Federico II University, 80138 Naples, Italy; pisano.simone@gmail.com
5. Department of Psychology, The University of Alabama, P.O. Box 870348, Tuscaloosa, AL 35487, USA; rsalekin@ua.edu
6. Department of Sciences of Education and Psychology, University of Florence, 50121 Firenze, Italy; annalaura.nocentini@unifi.it
* Correspondence: gabriele.masi@fsm.unipi.it; Tel.: +39-05-08861-11

Abstract: This study aimed to further validate the self-reported version of the Proposed Specifiers Conduct Disorder (PSCD) scale, testing the associations between the PSCD with a scale that measures emotional/behavioral difficulties and prosocial behaviors (Strength and Difficulties Questionnaire, SDQ). A total of 536 Italian students (47.76% male; 11–14 years) completed the PSCD, while their caregivers and teachers completed the SDQ. A series of confirmatory factor analyses to test the best fitting model were run. The internal consistency of the PSCD was evaluated, and the correlations between the PSCD self-reported scores and SDQ Parent and Teacher report scores were examined. A bi-factor model was fitted with a refined 19-item version of the scale, which showed adequate fit indices. The PSCD total score was strongly associated with higher parent- and teacher-rated conduct problems, hyperactivity, and lower prosocial behavioral symptoms. In conclusion, this study indicated that the self-report PSCD shows preliminary promise as a reliable, easy-to-use tool, for measuring psychopathic traits in Italian children and young adolescents.

Keywords: grandiose-manipulative; callous-unemotional; daring-impulsive; psychopathy; early adolescent; conduct problems; hyperactivity

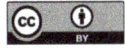

1. Introduction

Hare's Psychopathy Checklist (PCL-R; [1]), in its revised version, describes psychopathy as a multidimensional construct encompassing at least four components: Interpersonal (i.e., superficial charm, grandiose self, manipulative tendencies); Affective (i.e., lack of guilt and remorse, shallow affects); Lifestyle/Behavioral (i.e., parasitism, sensation seeking, impulsivity); and Antisocial (i.e., delinquency, criminality). This general multidimensional structure has been replicated in factor analysis-based studies in adults [2,3], and similar findings have been confirmed in children and adolescents [4,5].

Recent research has increasingly focused on one dimension of psychopathy in children and adolescent populations, namely Callous Unemotional traits (CU). Such a trend likely finds its roots in the several studies showing that the levels of CU traits (lack of guilt, shallow emotions, and proactive aggression) are associated with a more persistent and severe pattern of aggressive behavior and delinquency and a greater risk for adverse outcomes throughout the lifespan (e.g., antisocial behavior, substance use, violent crimes, and detentions; [6–10]).

Nevertheless, some recent evidence suggests that the combination of all dimensions of psychopathy is more strongly related to and predictive of conduct problems in childhood than CU traits alone, and childhood psychopathy would be preferably represented by all its dimensions (see [11,12]). Therefore, some tools have been developed for assessing all dimensions of psychopathy in childhood and adolescence.

A Youth Version (PCL:YV) of the PCL-R was developed by Forth, Kosson, and Hare [13] as a comprehensive assessment process to detect psychopathic traits in youths. Although detailed and exhaustive, this semi-structured interview is time-consuming since it requires 60 to 90 minutes to complete. Therefore, it is not easily accommodated in large-scale community studies. Moreover, Although its psychometric properties are generally strong [14,15], it does not allow for the direct opinion of the child being evaluated or parent report [15].

Among the most previously widely used clinical tools for psychopathic traits, the Antisocial Process Screening Device (APSD; [16]) is a 20-item parent-, teacher- or self-report rating scale based on the PCL-R. However, the alignment of its factor labels with the highest loading items on the corresponding subscale and their pathognomonic significance have been questioned [14–17]. Moreover, some concerns about its factors structure have been raised, with some studies finding a two-factor structure [18] and other studies finding a three-factor structure [19]. In addition, some authors have highlighted that the APSD clearly assesses negative behaviors, and its use as a self-report measure could lead to biased answers [20]; finally, some studies have found issues pertaining to its poor internal consistency, especially for the APSD's CU subscale [21].

With its more traditional factor structure with ten subscales loading onto the three main dimensions (Interpersonal, Affective, and Lifestyle) of psychopathy, the Youth Psychopathic Traits Inventory (YPI) [20] is a 50-item self-report questionnaire designed to assess psychopathic traits in community samples of adolescents. A Short Form (YPI-S; [22]) has been validated in children, with 18 items equally distributed across three subscales, thus being easier to be administered in clinical settings. Nonetheless, this scale does not consider the antisocial dimension of child psychopathy, including poor behavioral control and proactive aggression, which would likely represent the most maladaptive feature of the condition [12]. In addition, it does not include a scale for Conduct disorder (CD) symptoms which could be important to study with psychopathic traits. Finally, not all studies reported optimal internal consistency for the YPI [23]. Internal consistency issues have also been reported for the Childhood Psychopathy Scale (CPS) [21] and the most broadly used Child Problematic Traits Inventory (CPTI) [24], although generally the psychometric properties for the CPIT are good. Perhaps the broader issue is that the scales lack a CD scale for those interested in the assessment of psychopathy in relation to CD.

In order to overcome the abovementioned limitations of the previous measures, Salekin and Hare [11] developed the Proposed Specifiers for Conduct Disorder (PSCD). The original version of the PSCD is a theory-driven measure composed of 24-items. It was designed to assess all the components of youths' psychopathy, including grandiose-manipulative (GM) traits, callous-unemotional (CU) traits, daring-impulsive (DI) traits, plus CD/Oppositional Defiant Disorder (ODD) symptoms. A parent-report and a self-report version of the PSCD were then developed.

The first validation study of the PSCD was conducted by López-Romero and colleagues in 2019 [25]. The authors validated the parent-report version of the PSCD in a sample of 2,229 Spanish preschoolers aged 3 to 6 years. This was the first published study aimed to assess the psychometric properties of the PSCD. The version was adapted to be rated by parents and to include only age-appropriate items for preschoolers. The authors validated a four-factor model of the PSCD, including GM traits, CU traits, DI traits, and conduct problems. Associations with external criteria supported the validity of the

PSCD, including measures of child fearlessness, conduct problems, reactive and proactive aggressive behaviors, and emotional problems.

Recently, Luo and colleagues [26] assessed the psychometric and structural properties of the self-rated PSCD in a sample of 1,683 Chinese adolescents aged 11 to 17 years. A Confirmatory Factor Analysis (CFA) supported the four-factor bifactor model, showing good internal consistency. This model showed generally high convergent associations with alternative measures of psychopathy, namely, the APSD, the YPI, and the Inventory of Callous Unemotional traits (ICU) [27].

The Current Study

The PSCD construct validity has been established by a previous study by Luo et al. [26], as well as its associations with other measures of maladjustment. However, Luo et al. [26] examined the PSCD relation to the external criteria using only self-report measures. Some studies examined parent and child reports together and pointed out that parent measures had a greater magnitude of effect in predicting some outcomes [17,28]. Moreover, as the manifestations of the psychopathy dimensions are pervasive and not limited to a single context, teachers' reports of children's behavior at school could provide precious information. It is important to evaluate the relationships between the PSCD dimensions and low levels of youths' prosocial behaviors, often indicated as a risk sign for future negative outcomes [29,30]. Moreover, although some measures assessing youths' psychopathy are available in Italian, none of them have been validated. To sum up, the current study aimed to further validate the PSCD, testing the associations between the self-reported PSCD scores and parent- and teacher-reports of emotional/behavioral difficulties and prosocial behaviors. Given the similarities between Luo and colleagues' study and our sample, we hypothesized to find similar results regarding the PSCD factor structure and its internal consistency. We also hypothesized that the PSCD scores would be associated with higher Conduct Problems and Hyperactivity Behavior and lower Prosocial Behavior [12].

2. Materials and Methods

2.1. Subjects

We enrolled 536 Italian students (47.76% male) aged between 11–14 years (males mean age = 12.20, SD = 0.65; females mean age = 12.60, SD = 0.60), consisting of 87 (16.20%) 6th graders, 360 (67.20%) 7th graders and 89 (16.60%) 8th graders, among which 88% of participants were Caucasian (12% from Africa). Of the whole sample, 492 students agreed to participate in the study. Thirty-four language teachers and the students' caregivers were also involved. Regarding caregivers, most of the informants were mothers.

2.2. Procedures

Before completing any questionnaire, all the teachers, parents, and youths who agreed to participate in the study signed a written informed consent. Research assistants informed the participants that their participation in the study was voluntary, and they could withdraw from the study at any time. In addition, participants were assured of the confidentiality and anonymity of their answers. Throughout the study, research assistants were available to answer participants' questions. While sitting in a quiet classroom, students were asked to complete the PSCD, which required approximately 15 min. Teachers completed the SDQ for each student. The SDQ was provided by a researcher who returned the completed SDQs in approximately one week. During a school meeting, parents also completed the SDQ. The study was conducted according to the guidelines of the Declaration of Helsinki and approved by the Institutional Review Board of Istituto Comprensivo Milani (PTOF, prot. 456 2019) and by the Institutional Review Board of Istituto Comprensivo G. Sani (PTOF, prot. 8 2019).

2.3. Measures

Students completed the PSCD [11]. The PSCD includes four domains, namely: Grandiose-Manipulative - an interpersonal component, intended to measure grandiosity, superficial charm, manipulation, and deceitfulness (thus labeled "Grandiose–Manipulative" or GM traits); Callous-unemotional—an Affective dimension, assessing callousness, uncaring affect, and disregard to others (thus labeled "Callous–Unemotional" or CU traits); Daring-Impulsive—similar to a Lifestyle domain, including daringness, sensation seeking, recklessness and irresponsibility (thus "Daring–Impulsive" or DI traits); and Conduct Disorder—the antisocial component (also referred to as CD traits), designed to measure the four main categories of CD symptoms (aggression to people and animals, destruction of property, deceitfulness or theft and serious violation of rules). A four-factor structure was initially theoretically proposed by Salekin and Hare in 2016 [11] for the self-rated PSCD, and its 24 items were equally distributed across the four subscales, each including six items. Items are rated on a three-point Likert scale, with responses ranging from 0 (not true) to 2 (true); a Total Score includes all 24 items. A bilingual researcher (forward) translated the PSCD from English to Italian. Then, a different bilingual researcher back-translated the questionnaire from Italian to English. The final version was further discussed by the above-mentioned translators and one of the original authors of this measure (R. T. Salekin) until they reached an agreement. No cultural adaptations were needed.

We asked teachers and parents to complete the Italian version of the SDQ [31]. The SDQ includes 25 items, and answers are provided on a 3-point Likert scale. The SDQ includes five subscales assessing Conduct Problems (e.g., bullying); Hyperactivity (e.g., squirming); Emotional Problems (e.g., worrying), Peer Problems (e.g., disliked by other children), and Prosocial Behaviors (e.g., helping). When all the items are filled in, the subscales' scores range from 0 to 10. Higher scores indicate more behavioral problems, except for the prosocial behavior scores. In this study's sample, the SDQ reliability was generally satisfactory, as demonstrated by the mean internal consistency of subscales (Cronbach's α): 0.73 for Conduct Problems, 0.77 for Hyperactivity, 0.81 for Emotional Symptoms, 0.80 for Peer Problems, and 0.82 for Prosocial Behaviors.

2.4. Statistical Analysis

As a preliminary analysis, we performed descriptive statistics for all scales with SPSS 23.0. Analyses were conducted with 466 students with complete data (missing data, $N = 26$ about 5% of the sample, were excluded from the analyses). We calculated means and standard deviations for the PSCD total score, the PSCD subscales, and each item. A series of confirmatory factor analyses (CFAs) were conducted to test the best fitting model using MPLUS 7 and MLR as estimators with robust standard errors. The competing models of the PSCD structure were: Model 1: a one-factor model (all the 24 items loaded into a mono-factorial structure); Model 2: a four-factor model following the original definition as proposed by Salekin [12] (the 24 items of the PSCD as observed variables and the four factors as latent and correlated constructs-GM, CU, DI, and CD -, with each item specified to load on only one factor); Model 3: a second-order factor model with the four-factors as first-order constructs (see the previous model) and a second-order factor representing a general PSCD psychopathy syndrome; Model 4: a four factors bi-factor model where a general factor measured all the items directly and, at the same time, items loaded into their respective specific factors (GM, CU, DI, and CD). CFA fit indices included the comparative fit index (CFI) and root mean square error of approximation (RMSEA). Results were interpreted as follows: CFI values above 0.95, and RMSEA scores below 0.05, were considered indices of a good fit, whereas CFI larger than 0.90 and RMSEA smaller than 0.08 were considered indices of adequate model fit [32]. The comparison between competing factorial models has been analyzed using the AIC and the BIC values, and the ΔCFI.

We then evaluated the internal consistency of the PSCD score using the mean interitem correlations (MIC) and the ω_H for the general factor [33,34]. This index is usually used in short item scale, and it is used in Luo et al. [26]. The ω_H represents the ratio of the variance of the general factor compared to the total test variance, which reflects the percentage of systematic variance in unit-weighted total scores that can be attributed to the individual differences on the general factor. When ω_H values are high (≥ 0.80), relative to the percentage of variance explained by the group factors, it means that the total raw score could be interpreted as reflecting the target construct [35]. Moreover, the ideal range of MIC is 0.15 to 0.50; less than this, and the items are not well correlated and not measuring the same construct or idea very well. More than 0.50, and the items are close as to be almost repetitive. Multiple-Group analyses across gender were also conducted. Finally, we examined the correlations among the PSCD Subscales and Total Score, and Strengths and Difficulties Questionnaire Parent and Teacher report scores and independent samples t-tests were used to explore gender differences in the PSCD scores.

3. Results

3.1. Descriptive Statistics

Means and standard deviations of the 24 items of the original version of the scale are shown in Table 1.

Table 1. Means and standard deviations of the PSCD items.

Items	Min	Max	Skewness	Kurtosis	Mean	SD
1: I can turn on the charm in any situation	0	2	0.96	−0.12	0.47	0.62
2: I am a very important person	0	2	0.66	−0.62	0.60	0.66
3: I am very good at most things I do	0	2	−0.11	−0.44	1.21	0.59
4: Lying is easy for me	0	2	0.49	−0.95	0.71	0.72
5: I take advantage of others	0	2	2.20	4.19	0.21	0.47
6: I am a natural storyteller	0	2	0.42	−1.05	0.76	0.73
7: I don't waste time thinking about how I may have hurt others	0	2	1.11	0.07	0.46	0.65
8: I can turn and walk away from someone who is hurt	0	2	1.53	1.13	0.36	0.63
9: When people are happy or upset I do not seem to care	0	2	1.73	2.16	0.26	0.49
10: I like it when others are afraid of me	0	2	1.42	0.95	0.38	0.72
11: Some people consider me to be a mean person	0	2	1.05	−0.23	0.50	0.69
12: I rarely feel guilt or remorse	0	2	0.25	−1.11	0.85	0.73
13: I am daring	0	2	−0.04	−1.12	1.02	0.73
14: I like a lot of change or adventure	0	2	−0.45	−0.87	1.28	0.69
15: I get a thrill out of doing risky things	0	2	0.45	−1.20	0.76	0.77
16: I feel like I need a lot of stimulation	0	2	0.15	−1.25	0.91	0.76
17: I like to live in the moment	0	2	−0.62	−0.99	1.33	0.75
18: Some people think I am reckless	0	2	0.46	−1.23	0.75	0.78
19: I have stolen things	0	2	1.46	0.70	0.39	0.67
20: I have engaged in physical aggression against animals or people	0	2	1.02	−0.66	0.54	0.79
21: I have destroyed property	0	2	1.55	1.09	0.36	0.65
22: I break (violate) a lot of rules	0	2	1.06	−0.01	0.47	0.65
23: I started breaking rules before the age of 10 years	0	2	2.47	4.94	0.21	0.54
24: I can be argumentative and defiant (oppositional)	0	2	0.47	−1.01	0.74	0.75

Abbreviations: PSCD, Proposed Specifiers for Conduct Disorder; Min, minimum; Max, maximum; SD, standard deviation.

3.2. Psychometric Properties

Table 2 shows the fit indices of the competing models. The four models tested showed poor fit indices, although the best fitting model was the four factors bi-factor structure (Model 4). Besides, the comparison between models 1–4 considering AIC and BIC values and the ΔCFI (always > 0.02) suggested Model 4 as the best fitting, and thus it was accepted as the final model. Looking at the solution, we decided to delete the items that were non-significant in the general factor (items: 3, 12, 14, 16, 17) (see Model 4 revised). From GM traits, this included item 3. From CU traits, this included item 12; from DI traits, this included items 14, 16, and 17. Following the Modification Indices (MI = 12.927) we decided to set the loading of item 5 into the CU instead of the GM as in the original solution [12]. The final fit indices of this modified model showed acceptable fit indices.

Table 2. Fit indices of the competing models.

	χ^2	Df	p	CFI	RMSEA	AIC	BIC
Model 1: Mono-dimensional	732.540	252	<0.001	0.758	0.064 (0.059–0.069)	21,679.174	21,977.556
Model 2: Four Factors (original as Salekin, 2017)	606.143	246	<0.001	0.818	0.056 (0.050–0.062)	21,532.517	21,855.763
Model 3: Second Order	621.857	248	<0.001	0.812	0.057 (0.051–0.062)	21,543.189	21,858.147
Model 4: four factors bi-factor	495.433	228	<0.001	0.865	0.050 (0.044–0.056)	21,451.710	21,849.552
Model 4 revised: four factors bi-factor *	344.469	133	<0.001	0.910	0.059 (0.051–0.067)	16,556.136	16,871.094

* The items: 3-12-14-16-17 were deleted, and item 5 was loaded into the CU factor.

Figure 1 shows the factor loadings. This final model showed some similarities with the model found by Luo and colleagues [26]: in particular, item 17 resulted as not significant also in this Bifactor model. The general factor reflects quite well on the indicators of all the specific items. However, in line with other studies using bifactor models [36], unexpected results were found for five factor loadings measuring specific factors. The loadings of the items 10-11 (CU Factor), and 22-23-24 (CD Factor) resulted in not being significant in measuring these specific factors, although these items were theoretically assumed to be indicators of these factors. Overall, however, the findings demonstrate that covariance among observed indicators can be well accounted for by a latent general factor, reflecting common variance among all indicators, and four latent group factors, reflecting additional common variance for subsets of indicators.

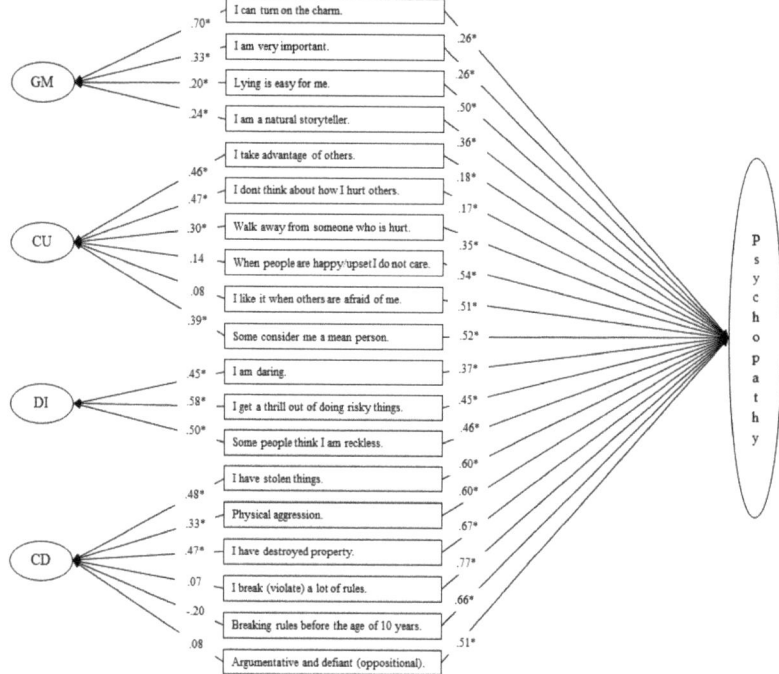

Figure 1. Factor loadings of the final four-factors Bifactor Model (standardized estimates). Abbreviations: GM, Grandiose–Manipulative; CU, Callous–Unemotional; DI, Daring–Impulsive; CD, Conduct Disorder. * $p < 0.001$.

As also made by Luo and colleagues [26], we compared the 24-item scale with the reduced 19-item version regarding their ability to identify youths with high psychopathy features (PSCD mean total score > 1). In our sample, the 24-item PSCD identified 46 youths (8.6%) with high psychopathy features, while the 19-item scale identified 42 youths (7.8%). The difference in proportion was significant ($\chi^2(1) = 412.54$, $p < 0.001$) and in favor of the original 24-item scale. However, it is important to mention that there was only a slight difference in the number of subjects identified and that the two versions of the PSCD are highly correlated ($r = 0.96$, $p < 0.001$).

Regarding internal consistency, the 19-item PSCD total score (items 3-12-14-16-17 eliminated and item 5 loaded into the CU factor) had a MIC value of 0.32. The subscales MIC values were all acceptable: 0.27 for GM, 0.26 for CU, 0.35 for DI, and 0.31 for CD. Moreover, the ω_H for the general factor was 0.80. We also tested for (in)variance across gender for the 19 items version of the PSCD. Configural and metric/scalar invariance were examined in sequence for gender groups. The model fit indices were acceptable for configural invariance (although the CFI was slightly lower than 0.90) (χ^2 (276) = 468.082, $p < 0.001$; CFI = 0.898; RMSEA = 0.057 (0.048–0.066), metric and scalar invariance model (χ^2 (313) = 461.817, $p < 0.001$; CFI = 0.905; RMSEA = 0.047 (0.038–0.056)). Besides, the difference test between configural and metric invariance models (χ^2 (15) = 15.541; $p = 0.413$) and the difference test between metric and scalar invariance models (χ^2 (37) = 11.885, $p = 1.00$) resulted non-significant, meaning that our final model of the PSCD was invariant across gender groups. Finally, Table 3 shows the descriptive statistics of the PSCD scores, with gender comparisons.

Table 3. Descriptive statistics of the PSCD subscales and total score, with gender comparisons.

	Range		Total Sample (N = 536) Mean (SD)	Males (N = 256) Mean (SD)	Females (N = 280) Mean (SD)	t	p	d
	Min	Max						
PSCD Total	0	31	10.01 (5.81)	11.35 (6.13)	8.68 (5.33)	−4.03	<0.001	0.46
GM	0	12	2.52 (1.68)	2.65 (1.66)	2.28 (1.67)	−4.66	<0.001	0.22
CU	0	6	2.18 (1.95)	2.60 (2.05)	1.88 (1.83)	−2.27	0.023	0.36
DI	0	11	2.54 (1.72)	2.80 (1.71)	2.20 (1.71)	−3.72	<0.001	0.35
CD	0	8	2.71 (2.64)	3.26 (2.80)	2.25 (2.37)	−3.57	<0.001	0.39

Abbreviations: PSCD Total, Proposed Specifiers for Conduct Disorder Total Score; GM, Grandiose–Manipulative; CU, Callous–Unemotional; DI, Daring–Impulsive; CD, Conduct Disorder.

3.3. Correlations with SDQ Scores

Table 4 shows the correlation between the PSCD scores and the SDQ parent- and teacher-report scores. The PSCD total score was strongly associated with parent- and teacher-rated conduct problems and hyperactivity symptoms; it was also negatively associated with parent- and teacher-reported prosocial behavior (moderate correlations). Scales of PSCD showed moderate or strong positive associations with conduct problems and hyperactivity symptoms. Among PSCD dimensions, only CU scores were associated with parent- and teacher-rated peer problems; only CU and CD scores were negatively associated with prosocial behaviors in the home and school contexts (moderate correlation indices).

Table 4. Bivariate correlations between the scores of the revised version of PSCD (19 items) and Strengths and Difficulties Questionnaire Parent and Teacher report scores.

	PSCD Total	GM	CU	DI	CD
PSCD Total	1				
GM	0.65 **	1			
CU	0.68 **	0.21 **	1		
DI	0.66 **	0.41 **	0.20 **	1	
CD	0.84 **	0.34 **	0.48 **	0.36 **	1
SDQ_P_EP	0.03	0.02	0.07	0.01	0.11
SDQ_P_CP	0.35 **	0.22 **	0.26 **	0.17 **	0.31 **
SDQ_P_HY	0.37 **	0.20 **	0.28 **	0.24 **	0.31 **
SDQ_P_PP	0.16 **	−0.03	0.31 **	−0.02	0.14 **
SDQ_P_PB	−0.21 **	−0.02	−0.28 **	−0.01	−0.22 **
SDQ_T_EP	0.07	0.02	0.10	−0.03	0.10
SDQ_T_CP	0.41 **	0.28 **	0.36 **	0.26 **	0.35 **
SDQ_T_HY	0.45 **	0.28 **	0.37 **	0.36 **	0.36 **
SDQ_T_PP	0.09	0.01	0.26 **	−0.01	0.02
SDQ_T_PB	−0.25 **	−0.13 *	−0.24 **	−0.19 **	−0.20 **

Abbreviations: PSCD Total, Proposed Specifiers for Conduct Disorder Total Score; GM, Grandiose–Manipulative; CU, Callous–Unemotional; DI, Daring–Impulsive; CD, Conduct Disorder; SDQ_P_EP, SDQ parent-report Emotional Problems; SDQ_P_CP, SDQ parent-report Conduct Problems; SDQ_P_HY, SDQ parent-report Hyperactivity Symptoms; SDQ_P_PP, SDQ parent-report Peer Problems; SDQ_P_PB, SDQ parent-report Prosocial Behavior; SDQ_T_EP, SDQ teacher-report Emotional Problems; SDQ_T_CP, SDQ teacher-report Conduct Problems; SDQ_T_HY, SDQ teacher-report Hyperactivity Symptoms; SDQ_T_PP, SDQ teacher-report Peer Problems; SDQ_T_PB, SDQ teacher-report Prosocial Behavior. * $p < 0.05$ ** $p < 0.01$. Correlation coefficients ≤ 0.10 are weak; 0.20 to 0.29 are moderate; ≥ 0.30 are good (Hemphill, 2003).

4. Discussion

As expected, and consistent with Luo et al. [26], findings from our sample of Italian young adolescents indicated that the self-report PSCD questionnaire supported an overall bi-factor model consisting of four factors (GM, CU, DI, and CD) and a general factor. It is important to note that recent evidence indicated that the bi-factor model presents some advantages compared to the higher-order model for describing the general psychopathy traits because it directly teases apart the unique contributions to the indicators of the general and specific factors [37].

Some modifications were necessary for the Italian version of the PSCD. Modification indices suggested that item 5 best loaded onto the CU factor instead of the GM, as in the original version of the PSCD. The Italian version of the PSCD does not include item 3 ("I am very good at most things") and item 12 ("I rarely feel guilt or remorse") of the original version of the PSCD. The item 3 mean score was generally high, suggesting that most of the subjects in our sample may have positively interpreted the statement (e.g., being competent and skillful). Item 12 assesses an emotional feature of CU traits, namely lack of remorse and guilt. Social desirability or dissimulation may have influenced the mean score of this item. Items 3 and 12 were also removed from the Chinese version of the PSCD, suggesting these items might not clearly represent the psychopathy dimensions in youths, or at least not in this sample. We also deleted items 14 ("I like a lot of change or adventure"), 16 ("I feel like I need a lot of stimulation"), and 17 ("I like to live in the moment"). It is unclear why these items did not load, and will need additional testing as with the PSCD. It is interesting to note that Luo et al. [26] maintained items 14 and 16 in the DI subscale. Waiting for new research that might shed novel light on the item distribution for the PSCD, we can also hypothesize that translation issues and/or cultural differences may explain the modifications needed for the Italian version of the PSCD. The PSCD total and factors internal consistency was acceptable, especially for MIC indices. Moreover, we did not find gender differences regarding the PSCD structure in this sample.

Our results showed that, based on the 19-item version of the PSCD, 7.8% of the students reported high psychopathy features. There are currently no data on the prevalence of psychopathy in Italian samples of early adolescents, and our study could provide some helpful information on this matter. Compared to Luo and colleagues [26], we found a higher rate of youths with high psychopathy features (7.8% vs. 5.8% for the refined versions; 8.6% vs. 5.2% for the 24-item versions). Cultural differences might explain this discrepancy in the prevalence of high psychopathy features. Findings showed that boys reported higher scores in all the PSCD scales and total scores than girls. Sex differences in levels of psychopathic traits have indeed been confirmed by previous studies using different measures. Frick, Bodin, and Barry [19] found that boys had significantly higher scores than females regarding Narcissism, Impulsivity, and CU traits assessed with the APSD. Similarly, Andershed, Hodgins, and Tengström [38] found that males reported higher scores in the Interpersonal, Affective, Behavioral, and Antisocial factors of the PCL:YV as well as higher CU traits assessed with the YPI (see also [39,40]).

Besides, this is the first study to explore the correlations between the self-report PSCD scores and the parent and teacher reports of emotional/behavioral difficulties and prosocial behaviors. The previous validation of the self-report PSCD [26] relied solely on self-report measures, which the authors themselves recognized as a major limitation of their study. As hypothesized, the correlations between PSCD scores and these external criterion variables supported associations between high levels of PSCD scores and high levels of behavioral problems, with some differences in the association between the PSCD single scales and the SDQ scores. The PSCD total score showed moderate and good positive associations with conceptually and clinically important variables, including conduct problems and hyperactivity behaviors in home and school contexts. Furthermore, the total score of the PSCD seemed to be also associated with low prosocial behaviors.

Among the PSCD dimensions it is particularly interesting to note that those individuals with elevated GM traits appeared to be rated by parents and teachers as not having difficulty with peers (SDQ-Peer Problems). That is, children with elevated GM traits generally seemed to be able to get along with their peers at least in the eyes of parents and teachers, or at least not be detected by parents and teachers, as having problems with their peers even though they engaged in antisocial behavior (conduct problems). Similarly, those youth with elevated DI traits were also able to get along with peers despite engaging in antisocial behavior although interestingly teachers for both GM and DI youth noted their lack of engagement in prosocial behavior indicating that they may not have completely evaded detection. Only the CU dimension appeared to be associated with noted Peer Problems and low Prosocial Behaviors. Different explanations can account for these unique associations, which deserve further investigation. Youth with GM traits are thought to be able to evade trouble more easily. Similarly, youth with elevated Di traits are not thought to suffer from the same cognitive problems as those with CU traits. Empathy impairments may be more core to high CU traits [41–43]. CU youths' inability to connect with other people' feelings and needs may result in general carelessness toward others, making youths with CU traits less prone to prosocial actions and with shorter, less stable [44], and satisfactory friendships [45].

Findings need to be interpreted considering some limitations. First, the sample size was relatively small. The final solution from the bi-factor model showed that the general factor reflects quite well indicators of all the specific dimensions; however, not significant factor loadings emerged for two items of the CU dimension and three items for the CD dimension. Although this pattern needs to be replicated, the finding suggested that caution needs to be considered when interpreting CU and CD scores. Moreover, even though beyond the primary aims of this study, we did not include other measures to assess psychopathic traits. The external criteria of the PSCD are limited to emotional and behavioral difficulties; other criteria relevant to the psychopathy construct should be considered in future studies, such as cognitive functioning [46], emotional intelligence and empathy [42,47], and proactive aggression [48]. We did not have temporal stability data on psychopathic traits for this group, although there are considerable data to show modest to high stability for children and adolescents [6,49].

5. Conclusions

Despite these limitations, we explored the associations between the PSCD scores and a wide range of behavioral and emotional difficulties. Behavioral problems are widely prevalent disorders in youths, and since their frequency is increasing, more reliable measures are constantly required. Self-report measures are particularly needed for an accurate assessment of early adolescents and older youths [50,51], since as their autonomy increases, parents are no longer completely aware of all the aspects of their child's life. The PSCD could help clinicians to identify youths who are at greatest risk and for whom targeted early interventions could be provided at a relatively low cost. The PSCD could also be an appealing instrument for different professional figures (e.g., social workers, pediatricians, psychologists): it has few items and could be easily added to screening batteries (e.g., large-scale epidemiological studies, evaluations in the school context). Moreover, the CD scale allows for assessing the four CD symptoms, as delineated in the DSM-5. However, further validation studies are needed before introducing the PSCD as a tool in clinical assessment procedures (e.g., test-retest reliability).

Author Contributions: Conceptualization, P.M., C.B. and R.T.S. Formal analysis, A.N.; Validation, A.G. and G.G.; Writing–original draft, P.M., V.L., A.M., S.P., G.S. and A.N.; Writing—review and editing, R.T.S. and G.M. All authors have read and agreed to the published version of the manuscript.

Funding: This work was supported by a grant from the IRCCS Fondazione Stella Maris (Ricerca Corrente (RC 2763771, 2.21_Tipizzazione genetico-clinica dei disturbi del comportamento in età evolutiva: implicazioni cliniche e di trattamento) and the '5 × 1000' voluntary contributions, Italian Ministry of Health).

Institutional Review Board Statement: The study was conducted according to the guidelines of the Declaration of Helsinki and approved by the Institutional Review Board of Istituto Comprensivo Milani (PTOF, prot. 456 2019) and by the Institutional Review Board of Istituto Comprensivo G. Sani (PTOF, prot. 8 2019).

Informed Consent Statement: Informed consent was obtained from all subjects involved in the study.

Data Availability Statement: The data are available from the corresponding author upon reasonable request.

Conflicts of Interest: Masi has received institutional research grants from Lundbeck and Humana, was in an advisory board for Angelini, and has been speaker for Angelini, FB Health, Janssen, Lundbeck, and Otsuka. All the other Authors do not have conflicts of interest to declare.

References

1. Hare, R. *Manual for the Revised Psychopathy Checklist*, 2nd ed.; Multi-Health Systems: Toronto, ON, Canada, 2003.
2. Hare, R.D.; Neumann, C.S. The role of antisociality in the psychopathy construct: Comment on skeem and cooke. *Psychol. Assess.* **2010**, *22*, 446–454. [CrossRef]
3. Neumann, C.S.; Hare, R.D.; Newman, J.P. The super-ordinate nature of the psychopathy checklist-revised. *J. Pers. Disord.* **2007**, *21*, 102–117. [CrossRef] [PubMed]
4. Colins, O.F.; Andershed, H.; Salekin, R.T.; Fanti, K.A. Comparing different approaches for subtyping children with conduct problems: Callous-unemotional traits only versus the multidimensional psychopathy construct. *J. Psychopathol. Behav. Assess.* **2018**, *40*, 6–15. [CrossRef]
5. Lee, S.S. Multidimensionality of youth psychopathic traits: Validation and future directions. *J. Psychopathol. Behav. Assess.* **2018**, *40*, 86–92. [CrossRef]
6. Pisano, S.; Muratori, P.; Gorga, C.; Levantini, V.; Iuliano, R.; Catone, G.; Coppola, G.; Milone, A.; Masi, G. Conduct disorders and psychopathy in children and adolescents: Aetiology, clinical presentation and treatment strategies of callous-unemotional traits. *Ital. J. Pediatr.* **2017**, *43*, 84. [CrossRef]
7. Frick, P.J.; Ray, J.V.; Thornton, L.C.; Kahn, R.E. Annual research review: A developmental psychopathology approach to understanding callous-unemotional traits in children and adolescents with serious conduct problems. *J. Child Psychol. Psychiatry Allied Discip.* **2014**, *55*, 532–548. [CrossRef]
8. Frick, P.J.; Ray, J.V.; Thornton, L.C.; Kahn, R.E. Can callous-unemotional traits enhance the understanding, diagnosis, and treatment of serious conduct problems in children and adolescents? *Compr. Rev.* **2013**, *140*, 1–57. [CrossRef]
9. Kahn, R.E.; Byrd, A.L.; Pardini, D.A. Callous-unemotional traits robustly predict future criminal offending in young men. *Law Hum. Behav.* **2013**, *37*, 87–97. [CrossRef] [PubMed]

10. Muratori, P.; Paciello, M.; Buonanno, C.; Milone, A.; Ruglioni, L.; Lochman, J.E.; Masi, G. Moral disengagement and callous–unemotional traits: A longitudinal study of Italian adolescents with a disruptive behaviour disorder. *Crim. Behav. Ment. Health* **2017**, *27*, 514–524. [CrossRef]
11. Salekin, R.T.; Hare, R.D. The Proposed Specifiers for Conduct Disorder (PSCD) Scale. Unpublished work. 2016.
12. Salekin, R.T. Research review: What do we know about psychopathic traits in children? *J. Child Psychol. Psychiatry Allied Discip.* **2017**, *58*, 1180–1200. [CrossRef] [PubMed]
13. Forth, A.E.; Kosson, D.S.; Hare, R.D. The hare psychopathy checklist: Youth version. *Psychol. Assess.* **2006**, *18*, 142–154. [CrossRef]
14. Dillard, C.L.; Salekin, R.T.; Barker, E.D.; Grimes, R.D. Psychopathy in adolescent offenders: An item response theory study of the antisocial process screening device-self report and the psychopathy checklist: Youth version. *Personal. Disord. Theory Res. Treat.* **2013**, *4*, 101–120. [CrossRef]
15. Kosson, D.S.; Cyterski, T.D.; Steuerwald, B.L.; Neumann, C.S.; Walker-Matthews, S. The reliability and validity of the psychopathy checklist: Youth version (PCL: YV) in nonincarcerated adolescent males. *Psychol. Assess.* **2002**, *14*, 97–109. [CrossRef]
16. Frick, P.; Hare, R. *Antisocial Process Screening Device: APSD*; Multi-Health Systems: Toronto, ON, Canada, 2001.
17. Falkenbach, D.M.; Poythress, N.G.; Heide, K.M. Psychopathic features in a juvenile diversion population: Reliability and predictive validity of two self-report measures. *Behav. Sci. Law* **2003**, *21*, 787–805. [CrossRef]
18. Frick, P.J.; O'Brien, B.S.; Wootton, J.M.; McBurnett, K. Psychopathy and conduct problems in children. *J. Abnorm. Psychol.* **1994**, *103*, 700–707. [CrossRef] [PubMed]
19. Frick, P.J.; Bodin, S.D.; Barry, C.T. Psychopathic traits and conduct problems in community and clinic-referred samples of children: Further development of the psychopathy screening device. *Psychol. Assess.* **2000**, *12*, 382–393. [CrossRef]
20. Andershed, H.; Kerr, M.; Stattin, H.; Levander, S. *Psychopathic Traits in Non-Referred Youths: A New Assessment Tool*; Elsevier: Den Haag, The Netherlands, 2002; pp. 131–158.
21. Lynam, D.R. Pursuing the psychopath: Capturing the fledgling psychopath in a nomological net. *J. Abnorm. Psychol.* **1997**, *106*, 425–438. [CrossRef]
22. van Baardewijk, Y.; Stegge, H.; Andershed, H.; Thomaes, S.; Scholte, E.; Vermeiren, R. Measuring psychopathic traits in children through self-report. The development of the youth psychopathic traits inventory-child version. *Int. J. Law Psychiatry* **2008**, *31*, 199–209. [CrossRef] [PubMed]
23. Poythress, N.G.; Dembo, R.; Wareham, J.; Greenbaum, P.E. Construct validity of the youth psychopathic traits inventory (YPI) and the antisocial process screening device (APSD) with justice-involved adolescents. *SAGE J.* **2006**, *33*, 26–55. [CrossRef]
24. Colins, O.F.; Andershed, H.; Frogner, L.; Lopez-Romero, L.; Veen, V.; Andershed, A.K. A new measure to assess psychopathic personality in children: The child problematic traits inventory. *J. Psychopathol. Behav. Assess.* **2014**, *36*, 4–21. [CrossRef]
25. López-Romero, L.; Romero, E.; Colins, O.F.; Andershed, H.; Hare, R.D.; Salekin, R.T. Proposed specifiers for conduct disorder (PSCD): Preliminary validation of the parent version in a spanish sample of preschoolers. *Psychol. Assess.* **2019**, *31*. [CrossRef]
26. Luo, J.; Wang, M.C.; Neumann, C.S.; Hare, R.D.; Salekin, R.T. Factor structure and construct validity of the proposed specifiers for conduct disorder (PSCD) scale in chinese adolescents. *Assessment* **2020**, *28*, 1765–1784. [CrossRef]
27. Frick, P.J. Inventory of Callous-Unemotional Traits, University of New Orleans. Unpublished rating scale. 2004.
28. White, S.F.; Cruise, K.R.; Frick, P.J. Differential correlates to self-report and parent-report of callous-unemotional traits in a sample of juvenile sexual offenders. *Behav. Sci. Law* **2009**, *27*, 910–928. [CrossRef]
29. Padilla-Walker, L.M.; Carlo, G.; Nielson, M.G. Does Helping Keep Teens Protected? Longitudinal Bidirectional Relations between Prosocial Behavior and Problem Behavior. *Child Dev.* **2015**, *86*, 1759–1772. [CrossRef] [PubMed]
30. Flynn, E.; Ehrenreich, S.E.; Beron, K.J.; Underwood, M.K. Prosocial Behavior: Long-term Trajectories and Psychosocial Outcomes. *Soc. Dev.* **2015**, *24*, 462–482. [CrossRef]
31. Tobia, V.; Marzocchi, G. Norme italiane dello strengths and difficulties questionnaire (SDQ): Il comportamento dei bambini italiani valutato dai loro insegnanti. *Disturbi Attenzione Iperattività* **2011**, *6*, 15–22.
32. Hu, L.T.; Bentler, P.M. Cutoff criteria for fit indexes in covariance structure analysis: Conventional criteria versus new alternatives. *Struct. Equ. Model.* **1999**, *6*, 1–55. [CrossRef]
33. Clark, L.A.; Watson, D. Constructing validity: Basic issues in objective scale development. *Psychol. Assess.* **1995**, *7*, 309–319. [CrossRef]
34. Zinbarg, R.E.; Revelle, W.; Yovel, I.; Li, W. Cronbach's, α Revelle's β and McDonald's ω H: Their relations with each other and two alternative conceptualizations of reliability. *Psychometrika* **2005**, *70*, 123–133. [CrossRef]
35. Reise, S.P.; Bonifay, W.E.; Haviland, M.G. Modeling psychological measures in the presence of multidimensionality. *J. Pers. Assess.* **2012**, *95*, 129–140. [CrossRef] [PubMed]
36. Eid, M.; Krumm, S.; Koch, T.; Schulze, J. Bifactor models for predicting criteria by general and specific factors: Problems of nonidentifiability and alternative solutions. *J. Intell.* **2018**, *6*, 42. [CrossRef] [PubMed]
37. Bornovalova, M.A.; Choate, A.M.; Fatimah, H.; Petersen, K.J.; Wiernik, B.M. Appropriate use of bifactor analysis in psychopathology research: Appreciating benefits and limitations. *Biol. Psychiatry* **2020**, *88*, 18–27. [CrossRef] [PubMed]
38. Andershed, H.; Hodgins, S.; Tengström, A. Convergent validity of the youth psychopathic traits inventory (YPI) association with the psychopathy checklist: Youth version (PCL:YV). *Assessment* **2007**, *14*, 144–154. [CrossRef]
39. Dadds, M.R.; Fraser, J.; Frost, A.; Hawes, D.J. Disentangling the underlying dimensions of psychopathy and conduct problems in childhood: A community study. *J. Consult. Clin. Psychol.* **2005**, *73*, 400. [CrossRef]

40. Baker, L.A.; Raine, A.; Liu, J.; Jacobson, K.C. Differential genetic and environmental influences on reactive and proactive aggression in children. *J. Abnorm. Child Psychol.* **2008**, *36*, 1265–1278. [CrossRef]
41. Brouns, B.H.J.; De Wied, M.A.; Keijsers, L.; Branje, S.; Van Goozen, S.H.M.; Meeus, W.H.J. Concurrent and prospective effects of psychopathic traits on affective and cognitive empathy in a community sample of late adolescents. *J. Child Psychol. Psychiatry Allied Discip.* **2013**, *54*, 969–976. [CrossRef] [PubMed]
42. Jones, A.P.; Happé, F.G.E.; Gilbert, F.; Burnett, S.; Viding, E. Feeling, caring, knowing: Different types of empathy deficit in boys with psychopathic tendencies and autism spectrum disorder. *J. Child Psychol. Psychiatry* **2010**, *51*, 1188–1197. [CrossRef] [PubMed]
43. Eisenberg, N.; Eggum, N.D.; Di Giunta, L. Empathy-related responding: Associations with prosocial behavior, aggression, and intergroup relations. *Soc. Issues Policy Rev.* **2010**, *4*, 143–180. [CrossRef]
44. Muñoz, L.C.; Frick, P.J.; Kimonis, E.R.; Aucoin, K.J. Types of aggression, responsiveness to provocation, and callous-unemotional traits in detained adolescents. *J. Abnorm. Child Psychol.* **2008**, *36*, 15–28. [CrossRef]
45. Haas, S.M.; Becker, S.P.; Epstein, J.N.; Frick, P.J. Callous-unemotional traits are uniquely associated with poorer peer functioning in school-aged children. *J. Abnorm. Child Psychol.* **2018**, *46*, 781–793. [CrossRef]
46. Salekin, R.T.; Neumann, C.S.; Leistico, A.R.; Zalot, A. A psychopathy in youth and intelligence: An investigation of Cleckley's hypothesis. *J. Clin. Child Adolesc. Psychol.* **2004**, *33*, 731–742. [CrossRef]
47. Milone, A.; Cerniglia, L.; Cristofani, C.; Inguaggiato, E.; Levantini, V.; Masi, G.; Paciello, M.; Simone, F.; Muratori, P. Empathy in youths with conduct disorder and callous-unemotional traits. *Neural Plast.* **2019**, *2019*, 9638973. [CrossRef] [PubMed]
48. Blader, J.C.; Pliszka, S.R.; Kafantaris, V.; Foley, C.A.; Crowell, J.A.; Carlson, G.A.; Sauder, C.L.; Margulies, D.M.; Sinha, C.; Sverd, J.; et al. Callous-unemotional traits, proactive aggression, and treatment outcomes of aggressive children with attention-deficit/hyperactivity disorder. *J. Am. Acad. Child Adolesc. Psychiatry* **2013**, *52*, 1281–1293. [CrossRef] [PubMed]
49. Andershed, H. Stability and change of psychopathic traits: What do we know? In *Handbook of Child Adolescent Psychopathy*; The Guilford Press: New York, NY, USA, 2010; pp. 233–250. ISBN 978-1-60623-682-6.
50. Masi, G.; Milone, A.; Brovedani, P.; Pisano, S.; Muratori, P. Psychiatric evaluation of youths with disruptive behavior disorders and psychopathic traits: A critical review of assessment measures. *Neurosci. Biobehav. Rev.* **2018**, *91*, 21–33. [CrossRef] [PubMed]
51. Paulhus, D.L.; Vazire, S. The self-report method. *Handb. Res. Methods Personal. Psychol.* **2007**, *1*, 224–239.

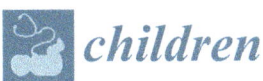

Article

Evaluation of an Early Intervention Model for Child and Adolescent Victims of Interpersonal Violence

Claudia Calvano [1,2,*], Elena Murray [1], Lea Bentz [1], Sascha Bos [1], Kathrin Reiter [1], Loretta Ihme [3] and Sibylle M. Winter [1]

[1] Department of Child and Adolescent Psychiatry, Charité—Universitätsmedizin Berlin, Corporate Member of Freie Universität Berlin, Humboldt-Universität zu Berlin and Berlin Institute of Health, Augustenburger Platz 1, 13353 Berlin, Germany; elena.murray@charite.de (E.M.); lea.bentz@charite.de (L.B.); sascha.bos@charite.de (S.B.); kathrin.reiter@charite.de (K.R.); sibylle.winter@charite.de (S.M.W.)
[2] Clinical Child and Adolescent Psychology and Psychotherapy, Freie Universität Berlin, Habelschwerdter Allee 45, 14195 Berlin, Germany
[3] Center for Chronically Sick Children, Charité—Universitätsmedizin Berlin, Corporate Member of Freie Universität Berlin, Humboldt-Universität zu Berlin and Berlin Institute of Health, Augustenburger Platz 1, 13353 Berlin, Germany; loretta.ihme@charite.de
* Correspondence: claudia.calvano@fu-berlin.de; Tel.: +49-30-838-58570

Abstract: Only the minority of youth exposed to traumatic events receive mental health care, as trauma-informed clinical services are lacking or are poorly accessible. In order to bridge this gap, the Outpatient Trauma Clinic (OTC) was founded, an easily accessible early, short-time intervention, with onward referral to follow-up treatment. This report presents the OTC's interventional approach and first outcome data. Using a retrospective naturalistic design, we analyzed trauma- and intervention-related data of the sample (n = 377, 55.4% female, mean age 10.95, SD = 4.69). Following drop-out analyses, predictors for treatment outcome were identified by logistic regression. The majority (81.9%) was suffering from posttraumatic stress disorder (PTSD) or adjustment disorders. Around one forth dropped out of treatment; these cases showed higher avoidance symptoms at presentation. In 91%, psychological symptoms improved. Experience of multiple traumatic events was the strongest predictor for poor treatment outcome (B = −0.823, SE = 0.313, OR = 0.439, 95% CI 0.238–0.811). Around two thirds were connected to follow-up treatment. The OTC realized a high retention rate, initial improvement of symptoms and referral to subsequent longer-term psychotherapeutic treatment in the majority. Further dissemination of comparable early intervention models is needed, in order to improve mental health care for this vulnerable group.

Keywords: children and adolescents; clinical practice; early intervention; interpersonal violence; sexual abuse

1. Introduction

According to epidemiological studies, around 30% of children and adolescents experience at least one form of interpersonal trauma [1,2]. In a substantial number of cases, this is associated with an increased risk for disturbances in mental and physical development [3–5]. Post-traumatic stress-disorder, affective and anxiety disorders as well as behavioral problems are among the most frequent trauma-related mental disorders in children and adolescents [1,6]. Besides a child's female gender [7–9] and a young age at the first traumatic event [10], victims of sexual abuse [4,11] and victims of multiple trauma [12] are particularly at risk for poor prognosis.

In light of the high prevalence, poor prognoses and the substantial costs for the health system [13], effective treatment is urgently needed. Comprehensive meta-analyses show that trauma-focused psychological interventions are effective for the reduction of PTSD, depression and anxiety in children and adolescents, across age groups and trauma types, in controlled and uncontrolled trials [14], with promising results for long-term effects [15].

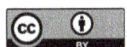

In light of this evidence, translation of trauma-informed intervention into clinical practice is warranted. In order to attain this goal and to improve the health care situation of trauma victims, different approaches and structures of trauma care have been established across Europe in recent years, with variations due to cultural backgrounds and (health-)economic situations [16,17]. However, the countries face similar challenges in the translation of evidence-based intervention into practice and in the promotion and dissemination of trauma-informed treatment models. In Germany, counseling services, crisis intervention and outpatient clinics for victims of interpersonal violence, often affiliated with psychiatric hospitals, have been emerging [16].

Despite these efforts, there is still a discrepancy between the need, the accessibility and the availability of trauma-informed clinical services [16]. For children and adolescents, there is an especially pronounced gap in health care provision and only the minority of children and adolescents exposed to traumatic events receive adequate treatment [18–21]. Data published in 2017 illustrate the situation of trauma care for children and adolescents in Germany: Münzer et al. analyzed the health care utilization of 241 children aged 4–17 years with a history of maltreatment in Germany and point out that 65% of the sample did not receive any psychotherapeutic intervention—and among the cases who did, only a few received trauma-focused psychotherapy [19]. Barriers for seeking and accessing mental health care for affected children and adolescents are by large part structural, e.g., lack of coordination and integration of services, service costs and long waiting times [22]. In a qualitative study [18], internet posts by young people in online trauma forums were analyzed. Their data suggest that structural barriers are not only at work when seeking care, but also at the end of treatment, when guidance for the patients through the pathways within the health care system seems warranted [18].

The Berlin Outpatient Trauma Clinic (OTC) for children and adolescents aims to bridge the void in both the availability of early trauma-informed care and in the connection to longer-term psychological intervention, if needed. In line with the approaches outlined in [16], the Berlin Outpatient Trauma Clinic is affiliated with the Department for Child and Adolescent Psychiatry, Charité—Universitätsmedizin Berlin, Germany. It was founded in 2012 in order to establish an easily accessible, early and specialized outpatient treatment setting for child and adolescent victims of interpersonal violence. Within a short-term early intervention setting, the OTC offers clinical assessment, stabilization and first psychotherapeutic support, as well as an onward referral to longer-term follow-up treatment. The OTC is the first treatment center the affected families consult after the traumatic event. Besides self-referrals by the families, a variety of institutions like the pediatric clinic, social services or the police refer the families to the clinic. The treatment in the OTC is independent of health insurance status as it is funded by the Crime Victims' Compensation Act, which defines the entitlement for compensation for victims of a violent crime [23]. So far, the OTC represents the only trauma-specific early intervention clinic for both children and adolescents in Berlin, financed by the Berlin Senate.

While the need for further implementation of trauma care for children and adolescents is consistently underlined in the literature [18–21], and approaches have been emerging [16], up to now, little is known about the unselected, treatment-seeking samples of children and adolescents [22,24]. However, knowledge on trauma characteristics, mental health, the need for treatment and the families' further pathways through the healthcare system among a naturalistic sample [16,17] will provide valuable contributions to the development and implementation of treatment approaches for this vulnerable group. While for adult populations, few studies with unselected clinical samples are available [25,26], for children and adolescents, comparable data are scarce.

This clinical report intents to fill the gaps in the existing literature by presenting the approach and the data from the health care seeking sample of the OTC in Berlin, Germany, affiliated with the Department of Child Psychiatry and Psychotherapy. The first aim of this clinical report is to systematically describe the sample of the OTC with respect to sociodemographic variables, trauma-related and intervention-related variables. The second aim is to explore the range of trauma-related mental disorders across all age groups. The third aim is to conduct systematic dropout analyses followed by a presentation of treatment outcome and an analysis of its predictors. In line with the literature, we hypothesized that female gender, younger age, a longer time span untreated, the experience of sexual abuse and the experience of multiple traumatic events were associated with poor outcome.

2. Materials and Methods

2.1. Procedure in the OTC

The formal requirements for treatment in the OTC are child age <18 years, Berlin residency and the experience of interpersonal violence. All cases are assessed and treated by child and adolescent psychotherapists specialized in trauma-focused psychotherapy. With a contingent of up to 18 sessions, the OTC conducts a comprehensive psychological assessment, provides psychosocial support (e.g., a clearance of the situation, and the support of the family with formal steps), and first psychological interventions (e.g., stabilization, psychoeducation, provision of coping skills, parental counseling and, depending on the progress and stability, trauma exposure resp. trauma narratives). The intervention in the OTC follows an adaptive, tailored approach, mirroring the concept of trauma-informed care [22]. At the end of the treatment, individual recommendations for further interventions are stated and longer-term follow-up-intervention for the patients is initiated, if needed.

For this paper, data of all the cases who have consulted the clinic since its foundation are presented (April 2012–March 2020). Data are derived from the internal documentation and from the final letter, which is required for funding. The letter needs to include the anamnesis, results of the psychological assessment together with an evaluation whether or not the psychological symptoms are causally related to the experience of the traumatic event(s), descriptions of the interventions, of treatment outcome and, if applicable, a description of specific recommendations for further treatment.

The concomitant research of the OTC has been approved by the Ethics Committee of the Charité—Universitätsmedizin Berlin (number EA2/145/18, date of approval 30 July 2018).

2.2. Measures

2.2.1. Sociodemographic and Trauma-Related Data

With the use of a structured questionnaire, sociodemographic data and descriptive data on the traumatic event (type of trauma, single vs. multiple events, offender, time span until first visit in the clinic) were collected. The types of traumatic events represented in the clinic are predefined by the Crime Victim Compensation Act and are categorized into sexual abuse, physical violence, witnessing violence, being victim of an attack, and other interpersonal trauma like psychological distress due to indirect involvement in violence, e.g., the information of a sudden death of a close person.

2.2.2. Mental Disorders According to ICD-10, Axis 1

For each case, at the beginning of treatment, comprehensive clinical interviews are carried out in order to evaluate (1) the absence or presence of a mental disorder according to the ICD-10 classification system and (2) whether or not the symptoms were related to the traumatic event.

2.2.3. Intervention-Related Data

We analyzed the number of sessions, the time range of the intervention and the recommendations concerning follow-up treatment on a descriptive level. For each case, the clinicians evaluated whether or not further follow-up intervention was required and if so, whether it should focus on the trauma, on other psychological or psychosocial problems or on a combination of both.

2.2.4. Improvement of Psychological Symptoms

The measure for the improvement of psychological symptoms used in the OTC is derived from the standardized, therapist-reported documentation system for all patients in inpatient and outpatient treatment in the Department of Child and Adolescent Psychiatry. Thus, at the end of treatment in the OTC, the overall change of psychological symptoms was assessed in therapist report by the item "improvement of psychological symptoms", rated on a standardized 5-point scale (fully improved, strongly improved, improved a little, no change, worsened). In logistic regression analyses, good outcome was defined as 1 = fully improved or clearly improved.

2.3. Data Analysis

Data were analyzed with SPSS, Version 25. Descriptive data analyses were used for the presentation of sample characteristics as well as trauma-related- and intervention-related characteristics. As the samples cover a broad age group, sensitivity analyses for age were conducted. For the drop out analyses, three groups (completers vs. referrals vs. decliners) were defined and compared on sociodemographic-, trauma- and intervention-related variables. In case of statistical trends ($p < 0.10$) on an overall level, post-hoc-analyses were conducted. Predictors for treatment outcome were first analyzed by univariate logistic regression, providing information on the importance of each predictor by itself. Following an explorative approach, we systematically tested sociodemographic predictors (child age, gender), trauma type (sexual abuse yes/no), other trauma-related characteristics (offender, multiple events yes/no), intervention-related data (number of sessions, time span until first visit) and baseline symptoms of posttraumatic stress (intrusions and avoidance scores derived from the CRIES-8 [27] as predictors. The significant predictors on univariate level were entered in a multivariate regression to gain a more comprehensive picture. For the regression analyses, only data of the completers were used.

3. Results

3.1. Participants

In total, 377 patients were treated in the OTC till 3/2020, with a mean age of M = 10.95 years (SD = 4.69, range 0.58–18.50 years). 80.3% of the sample was above the age of 6 years (0–5 years n = 74, 19.6%; 6–13 years n = 169, 44.8%; 14–18 years n = 134, 35.5%). 55.4% of the patients were girls. Table 1 summarizes trauma-related descriptive data of the sample. There were no statistically significant differences between the age groups in the trauma-related variables.

In the total sample, the majority presented with one (n = 230, 61.0%) or two different trauma types (n = 113, 30.0%). The rate of co-occurrence varied across the trauma types (see Figure 1). With the exception of sexual abuse, the co-occurrence of two different trauma types were the most frequent pattern.

3.2. Mental Disorders According to ICD-10

Structured anamnesis and psychiatric assessment provided an Axis 1-diagnosis according to ICD-10 in 310 cases (82.2%). The clear majority of diagnoses were trauma-related, i.e., the symptoms occurred after the traumatic event(s) (n = 288; 92.9%). In 22 cases (7.1%) only, the diagnosis was present already before the trauma. The onset of a broad range of mental disorders was observed. Adjustment disorders and PTSD were the primary trauma-related mental disorder in the majority of cases, across all age groups (81.9% of the total sample). In the age group 14–18 years, depressive disorders were the third most frequent primary trauma-related disorder; while in the age group 6–13 years, externalizing disorders were the third most frequent disorder and in the age group 0–5 years, emotional disorders, respectively. On average, comorbidity was relatively low, with 1.37 diagnoses per patient (SD = 0.70, Median = 1, Modus = 1; range 1–4). Table 2 summarizes the diagnoses on Axis 1 according to ICD-10.

Table 1. Descriptive data in relation to the traumatic event.

	Total Sample n = 377		Age Groups					
			0–5 Years n = 74		6–13 Years n = 169		14–18 Years n = 134	
	n	(%)	n	(%)	n	(%)	n	(%)
Type of traumatic event [†]								
Sexual abuse	133	35.50%	15	23.40%	56	33.10%	62	46.30%
Physical violence	126	33.60%	31	48.40%	45	26.60%	50	37.30%
Witness of violence	139	37.10%	43	67.20%	71	42.00%	25	18.70%
Interpersonal attack	71	18.90%	5	7.80%	21	12.40%	45	33.60%
Other [‡]	87	23.30%	18	28.10%	41	24.30%	28	20.90%
Frequency of trauma [§]								
Single event	232	61.50%	27	42.20%	97	57.40%	108	80.60%
Multiple events	142	37.70%	45	70.30%	71	42.00%	26	19.40%
Offender								
Close environment	179	47.50%	60	93.80%	88	52.10%	31	23.10%
Broad environment	59	15.60%	4	6.30%	26	15.40%	29	21.60%
Unknown person	130	34.50%	7	10.90%	52	30.80%	71	53.00%
Unidentified	9	2.40%	3	4.70%	3	1.80%	3	2.20%
Time span between trauma and first visit [¶]								
M (SD)	16.22 (23.79)		14.40(18.5)		14.03(17.7)		19.14(29.97)	
Median	6		7.14		6		5.5	
Modus	1.43		1.57		0.57		1.29	
range	0.14–178.9		1–71.43		0.29–72.14		0.14–178.86	

Notes. [†] multiple answers possible; [‡] e.g., psychological distress due to indirect involvement in violence, e.g., the information of a sudden death of a close person; [§] in 3 cases data were missing; [¶] time span between trauma and first visit in weeks.

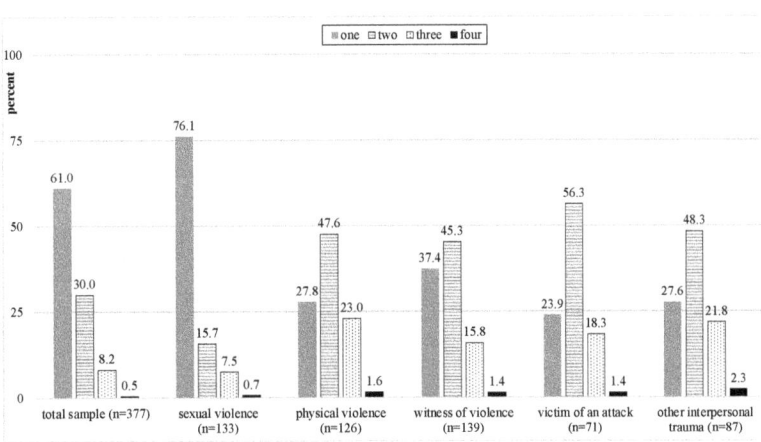

Figure 1. Co-occurrence between trauma types. The bars refer to the numbers of other trauma types present for each primary trauma type.

3.3. Drop out Analyses

In total, 242 cases (64.2%) completed the treatment in the OTC ("completers"). 26 cases (6.9%) were referred to inpatient treatment due to the high severity of psychological symptoms ("referrals"). While in 13 cases (3.4%) organizational reasons (e.g., no Berlin residency) prohibited further treatment, 92 cases (24.4%) did not continue their sessions and were lost in follow-up ("decliners"). There was a trend that the time span between trauma and first visit differed between groups (F(2, 257) = 2.972, p = 0.053), with the highest time span until the first visit at the OTC for the referrals to inpatient treatment (M = 24.85, SD = 28.24) and the shortest for the completers (M = 13.67, SD = 18.56). There were significant differences between the three groups on the level of avoidance ($F(2, 128) = 4.42$, $p = 0.014$) and the total PTSD score at baseline ($F(2, 140) = 3.909$, $p = 0.022$) as measured with the CRIES-8 [27]. Post-Hoc tests showed significant higher avoidance scores in the decliners (M = 3.93, 0.88) than in the completers (M = 3.12, SD = 1.18; see Table 3). Concerning the duration of the intervention till drop out, decliners (M=2.72 months, SD = 4.13) and referrals to inpatient treatment (M = 3.85 months, SD = 4.76) showed a comparable time in intervention, but significantly shorter than the completers (M = 7.51 months, SD = 5.85, $p = 0.003$ and $p < 0.001$, respectively). The three groups did not differ with respect to gender ($\chi^2(2) = 2.160$, $p = 0.340$), age ($F(2, 357) = 0.280$, $p = 0.756$) nor trauma type (sexual violence ($\chi^2(2) = 5.239$, $p = 0.073$; physical violence ($\chi^2(2) = 1.024$, $p = 0.599$; witness of violence ($\chi^2(2) = 1.183$, $p = 0.554$; victim of an attack ($\chi^2(2) = 1.211$, $p = 0.546$). Table 3 summarizes the results of post-hoc tests for those variables with significant overall effects.

Table 2. Mental disorders in relation to the traumatic event on axis-1 according to ICD-10, summarized in categories of disorders, for the total sample and the age groups.

	Total Sample n=278		Age 0–5 Years n = 49		Age 6–13 Years n = 121		Age 14–18 Years n = 108	
	n	(%)	n	(%)	n	(%)	n	(%)
Stress-related disorders								
PTSD (F43.1)	115	(41.7%)	12	(24.5%)	49	(40.5%)	54	(50.0%)
Adjustment disorder (F43.2x)	111	(40.2%)	17	(34.7%)	57	(47.1%)	37	(34.3%)
Acute reaction disorder (F43.0)	7	(2.5%)	1	(2.0%)	0	(0.0%)	6	(5.6%)
Internalizing disorders								
Depressive disorders (F32.x, F33.x, F34.x)	28	(10.1%)	0	(0.0%)	11	(9.1%)	17	(15.7%)
Anxiety disorder (F40.x, F41.x)	4	(1.4%)	0	(0.0%)	1	(0.8%)	3	(2.8%)
Emotional disorders (F93.x)	19	(6.9%)	12	(24.5%)	6	(5.0%)	1	(0.9%)
Externalizing disorders								
ADHD (F90.x)	15	(5.4%)	4	(8.2%)	11	(9.1%)	0	(0,0%)
Conduct disorder (F91.x)	19	(6.9%)	4	(8.2%)	11	(9.1%)	4	(3.7%)
Other disorders								
Psychoactive substance use (F1x.x)	9	(3.3%)	0	(0.0%)	3	(2.5%)	6	(5.6%)
Obsessive compulsive disorder (F42.x)	3	(1.1%)	0	(0.0%)	1	(0.8%)	2	(1.9%)
Dissociation disorder (F44.x)	3	(1.1%)	0	(0.0%)	1	(0.8%)	2	(1.9%)
Somatoform disorder (F45.x)	5	(1.8%)	0	(0.0%)	1	(0.8%)	4	(3.7%)
Eating disorder (F50.x, F51.x)	4	(1.4%)	0	(0.0%)	0	(0.0%)	4	(3.7%)
Personality disorder (F60.x)	10	(3.6%)	0	(0.0%)	1	(0.8%)	9	(8.3%)
Attachment disorder (F94.1, F94.2)	7	(2.5%)	3	(6.1%)	4	(3.3%)	0	(0.0%)
Other disorder of social functions (F95)	2	(0.7%)	0	(0.0%)	2	(1.7%)	0	(0.0%)
Enuresis/Encopresis (F98.0, F98.1)	11	(4.0%)	2	(4.1%)	9	(7.4%)	0	(0.0%)
Other behavioral or emotional disorder (F98.8)	6	(2.2%)	4	(8.2%)	1	(0.8%)	1	(0.9%)

Notes. n in the table refers to the number of cases with the specific diagnosis, %-score refers to the percentage within the total sample resp. within the age group for each category of diagnoses. The highest proportion of a specific disorder across the three age groups is marked in bold. Table includes comorbidities.

3.4. Intervention-Related Data

3.4.1. Number of Sessions

Analyses on the completers revealed that on average, 10.18 (SD = 6.04) sessions were conducted (Median = 9, Modus = 18, range 1–18). While there were no age or gender effects, victims of sexual abuse received a significantly higher number of sessions than the other trauma types (M = 11.72, SD = 6.45 versus M = 9.05, SD = 5.55, $p = 0.001$). The average time span of intervention was 23.93 weeks (SD = 23.02, range 0–126 weeks, Median = 17 weeks). There were no differences for gender, age or trauma type for the time span of intervention.

Table 3. Results of posthoc-tests for variables with a significant overall effect in the drop-out analyses.

Variable	Subgroup †	n	M	SD	Post Hoc 1 vs. 2			Post Hoc 1 vs. 3			Post Hoc 2 vs. 3		
					MD	SE	95% CI	MD	SE	95% CI	MD	SE	95% CI
Time till first visit in weeks	1 Completers	187	13.67	18.56	11.18	5.78	−25.10–2.74	−5.93	3.37	−14.05–2.19	5.24	6.23	−9.78–20.27
	2 Referrals	18	24.85	28.24									
	3 Decliners	65	19.60	32.78									
Number of sessions	1 Completers	242	10.15	6.04	**4.65 ***	**1.12**	**1.96–7.34**	**5.75 ***	**0.67**	**4.15–7.36**	1.10	1.21	−1.80–4.00
	2 Referrals	26	5.50	3.46									
	3 Decliners	91	4.40	3.93									
Time in treatment (months)	1 Completers	243	7.51	5.85	**3.67 **	**1.11**	**0.99–6.34**	**4.79 ***	**0.66**	**3.21–6.38**	1.12	1.20	−1.75–4.01
	2 Referrals	26	3.84	4.76									
	3 Decliners	92	2.72	4.13									
Avoidance symptoms ‡	1 Completers	96	12.50	5.57	−2.68	1.66	−6.70–1.34	**−3.21 ***	**1.19**	**−6.09—−0.33**	−0.53	1.89	−5.12–4.07
	2 Referrals	11	15.18	4.22									
	3 Decliners	24	15.71	3.85									
PTSD total score ‡	1 Completers	109	23.16	9.98	−6.48	2.97	−13.67–0.71	−4.32	2.15	−9.53–0.89	2.15	3.44	−6.17–10.49
	2 Referrals	11	29.64	5.78									
	3 Decliners	23	27.48	7.49									

Notes. † Referrals include the cases with high severity, referred to inpatient treatment; decliner include the cases who dropped out of treatment; ‡ as measured with CRIES-8 at baseline [27]; MD = mean difference, SE = standard error, CI = confidence interval for MD. Significant differences in bold. * $p < 0.05$, ** $p < 0.01$, *** $p < 0.001$.

3.4.2. Recommendation for Further Treatment

Regarding the 239 completers, in about two thirds ($n = 153$, 64.0%), follow-up treatment was recommended. Outpatient psychotherapy ($n = 113$, 73.9%) was the most frequent recommendation at the end of the intervention, followed by recommendations for outpatient child psychiatry in 35 cases (22.9%), inpatient psychiatric treatment in one case (0.6%) and social measures for child protection in four cases (2.6%). For the clear majority ($n = 142$, 95.3%), further trauma-related psychotherapeutic intervention was recommended. Age groups did not differ in terms of recommendations (results not shown). The majority (69.4%) of the victims of sexual abuse needed further treatment, which was in contrast to victims of an attack (35.4% were recommended further treatment). For the other trauma types, about half of the cases were in need for further intervention (51.7–55.4%).

3.5. Analyses of Treatment Outcome

For the cases completing the intervention ($n = 235$), about half of the cases showed good outcome ($n = 121$, 51.5%), defined as full improvement ($n = 28$), or strong improvement ($n = 93$) of psychological symptoms. The other large part improved a little ($n = 94$; 40.0%). For 19 cases, no change was observed (8.1%) and in one case, worsening of psychological symptoms was stated (0.4%). There were no age or gender effects in the rating (results not shown).

Table 4 summarizes the significant predictors derived from the univariate regression analyses on good treatment outcome (coded with 1 = strong or full improvement of psychological symptoms). Female gender, victims of multiple traumatic events and victims of sexual violence as well as the cases with a higher number of intervention sessions were at risk for poor treatment outcome. The other sociodemographic, trauma-or intervention-related predictors were not significantly related with the outcome (results not shown).

Table 4. Summary of significant predictions in univariate logistic regression on good treatment outcome, defined as "improvement of psychological symptoms" at the end of the intervention (coded with 1, $n = 121$).

	Improvement of Psychological Symptoms				
	B	SE	p	OR	95% CI OR
Sociodemographic predictors					
Female gender	−0.544	0.266	0.041	0.581	0.345–0.978
Trauma-related predictors					
Multiple traumatic events	−0.976	0.282	0.001	0.377	0.217–0.655
Sexual abuse	−0.852	0.287	0.003	0.427	0.243–0.750
Intervention-related predictors					
Number of sessions	−0.069	0.023	0.002	0.934	0.893–0.976

Notes. The categorial predictors female gender, multiple traumatic events and sexual abuse all included with 1 = yes in the regression analyses.

Additionally. in multivariate regression, the presence of multiple traumatic events at presentation (B = −0.823, SE = 0.313, $p = 0.009$, OR = 0.439, 95% CI 0.238–0.811) and, with a weaker effect, a higher number of sessions (B = −0.070, SE = 0.025, $p = 0.006$, OR = 0.933, 95% CI 0.887–0.980) were inversely related with good treatment outcome.

4. Discussion

This report presented the interventional approach and clinical data from the OTC for child and adolescent victims of interpersonal violence. In this paper, we aimed to (1) provide a comprehensive account of trauma-specific characteristics of the treatment-seeking sample, (2) assess the onset and rates of trauma-related mental disorders, (3) describe intervention-related data and (4) evaluate in how far improvements in psychological symptoms can be achieved within the scope of the first-care, short-term naturalistic intervention. Furthermore, factors related to drop out were explored.

Summing up the descriptive analyses, the trauma types were equally distributed across the age groups, an average co-occurrence of one to two trauma types was observed and over one third of the sample experienced multiple events within one trauma type. A high proportion was acutely presenting at the clinic within the first two weeks after trauma. In the majority of cases, the offenders were known from the personal environment, which implies that within this first-care setting, additional measures for safety and child protection were regularly warranted.

The second aim was to give an account on the mental health in the clinical sample. In total, 82.2% were diagnosed with a mental disorder, and of these, in 92.9%, the onset was related to the experience of the trauma. Adjustment disorders and PTSD were the most prevalent diagnoses, in line with epidemiological data [1,6,28]. While adjustment disorders were more frequently diagnosed up to the age of 13 years, the majority of adolescents suffered from PTSD. School-aged children additionally showed externalizing symptoms and onset of enuresis or encopresis while the preschoolers showed a higher rate of childhood emotional disorders like separation anxiety. The broad range of clinical diagnoses and especially the higher variety of comorbid diagnoses like substance abuse and personality disorders in the adolescent subgroup mirror the relevance of transdiagnostic approaches in trauma-focused care [29] and the need for a broad psychiatric assessment. The complexity of the acutely presenting cases also underline the need for an adapted clinical approach with an increased share of psychosocial and psychological stabilization [30].

The third aim was to explore intervention-related data and treatment outcome. The average treatment duration, independent of age, gender or trauma type, covered approximately four to six months and on average, ten sessions were provided. The regression analyses aimed to get a better picture of the characteristics related to treatment outcome. Results replicated findings in the literature, as in our sample, girls [7–9] and victims of sexual abuse [4,11] were at risk for poor treatment outcome. Beyond all other predictors, children and adolescents with a history of multiple traumatic events, independent of the type of trauma, were at highest risk for poor improvement of psychological symptoms, which adds to previous findings as well [12,31]. Noteworthy, in this report, the outcomes only refer to therapists' rating at the end of the intervention. While this measure is an established part of the internal documentation and quality assurance in the university clinic, the one-item measure only captures improvement on an overall level, limiting generalizability for further, more specific psychological symptoms. Further, only therapist ratings are collected and patient-reported data are currently not available. Therefore, for further proceedings of the OTC's and other clinical services' concomitant research, the use of validated and more differentiated measures for treatment outcome, both in therapist and in patient-report need to be implemented. This will increase validity and generalizability, and will facilitate future replication of our findings.

Dropout analyses indicated that the majority of cases regularly finished their treatment in the OTC. At 24%, the rate of decliners in our naturalistic setting was comparable to that of completers in large randomized-controlled trials for the evaluation of trauma-focused cognitive behavioral therapy [32,33]. However and noteworthy, the context conditions (e.g., naturalistic clinical setting vs. standardized research setting; treatment seeking sample vs. participation in a clinical trial) are differing to a high degree, therefore comparisons are limited. Further naturalistic studies are warranted in order to gain more insight into attrition and more knowledge on how to best prevent early drop out. In our sample, the cases who dropped out of treatment showed the highest level of avoidance symptoms. This highlights the relevance of early screening particularly for avoidance symptoms, which will provide valuable information and individual target points for preventive actions. Thus, the screening needs to be followed by an early provision of strategies to target avoidance, e.g., symptom and trigger monitoring and provision of coping skills. These measures may help to identify cases at risk at an early stage and to reduce dropout from trauma-focused intervention. Besides avoidance symptoms, the time span between the traumatic event and presentation in the clinic emerged as relevant factor, too: the decliners showed a significantly longer time span till their first visit than the completers. In order to reduce the time span untreated, barriers need to be addressed. This calls for better access to care [18], increased availability of clinics [19,20] and trauma-informed approaches [22], in order to reach out to those in need for treatment.

The overlap between trauma types was comparable with the rate reported for other community samples [31,32]. While this is a common phenomenon, conclusions of the trauma type-specific analyses in this paper are limited. Nevertheless, for victims of sexual abuse a more distinct pattern was observed on a descriptive level. While the rate of co-occurrence with other trauma types was comparably low, a higher number of sessions was required than for the other trauma types and the majority was in need for follow-up-intervention. The data therefore suggest that a tailored approach for the specific requirement of victims of sexual abuse might be warranted, e.g., by offering an extended quota of sessions.

The data from this report entail public health relevancy. First, the need for a specialized and accessible outpatient clinic for traumatized children and adolescents is evidenced by the high number of patients since the foundation of the trauma clinic, with about one new referral per week. Second, by the accessibility of the clinic, the burdened cases did receive an early trauma-informed and individualized intervention, contrasting the otherwise high probability that they were left untreated and not connected to any health services, for a longer time span at least [19,20]. Therefore trauma-informed facilities such as the OTC can play an important bridging role between onset of the trauma and the access to early intervention and the mental health care system: For one third of the patients, the provision of an initial clinical assessment, clearing and stabilization at the OTC led to reduction of psychological distress to the extent that no further follow-up treatment was required (and thereby helping to reduce the pressure on health care overload and costs). For the other two thirds, targeted follow-up treatment could be recommended and initiated by the clinic to contribute to sustained care. Further data on mental health care use and longer-term outcome are not yet available; however, a 3–12-months follow-up study is currently running.

In conclusion, early trauma-informed treatments, like described in the literature [22] and like the early intervention approach of the OTC described in this paper, are able to provide comprehensive and specialized support the families during early stages after the traumatic event; this may mitigate the risk for persistence of symptoms in the vulnerable group of children and adolescents.

Nationwide policies within the health care system need to ensure that trauma care for this vulnerable group is available and accessible [17] in order to facilitate assessment and intervention. Furthermore, knowledge on treatment centers' procedures and on their implementation of care will help to disseminate treatment approaches, which is especially warranted in the area of child and adolescent trauma, where a lack of treatment has been observed [19]. Therefore, enabling fast referral to specialized trauma-informed treatment centers like the OTC, and building up regional networks of trauma-informed care to foster direct follow-up treatment for the affected families are the key efforts which must urgently and widely be undertaken in clinical practice. Thus, we call other psychiatric and pediatric clinics to adapt this early treatment approach for the sake of improving and expanding the care for traumatized children and adolescents.

Author Contributions: Conceptualization, C.C., E.M., S.B., K.R., L.I. and S.M.W.; Data curation, E.M., L.B., S.B. and K.R.; Formal analysis, C.C.; Methodology, C.C.; Project administration, C.C., E.M., L.B., S.B., K.R., L.I. and S.M.W.; Supervision, C.C. and S.M.W.; Writing—original draft, C.C.; Writing—review & editing, C.C., E.M., L.B., S.B., K.R., L.I. and S.M.W. All authors have read and agreed to the published version of the manuscript.

Funding: This research received no external funding.

Institutional Review Board Statement: The study was approved by the Ethics Committee of the Charité—Universitätsmedizin Berlin (EA2/145/18, date of approval 30 July 2018).

Informed Consent Statement: The retrospective study was carried out as part of the accompanying clinical research of the Charité—Universitätsmedizin Berlin, which is why no separate consent was obtained for this study.

Data Availability Statement: The data that support the findings of this study are available upon reasonable request from the corresponding author. The data are not publicly available due to privacy or ethical restrictions.

Acknowledgments: We wish to thank Anneke Lipinski, Sophie Seja and Jana Kindermann for their encouragement and support in data collection and data entry. We acknowledge support by the Open Access Publication Fund of the Freie Universität Berlin.

Conflicts of Interest: The authors declare no conflict of interest.

References

1. Copeland, W.E.; Keeler, G.; Angold, A.; Costello, E.J. Traumatic events and posttraumatic stress in childhood. *Arch. Gen. Psychiatry* **2007**, *64*, 577–584. [CrossRef] [PubMed]
2. Witt, A.; Brown, R.C.; Plener, P.L.; Brähler, E.; Fegert, J.M. Child maltreatment in Germany: Prevalence rates in the general population. *Child Adolesc. Psychiatry Ment. Health* **2017**, *11*, 47. [CrossRef]
3. Clemens, V.; Huber-Lang, M.; Plener, P.L.; Brähler, E.; Brown, R.C.; Fegert, J.M. Association of child maltreatment subtypes and long-term physical health in a German representative sample. *Eur. J. Psychotraumatol.* **2018**, *9*, 1510278. [CrossRef] [PubMed]
4. Hodgdon, H.B.; Spinazzola, J.; Briggs, E.C.; Liang, L.-J.; Steinberg, A.M.; Layne, C.M. Maltreatment type, exposure characteristics, and mental health outcomes among clinic referred trauma-exposed youth. *Child Abus. Negl.* **2018**, *82*, 12–22. [CrossRef]
5. Price, M.; Higa-McMillan, C.; Kim, S.; Frueh, B.C. Trauma experience in children and adolescents: An assessment of the effects of trauma type and role of interpersonal proximity. *J. Anxiety Disord.* **2013**, *27*, 652–660. [CrossRef] [PubMed]
6. Spinazzola, J.; Hodgdon, H.; Liang, L.-J.; Ford, J.D.; Layne, C.M.; Pynoos, R.; Briggs, E.C.; Stolbach, B.; Kisiel, C. Unseen wounds: The contribution of psychological maltreatment to child and adolescent mental health and risk outcomes. *Psychol. Trauma Theory Res. Pract. Policy* **2014**, *6*, S18. [CrossRef]
7. Alisic, E.; Zalta, A.K.; van Wesel, F.; Larsen, S.E.; Hafstad, G.S.; Hassanpour, K.; Smid, G.E. Rates of post-traumatic stress disorder in trauma-exposed children and adolescents: Meta-analysis. *Br. J. Psychiatry* **2014**, *204*, 335–340. [CrossRef]
8. De Haan, A.; Tutus, D.; Goldbeck, L.; Rosner, R.; Landolt, M.A. Do dysfunctional posttraumatic cognitions play a mediating role in trauma adjustment? Findings from interpersonal and accidental trauma samples of children and adolescents. *Eur. J. Psychotraumatol.* **2019**, *10*, 1596508. [CrossRef]
9. Lindebo Knutsen, M.; Sachser, C.; Holt, T.; Goldbeck, L.; Jensen, T.K. Trajectories and possible predictors of treatment outcome for youth receiving trauma-focused cognitive behavioral therapy. *Psychol. Trauma Theory Res. Pract. Policy* **2019**, *12*, 336–346. [CrossRef]
10. Witt, A.; Munzer, A.; Ganser, H.G.; Goldbeck, L.; Fegert, J.M.; Plener, P.L. The impact of maltreatment characteristics and revictimization on functioning trajectories in children and adolescents: A growth mixture model analysis. *Child Abus. Negl.* **2019**, *90*, 32–42. [CrossRef]
11. Münzer, A.; Fegert, J.M.; Goldbeck, L. Psychological Symptoms of Sexually Victimized Children and Adolescents Compared with Other Maltreatment Subtypes. *J. Child Sex. Abus.* **2016**, *25*, 326–346. [CrossRef] [PubMed]
12. Greger, H.K.; Myhre, A.K.; Lydersen, S.; Jozefiak, T. Previous maltreatment and present mental health in a high-risk adolescent population. *Child Abus. Negl.* **2015**, *45*, 122–134. [CrossRef] [PubMed]
13. Habetha, S.; Bleich, S.; Weidenhammer, J.; Fegert, J.M. A prevalence-based approach to societal costs occurring in consequence of child abuse and neglect. *Child Adolesc. Psychiatry Ment. Health* **2012**, *6*, 35. [CrossRef]
14. Gutermann, J.; Schreiber, F.; Matulis, S.; Schwartzkopff, L.; Deppe, J.; Steil, R. Psychological Treatments for Symptoms of Posttraumatic Stress Disorder in Children, Adolescents, and Young Adults: A Meta-Analysis. *Clin. Child Fam. Psychol. Rev.* **2016**, *19*, 77–93. [CrossRef] [PubMed]
15. Gutermann, J.; Schwartzkopff, L.; Steil, R. Meta-analysis of the Long-Term Treatment Effects of Psychological Interventions in Youth with PTSD Symptoms. *Clin. Child Fam. Psychol. Rev.* **2017**, *20*, 422–434. [CrossRef]
16. Schafer, I.; Hopchet, M.; Vandamme, N.; Ajdukovic, D.; El-Hage, W.; Egreteau, L.; Javakhishvili, J.D.; Makhashvili, N.; Lampe, A.; Ardino, V.; et al. Trauma and trauma care in Europe. *Eur. J. Psychotraumatol.* **2018**, *9*, 1556553. [CrossRef]
17. Kazlauskas, E.; Javakhishvilli, J.; Meewisse, M.; Merecz-Kot, D.; Sar, V.; Schafer, I.; Schnyder, U.; Gersons, B.P.R. Trauma treatment across Europe: Where do we stand now from a perspective of seven countries. *Eur. J. Psychotraumatol.* **2016**, *7*, 29450. [CrossRef]
18. Ellinghaus, C.; Truss, K.; Liao Siling, J.; Phillips, L.; Eastwood, O.; Medrano, C.; Bendall, S. "I'm tired of being pulled from pillar to post": A qualitative analysis of barriers to mental health care for trauma-exposed young people. *Early Interv. Psychiatry* **2020**, *15*, 113–122. [CrossRef]
19. Münzer, A.; Rosner, R.; Ganser, H.G.; Naumann, A.; Plener, P.L.; Witt, A.; Goldbeck, L. Usual care for maltreatment-related pediatric posttraumatic stress disorder in Germany. *Z. Kinder Jugendpsychiatr. Psychother.* **2017**, *46*, 135–141. [CrossRef]

20. Pawils, S.; Nick, S.; Metzner, F.; Lotzin, A.; Schäfer, I. Versorgungssituation von Kindern, Jugendlichen und Erwachsenen mit sexuellen Gewalterfahrungen in Deutschland. *Bundesgesundheitsblatt Gesundh. Gesundh.* **2017**, *60*, 1046–1054. [CrossRef]
21. Toth, S.L.; Manly, J.T. Bridging research and practice: Challenges and successes in implementing evidence-based preventive intervention strategies for child maltreatment. *Child Abus. Negl.* **2011**, *35*, 633–636. [CrossRef]
22. Bendall, S.; Eastwood, O.; Cox, G.; Farrelly-Rosch, A.; Nicoll, H.; Peters, W.; Bailey, A.P.; McGorry, P.D.; Scanlan, F. A systematic review and synthesis of trauma-informed care within outpatient and counseling health settings for young people. *Child Maltreat.* **2020**, *26*, 313–324. [CrossRef] [PubMed]
23. Federal Ministry of Labour and Social Affairs. Compensation and Assistance for Victims of Violent Crime. 2016. Available online: https://www.bmas.de/EN/Social-Affairs/Socialcompensation-law/compensation-and-assistance-for-victims-of-violent-crime.html (accessed on 10 September 2021).
24. Kolko, D.J.; Hoagwood, K.E.; Springgate, B. Treatment research for children and youth exposed to traumatic events: Moving beyond efficacy to amp up public health impact. *Gen. Hosp. Psychiatry* **2010**, *32*, 465–476. [CrossRef]
25. Ehlers, A.; Grey, N.; Wild, J.; Stott, R.; Liness, S.; Deale, A.; Handley, R.; Albert, I.; Cullen, D.; Hackmann, A.; et al. Implementation of cognitive therapy for PTSD in routine clinical care: Effectiveness and moderators of outcome in a consecutive sample. *Behav. Res. Ther.* **2013**, *51*, 742–752. [CrossRef]
26. Ghafoori, B.; Wolf, M.G.; Nylund-Gibson, K.; Felix, E.D. A naturalistic study exploring mental health outcomes following trauma-focused treatment among diverse survivors of crime and violence. *J. Affect. Disord.* **2019**, *245*, 617–625. [CrossRef]
27. Perrin, S.; Meiser-Stedman, R.; Smith, P. The Children's Revised Impact of Event Scale (CRIES): Validity as a Screening Instrument for PTSD. *Behav. Cogn. Psychother.* **2005**, *33*, 487–498. [CrossRef]
28. Ackerman, P.T.; Newton, J.E.; McPherson, W.B.; Jones, J.G.; Dykman, R.A. Prevalence of post traumatic stress disorder and other psychiatric diagnoses in three groups of abused children (sexual, physical, and both). *Child Abus. Negl.* **1998**, *22*, 759–774. [CrossRef]
29. Sachser, C.; Goldbeck, L. Angst, Depression und Trauma–transdiagnostische Effekte der traumafokussierten kognitiven Verhaltenstherapie (TF-KVT). *Kindh. Entwickl.* **2017**, *26*, 93–99. [CrossRef]
30. Cohen, J.A.; Mannarino, A.P.; Kliethermes, M.; Murray, L.A. Trauma-focused CBT for youth with complex trauma. *Child Abus. Negl.* **2012**, *36*, 528–541. [CrossRef]
31. Smith, P.; Dalgleish, T.; Meiser-Stedman, R. Practitioner Review: Posttraumatic stress disorder and its treatment in children and adolescents. *J. Child Psychol. Psychiatry* **2019**, *60*, 500–515. [CrossRef] [PubMed]
32. Goldbeck, L.; Muche, R.; Sachser, C.; Tutus, D.; Rosner, R. Effectiveness of Trauma-Focused Cognitive Behavioral Therapy for Children and Adolescents: A Randomized Controlled Trial in Eight German Mental Health Clinics. *Psychother. Psychosom.* **2016**, *85*, 159–170. [CrossRef] [PubMed]
33. Jensen, T.K.; Holt, T.; Ormhaug, S.M.; Egeland, K.; Granly, L.; Hoaas, L.C.; Hukkelberg, S.S.; Indregard, T.; Stormyren, S.D.; Wentzel-Larsen, T. A randomized effectiveness study comparing trauma-focused cognitive behavioral therapy with therapy as usual for youth. *J. Clin. Child. Adolesc. Psychol.* **2014**, *43*, 356–369. [CrossRef] [PubMed]

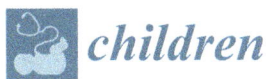

Article

Parental Internalizing Psychopathology and PTSD in Offspring after the 2012 Earthquake in Italy

Barbara Forresi [1,*,†], Marcella Caputi [2,†], Simona Scaini [1], Ernesto Caffo [3], Gabriella Aggazzotti [3] and Elena Righi [3]

1 Department of Psychology, Sigmund Freud University (Milan), Ripa di Porta Ticinese, 77-20143 Milan, Italy; s.scaini@milano-sfu.it
2 Department of Life Sciences, University of Trieste, Via E. Weiss, 2-34128 Trieste, Italy; marcella.caputi@units.it
3 Department of Biomedical, Metabolic, and Neural Sciences, University of Modena and Reggio Emilia, 287-41125 Via Campi, Italy; ernesto.caffo@unimore.it (E.C.); gabriella.aggazzotti@unimore.it (G.A.); elena.righi@unimore.it (E.R.)
* Correspondence: b.forresi@milano-sfu.it
† These authors contributed equally to this work.

Abstract: Post-traumatic stress disorder (PTSD) is common in youths after earthquakes, with parental psychopathology among the most significant predictors. This study investigated the contribution and the interactional effects of parental internalizing psychopathology, the severity of exposure to the earthquake, and past traumatic events to predict PTSD in offspring, also testing the reverse pattern. Two years after the 2012 earthquake in Italy, 843 children and adolescents (9–15 years) living in two differently affected areas were administered a questionnaire on traumatic exposure and the UCLA PTSD Reaction Index. Anxiety, depression, and somatization were assessed in 1162 parents through the SCL-90-R. General linear model showed that, for offspring in the high-impact area, predictors of PTSD were earthquake exposure, past trauma, and parental internalizing symptoms, taken individually. An interaction between earthquake exposure and parental depression or anxiety (not somatization) was also found. In the low-impact area, youth PTSD was only predicted by earthquake exposure. The reverse pattern was significant, with parental psychopathology explained by offspring PTSD. Overall, findings support the association between parental and offspring psychopathology after natural disasters, emphasizing the importance of environmental factors in this relationship. Although further research is needed, these results should be carefully considered when developing mental health interventions.

Keywords: earthquake; trauma; PTSD; parental psychopathology; internalizing disorders; youths; children; adolescents

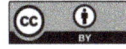

1. Introduction

As the frequency of large-scale disasters and emergencies is increasing around the globe, children and adolescents are among the most vulnerable populations for the development of negative mental health consequences. Several studies confirmed that youths exposed to disasters show an increased prevalence of psychological disorders such as post-traumatic stress disorder (PTSD), depression, anxiety/somatization disorders, substance abuse, and sleep problems [1–6]. One of the most common sequelae is represented by PTSD [3,7–14], with a prevalence in youths ranging between 5% and 60% [15]. High rates of PTSD have been detected among children and adolescents not only in the aftermath but also several years after earthquakes [7,10,11,16–27]. According to a recent meta-analysis of studies conducted among children and adolescents exposed to earthquakes and floods [28], the pooled prevalence of PTSD was 19.2%, 30%, 24.4%, and 20.4% in the first, second, third, and fourth six-month intervals after the event.

Considering the long-lasting effects of PTSD and its negative impact across development, identification of its predictors is of primary importance. Several pre-traumatic and peritraumatic predictors of PTSD in children and adolescents after disasters have been identified [15,28–30], such as demographic characteristics (e.g., being female), pre-disaster events and functioning (e.g., previous traumatic events and psychological difficulties), and severity of disaster exposure (e.g., being trapped, experiencing injuries and losses). While prior trauma was identified as a small to medium risk factor, the severity of exposure appeared as the strongest risk factor [29]. According to the meta-analytic examination by Furr and colleagues [30], for example, higher death toll, proximity, and personal loss were each associated with increased post-traumatic stress symptoms (PTSS) in youths.

Among post-traumatic factors, the meta-analysis by Trickey and colleagues [29] highlighted the important role played by parental psychological problems and family functioning in youth PTSD. This association between psychological difficulties in parents and offspring can be referred not only to a genetic predisposition and therefore to common biological bases for emotional processing but also to difficult parenting or other family challenges [31,32]. Parents represent the primary support for children and adolescents after traumatic events and disasters [33], and their psychopathology may have a cascade effect on several other variables such as parenting styles [34], parent-youth communication, and relationships [35]. Moreover, according to the model of Pynoos and colleagues [36], parents can moderate the impact of the event, of proximal reminders and secondary stressors, supporting the cognitive appraisal of what occurred, as well as the ongoing adjustment. It is therefore evident that youth mental health after traumatic events and disasters can be best understood only considering their family context, according to a socio-ecological model (e.g., the work of [31,37–41]).

The relevance of parental psychopathology as a risk factor for PTSD in offspring has been extensively studied after several potentially traumatic events, ranging from hospitalization and pediatric burn [42–49] to traffic injuries, community violence, industrial disasters, war, and terrorist attacks [32,50–58]. The association has also been detected after earthquakes [12,16,59–64] and other natural disasters [41,65–68]. However, existing research is still scant and affected by many methodological flaws, including poor in-depth analysis of the role of parental distress on child outcomes, a limited consideration of bidirectional associations, the use of a single source of information (parent or child) [69,70].

In their cross-sectional study, Spell and colleagues [41] found that maternal distress predicted PTSS in children exposed to Hurricane Katrina. Instead, Kiliç and colleagues [62,63] found that six months after the Bolu earthquake in Turkey, PTSD in children was affected by their father's traumatic stress and depression. Similarly, in their survey of survivors from three disasters, North and colleagues [69] found that parental psychopathology was associated with child emotional and behavioral problems. A recent meta-analysis [31] confirmed that parental PTSD is associated with children's psychological distress.

The same topic was explored in a longitudinal perspective [60,71]. After the Great East Japan Earthquake, Honda and colleagues [60] investigated the impact of parental PTSD on children's mental health using multivariate logistic regression analysis. While cross-sectionally no significant association was found, parental PTSD symptoms at baseline were a significant predictor of children's internalizing problems measured three years later. In another study, children exposed to Hurricane Katrina whose mothers had a chronic PTSD trajectory also presented severe post-traumatic stress symptoms two years later [71].

A smaller number of studies focused on the opposite relationship, investigating whether children's PTSD has an impact on parental mental health. In a recent article, Pfefferbaum and North [72] explored cross-sectionally the influence of children's psychopathology on their parents' mental health in a large sample including 1066 children and 556 parents exposed to different disasters and terrorist attacks, with findings supporting the direction from child psychopathology to parental PTSD.

Similarly, in their longitudinal study, Shi and colleagues [64] studied 688 parent-adolescent dyads after the 2008 Wenchuan earthquake, finding that parental PTSS at 1 year prospectively predicted teens' PTSS after 18 months; on the other side, youth PTSS at 1 year predicted maternal but not paternal PTSS 18 months later. This study indeed highlights a causal role of parental PTSS on PTSS in offspring and a bidirectional pattern of influence between maternal and youth psychopathology.

Inconsistent conclusions were drawn by Juth and colleagues [61]. Using the interesting Actor-Partner Interdependence Model (APIM) after a major earthquake in Indonesia, researchers observed cross-sectionally that parental post-traumatic symptoms resulted in being associated with children's distress: the reverse was not true, suggesting the existence of a unidirectional path of influence.

In conclusion, notwithstanding a strong consensus on the relationship between parental psychopathology and youth PTSD after disasters, research in this field is still scant and mostly focused on parental PTSD [41,60,65,67,73], parental depression [62,63,67], or general psychological distress [41]. To our knowledge, no study focused on a broader pattern of parental internalizing psychopathology, including somatization, anxiety, and depression.

Furthermore, while the relationship between parental psychopathology and offspring PTSD found significant support, a reciprocal pattern of influence has been suggested with preliminary evidence [64,72], without clear conclusions. Notably, none of the previous studies looked at parental psychopathology in interaction with the severity of exposure to the earthquake and past trauma to determine PTSD in offspring.

The present cross-sectional study aimed at contributing to the literature on natural disasters in the light of the important role played by parental mental health in offspring PTSD [74–76].

The overall purpose was to examine the relationship between parental internalizing psychopathology and PTSD in offspring two years after the earthquake that hit Northern Italy in 2012, comparing students living in the area most affected by the earthquake with others living in a nearby control area. As to our knowledge, no previous study was able to compare the psychopathology of parents and their offspring in two differently exposed samples.

In the first place, we were interested in exploring the correlational patterns between parental and youth psychopathology, especially considering parental internalizing symptoms (somatization/anxiety/depression) and offspring PTSD. Secondly, we investigated the relative contribution of parental internalizing psychopathology, the severity of exposure to earthquake, and prior trauma in affecting youth PTSD scores. Interactional effects between these variables were also explored. Finally, the relative contribution of offspring PTSD, earthquake exposure, and past trauma on parental internalizing psychopathology was analyzed. As for the previous hypothesis, interactional effects were examined.

Based on the scientific literature, an association between parental internalizing psychopathology and offspring PTSD was hypothesized. Specifically, we expected a significant contribution of parental psychopathology, the severity of exposure, and prior trauma in explaining PTSD variance in youths. Moreover, we expected offspring PTSD to have a role in parental psychopathology. Regarding the interactional analysis, no a priori hypothesis was generated due to the lack of previous studies of this kind on natural disasters.

2. Materials and Methods

2.1. Participants

Sampling included youths living in the province of Modena hit by the 2012 earthquake, and recruitment was conducted in primary and secondary schools randomly selected from the comprehensive School Regional Office register, published by the Italian Ministry of Education. To recruit participants, the province of Modena was divided into two areas: an "earthquake area" (EA), including the epicenter and the most affected zones, and a "control area" (CA), characterized by no human losses or damages to buildings due to the earthquake.

The sample of the present study, therefore, included 518 children and adolescents living in the most affected area, with a mean age of 11.21 ± 1.51 years (range 8–15 years; 48.9% males), and 325 children (mean age 11.26 ± 1.29; 52.6% males) living in the control area. With respect to sex, age, or nationality, no significant differences between the two areas were found.

A total of 1162 parents also agreed to provide information on their mental health. Parental psychopathology was examined for 474 children and adolescents in the EA (age range 29–65 ys, mean age = 43.17, SD = 5.43) and for 308 in the CA (age range 28–61 ys, mean age = 43.49, SD = 6.44). None of the youths had been previously in contact with mental health services.

2.2. Measures

Children and adolescents were administered an assessment protocol including:

An exposure questionnaire created ad hoc to collect demographic data, information on the degree of exposure to the earthquake (occurrence of personal, familiar, or friend injuries or death, house damages or displacement), exposure to past traumatic events (e.g., parental divorce, personal or relatives' accidents, previous illnesses, or losses). Each item had a yes/no response format, and two indexes of exposure (earthquake exposure and lifetime traumatic exposure) were calculated. These were used as continuous in correlation analyses, while they have been dichotomized in the GLM. In the last case, a score of "1" was attributed to each youth with the severity of exposure to earthquake or a lifetime exposure over $50°$ percentile of the observed distribution.

The UCLA Post-traumatic Stress Disorder Reaction Index *(PTSD-RI)* for DSM-IV [77]: the most widely used instrument to assess trauma exposure and PTSD in children and adolescents exposed to any type of trauma. The 20-item version has a 5-point Likert response scale, and a total severity score can be calculated. Cronbach's alpha was 0.90 for internal consistency across versions, and test–retest reliability was 0.84 [77]. According to the official scoring system, a cutoff > 38 was used to identify probable PTSD cases. For the purposes of this study, we derived a continuous score that was used in the analyses.

Although the Italian version of this questionnaire has not been validated, the translation process followed published guidelines, including a back-translation independently conducted by two translators.

Parents were administered the following instrument:

Symptom Checklist-90-R (SCL-90-R) [78,79], Italian version [80]. This 90-item self-report measure using a 5-point Likert scale is aimed at assessing a broad range of psychopathological disorders (according to the DSM-IV-TR). Primary dimensions include somatization, obsessive-compulsive disorder, interpersonal sensitivity, depression, anxiety, hostility, phobic anxiety, paranoid ideation, and psychoticism. For the scope of the present research, analyses focused on internalizing scales (somatization, depression, anxiety). The sum of each domain score provides a Global Severity Index, whose clinical cutoff is 63. In the Italian version, internal coherence was good for all subscales ranging between 0.70 and 0.96 [81].

2.3. Procedure

The study was conducted according to the guidelines of the Declaration of Helsinki and approved by the Ethical Committee of the Province of Modena (protocol n. 268/12). Two years after the earthquake, trained child psychiatrists and psychologists conducted the assessment following the authorization of the school governance (principal and board). Only children whose parents signed the informed consent and who provided their personal consent were enrolled. Subjects with likely PTSD were referred to the local child neuropsychiatric services.

2.4. Statistical Analysis

Means, standard deviations, frequencies, and percentages were used for descriptive data analysis. Pearson's correlation coefficients were implemented to examine the relationship between PTSD scores, number of earthquake-related stressful events, number of prior traumatic events, and parental psychopathology scores. Finally, general linear model (GLM) was applied to explore the relative contribution of parental psychopathology, earthquake exposure, and past trauma to predict child PTSD scores. Due to the high level of collinearity among the three SCL-90-R subscales (somatization, depression, anxiety), we implemented separate models. Firstly, interaction and simple slope analyses were implemented to evaluate the interactive effects between parental psychopathology (somatization/anxiety/depression) and the variables concerning earthquake exposure and past trauma. Then, GLM was used to analyze the interactive effects between offspring PTSD scores and, respectively, the severity of exposure and past traumatic events to predict parental psychopathology (somatization/anxiety/depression). All the variables were z-transformed, and analyses were adjusted for child age and sex. Statistical analyses were performed using IBM SPSS Statistics package version 24. For all statistical tests, a $p < 0.05$ was considered statistically significant.

3. Results

3.1. Descriptive Analyses

The prevalence of probable PTSD in children and adolescents living in the area most affected by the earthquake was 1.9% (4.4% near the epicenter), and it was significantly higher than in the control zone (0.4%; $p < 0.001$). In the EA, the mean total PTSD score was also significantly higher than in the CA (15.62 ± 9.52 vs. 11.08 ± 7.50; $p < 0.001$).

While lifetime stressful events showed similar frequencies in the two areas (EA = 33.7% and CA = 37.8%, $p = 0.16$), rates (88.4%) of earthquake-related traumatic experiences in youths living in the EA were significantly higher than in the CA (19.5%; $p < 0.001$): 73.7% of children and adolescents in the EA had to leave the house for a period due to extensive damages, more than 30% had relatives or close friends who were injured or killed by the earthquake, and 4.2% experienced personal physical injuries. Moreover, about half of the youths in the EA experienced two or more events.

Nearly 1/3 of parents had high levels of psychopathology, with 28% in the EA having a global score at the SCL-90-R over the cutoff. This prevalence was higher than in the control sample (17.5%; $p < 0.001$). Significant differences were also observed in the subscales of interest for the present study: depression (22% vs. 11%; $p < 0.001$), somatization (20% vs. 16.2%; $p = 0.0049$), and anxiety (18.2% vs. 7.7%; $p < 0.001$) [82]. Mean values of all these variables are shown in Table 1, while correlations are shown in Table 2.

Table 1. Descriptive analyses of the main study variables.

	Earthquake Area M (SD)	Control Area M (SD)	t-Test	p
Offspring PTSD (CPTSD-RI)	15.62 (±9.52)	11.08 (±7.50)	−6.891	<0.001 ***
Parental somatization (SCL-90-R)	0.57 (±0.58)	0.52 (±0.47)	−1.341	0.180
Parental depression (SCL-90-R)	0.57 (±0.55)	0.45 (±0.45)	−3.371	=0.001 ***
Parental anxiety (SCL-90-R)	0.53 (±0.54)	0.40 (±0.38)	−3.923	<0.001 ***
Offspring severity of exposure to earthquake	2.24 (±0.1.17)	0.26 (±0.61)	−25.998	<0.001 ***
Offspring past traumatic events	0.52 (±0.90)	0.61 (±0.91)	1.232	0.218

Note. Significance levels *** $p < 0.001$; PTSD-RI = Post-Traumatic Stress Disorder—Reaction Index; SCL-90-R = Symptom Checklist-90-R.

Table 2. Correlations among the study variables in the EA and CA.

	2	3	4	5	6
1. Offspring PTSD (EA)	0.281 ** +	0.274 ** +	0.283 ** +	0.272 **	0.210 **
Offspring PTSD (CA)	0.068	−0.008	0.061	0.223 ***	0.126 *
2. Parental somatization (EA)	-	0.681 **	0.731 **	0.102	0.043
Parental somatization (CA)	-	0.649 ***	0.698 ***	0.055	0.025
3. Parental depression (EA)		-	0.838 ** +	0.095	0.019
Parental depression (CA)		-	0.753 ***	0.079	0.041
4. Parental anxiety (EA)			-	0.111	0.025
Parental anxiety (CA)			-	0.117	0.052
5. Offspring severity of exposure to earthquake (EA)				-	0.091
Offspring severity of exposure to earthquake (CA)				-	0.146 *
6. Offspring lifetime traumatic events (EA)					-
Offspring lifetime traumatic events (CA)					-

Note. Significance levels * $p < 0.05$, ** $p < 0.01$, *** $p < 0.001$. + indicates statistically significant difference between EA and CA correlations.

While in the most affected area PTSD in offspring was significantly related to their severity of exposure, past trauma, and parental psychopathology scores, in the low-affected control area PTSD did not correlate with parental internalizing psychopathology. Moreover, in both samples, parental psychopathology did not correlate with earthquake exposure and past trauma in their offspring.

3.2. Multivariate Analyses

In the earthquake area, GLM results (see Table 3) using youth PTSD-RI as the outcome variable revealed that parental somatization, depression, and anxiety together with earthquake exposure and past traumatic events are relevant risk factors for PTSD in children and adolescents.

In addition, we found a significant negative interaction between severity of exposure to the earthquake and parental depression or anxiety in predicting offspring PTSD symptoms. This interaction was not significant for somatization.

Table 3. General linear model for the PTSD-RI in the EA.

Dependent Variable: Offspring PTSD						
R^2 (adjusted) = 0.145						
Parameter	B	Std. Error	T	p	Lower Bound	Upper Bound
Offspring past traumatic events	0.416	0.109	3.821	0.000	0.201	0.603
Offspring severity of exposure to earthquake	0.297	0.105	2.818	0.005	0.089	0.504
Parental somatization	0.306	0.075	4.073	0.000	0.158	0.454
Offspring severity of exposure to earthquake * Parental somatization	−0.079	0.114	−0.691	0.490	−0.304	0.146
Offspring past traumatic events * Parental somatization	−0.060	0.112	−0.535	0.593	−0.281	0.161
Offspring sex	−0.035	0.102	−0.339	0.735	−0.236	0.167
Offspring age	0.010	0.034	0.295	0.768	−0.057	0.077

Table 3. Cont.

Dependent Variable: Offspring PTSD						
R^2 (adjusted) = 0.141						
Parameter	B	Std. Error	T	p	Lower Bound	Upper Bound
Offspring past traumatic events	0.426	0.106	4.001	0.000	0.216	0.636
Offspring severity of exposure to earthquake	0.350	0.103	3.384	0.001	0.146	0.554
Parental anxiety	0.317	0.076	4.150	0.000	0.167	0.468
Offspring severity of exposure to earthquake * Parental anxiety	−0.245	0.107	−2.2923	0.023	−0.455	−0.035
Offspring past traumatic events * Parental anxiety	−0.031	0.105	−0.300	0.765	−0.238	0.175
Offspring sex	−0.047	0.100	−0.469	0.639	−0.245	0.151
Offspring age	0.010	0.033	0.321	0.749	−0.054	0.075
Dependent Variable: Offspring PTSD						
R^2 (adjusted) = 0.159						
Parameter	B	Std. Error	T	p	Lower Bound	Upper Bound
Offspring past traumatic events	0.432	0.109	3.964	0.000	0.217	0.646
Offspring severity of exposure to earthquake	0.351	0.105	3.343	0.001	0.144	0.558
Parental depression	0.381	0.080	4.758	0.000	0.224	0.539
Offspring severity of exposure to earthquake * Parental depression	−0.313	0.111	−2.827	0.005	−0.531	−0.095
Offspring past traumatic events * Parental depression	−0.063	0.107	−0.588	0.557	−0.273	0.147
Offspring sex	−0.070	0.102	−0.684	0.495	−0.271	0.131
Offspring age	0.017	0.033	0.499	0.618	−0.049	0.083

Note: * indicates interactions between variables.

In the second set of models implemented with parental psychopathology as outcome (see Table 4), results showed that this was predicted by PTSD, and not by earthquake exposure nor past traumatic events experienced by their offspring. However, a negative interaction was observed between earthquake exposure and offspring PTSD in predicting depression and anxiety in parents.

The same analyses were conducted for children and adolescents living in the less affected control area (data not shown), and the severity of exposure to the earthquake resulted in the only significant predictor in all the models. No significant interactional effects were found.

In both areas, age and sex did not reach any statistical significance.

Table 4. General linear model for the SCL-90-R in the EA.

Dependent Variable: Parental Somatization (SCL-90-R)						
R^2 (adjusted) = 0.086						
Parameter	B	Std. Error	T	p	Lower Bound	Upper Bound
Offspring past traumatic events	0.051	0.119	0.428	0.669	−0.184	0.286
Offspring severity of exposure to earthquake	0.056	0.114	0.490	0.624	−0.169	0.281
PTSD-RI	0.416	0.094	4.451	0.000	0.232	0.600
Offspring severity of exposure to earthquake * Youth PTSD	−0.174	0.123	−1.410	0.160	−0.417	0.069
Offspring past traumatic events * Offspring PTSD	−0.101	0.125	−0.809	0.419	−0.348	0.145
Offspring sex	0.066	0.110	0.599	0.550	−0.151	0.282
Offspring age	0.064	0.036	1.789	0.075	−0.006	0.135

Table 4. Cont.

Dependent Variable: Parental Anxiety (SCL-90-R)						
R^2 (adjusted) = 0.064						
Parameter	B	Std. Error	T	p	Lower Bound	Upper Bound
Offspring past traumatic events	−0.013	0.122	−0.110	0.913	−0.253	0.226
Offspring severity of exposure to earthquake	−0.039	0.118	−0.330	0.742	−0.271	0.193
Offspring PTSD	0.400	0.098	4.089	0.000	0.207	0.593
Offspring severity of exposure to earthquake * PTSD-RI	−0.304	0.128	−2.377	0.018	−0.555	−0.052
Offspring past traumatic events * PTSD-RI	0.005	0.129	0.039	0.969	−0.248	0.258
Offspring sex	0.092	0.112	0.822	0.412	−0.129	0.314
Offspring age	0.049	0.037	1.334	0.183	−0.023	0.121
Dependent Variable: Parental Depression (SCL-90-R)						
R^2 (adjusted) = 0.096						
Parameter	B	Std. Error	T	p	Lower Bound	Upper Bound
Offspring past traumatic events	0.034	0.120	0.281	0.779	−0.203	0.271
Offspring severity of exposure to earthquake	−0.066	0.116	−0.568	0.570	−0.293	0.162
Offspring PTSD	0.443	0.094	4.736	0.000	0.259	0.628
Offspring severity of exposure to earthquake * Youth PTSD	−0.391	0.124	−3.149	0.002	−0.636	−0.147
Offspring past traumatic events * Offspring PTSD	0.025	0.125	0.202	0.840	−0.221	0.272
Offspring sex	0.140	0.111	1.262	0.208	−0.078	0.357
Offspring age	0.064	0.036	1.768	0.078	−0.007	0.135

Note: * indicates interactions between variables.

4. Discussion

The main aim of the present research was to explore the association between parental internalizing psychopathology and youth PTSD scores two years after the 2012 earthquake in Italy. Two subgroups of children and adolescents were compared: the first living in the most affected area and the other in a nearby control area with no human losses and damages to buildings.

As expected, correlations were found among PTSD total score in offspring and parental psychopathology, the severity of exposure, and previous traumatic events. These correlations were significant in the high-impact area but did not hold for children and adolescents living in the low-impact zone. Therefore, living in areas where losses and damages to buildings are extensive appears highly discriminant with respect to the long-term psychopathological impact of an earthquake.

These results were supported by multivariate analyses focusing on the relative contribution of parental internalizing psychopathology, the severity of exposure, and past trauma in predicting offspring PTSD. All these factors, in fact, explained a significant portion of the variance in PTSD total score, but only in the most affected area. In the other area, the only significant predictor was the degree of exposure to the earthquake. It is therefore confirmed, in accordance with recent systematic reviews and meta-analyses [15,28,29], the important role of previous traumatic events and severity of exposure to the earthquake in the development of children's and adolescents' PTSD. Our data collected two years after the earthquake are also in line with other studies evidencing that disaster exposure highly contributes to youth PTSD [7] up to three years later [38,60].

Evidence collected adds to a growing literature documenting the relationship between parental psychiatric difficulties and their offspring PTSD after earthquakes [41,60–64]. As highlighted in previous studies, parents struggling with their own psychopathology may have a limited ability to provide children and adolescents with adequate support in coping efforts and to construct a meaning for the trauma [36,47,64,66], as well as an adequate parenting style [38,67,83–85]. It can be therefore assumed that, for youth living close to the epicenter, exposed to human losses, personal injuries, and relocations, the impact of an earthquake is not only direct but also strengthened by the effects of other family members' psychopathology. Although it is not possible to draw any conclusions about the mechanisms underlying the association between parental psychopathology and offspring PTSD, the absence of a significant relationship in the low-impact areas seems to suggest the important role played by environmental factors in addition to a genetic liability.

Notably, the focus on parental internalizing symptoms in the present study extends previous literature on natural disasters, mostly limited to the investigation of parental PTSD [41,61,64] or depression [62,63]. To our knowledge, none of the previous studies investigated the relationship between parental somatization and youth PTSD after natural disasters, except for one study focusing on depression in children [86].

GLM analyses highlighted a negative interactional effect between the severity of earthquake exposure and parental anxiety or depression in explaining offspring PTSD. This result suggests that the relationships among predictors of youth PTSD could be complex, not limited to the impact of single variables per se or to an additional effect. While a boosted effect between these two factors could have been hypothesized, the result of interaction analyses seems to suggest a weakening effect of one variable on the other. It might be, for example, that in case of high exposure to the earthquake, parental anxiety or depression may have a minor role in explaining PTSD variance. Vice-versa, in the presence of severe anxiety or depression in parents, the severity of exposure might provide a lower contribution in explaining variance in offspring' psychological difficulties.

Furthermore, it is of clinical interest that the severity of exposure does not interact with parental somatization in affecting youth PTSD and that two years after the earthquake, these two variables keep an independent role. As no previous studies focused on the specific role of parental somatization on offspring PTSD, we can only suggest that, while parental anxiety and depression may interact with the severity of youth exposure to traumatic events through different cognitive processes [87], the mechanisms might be different for somatization. Future studies are needed to further explore and clarify this issue.

The third aim of the present study is found to support the hypothesis that parental psychopathology scores are predicted by offspring PTSD scores. This result is coherent with recent cross-sectional and longitudinal studies [64,72], suggesting the existence of a bidirectional pattern of influence between parental and youth psychopathology.

According to these results, not only does youth mental health rely on parents' functioning, but also PTSD in offspring may represent a maintaining variable for parental psychopathology. As highlighted by previous studies, psychopathology in children and adolescents can be extremely stressful for parents [88–90]. A meta-analysis including 32 studies, for example, found a significant association between child PTSS and both parent PTSS and depression [39]. The present study suggests the need to extend these findings to parental anxiety and somatization.

Finally, GLM analyses evidenced that even though parental psychopathology is not independently predicted by youth severity of exposure and lifetime traumatic events, an interaction effect can be observed between earthquake exposure and offspring PTSD on internalizing disorders in parents: even in this model, the interactional effect was not significant for parental somatization. In the case of low or high levels of traumatic events, therefore, the contribution of offspring PTSD in explaining parental psychopathology might be different. It could be hypothesized, for example, that when a youth is severely exposed to an earthquake, his/her PTSD gives a lower contribution in explaining variance in parental depression and anxiety. This result seems in line with studies showing that, after children's exposure to traumatic events, parents may feel guilt, shame, and a sense of hopelessness [91]. When parents feel that they failed "as a protective shield" [36], not being able to keep their child away from exposure to harm, they may develop negative emotions and concerns [87]. This "sense of failure" could manifest even in the presence of low levels of PTSD in offspring. The nature of the present study and the current state of knowledge invites cautious interpretations. The complexity of interactions among variables in traumatic situations deserves continued investigation and thoughtful study.

Strengths, Limitations, and Future Research

This study has several strengths and limitations. It is one of the few studies carried out in Italy after an earthquake, with a large sample of children, adolescents, and parents. Furthermore, it extends findings of previous studies considering internalizing difficulties (anxiety, depression, and somatization) and having a comparison sample living in a less affected area.

In addition, both children and parents self-assessed their symptoms. As highlighted in previous studies [64,70], one of the most common methodological flaws in research assessing the effects of disasters on children's mental health is represented by relying on parents as the only informant (with parental problems influencing the ratings of their children's problems).

Among the methodological shortcomings, the first and most important is represented by the cross-sectional design of the study, which limits conclusions about the directionality of the effects. Another is the use of short and self-report instruments, albeit extensively used in the aftermath of natural disasters. A clinical interview would have been more appropriate than a self-report instrument in assessing offspring PTSD. Finally, trauma exposure severity and past trauma were only reported by children and adolescents (and they did not correlate with adults' psychopathology): a more detailed assessment of parental exposure to earthquake, as well as pre-disaster data on parental and offspring psychopathology, would have allowed a better interpretation of the results.

New lines of research are needed to improve knowledge about the interactions among different variables as well as among different subjects exposed to disasters. Most importantly, longitudinal studies are needed, as the process of influence between parents and their offspring psychopathology is likely to be dynamic and not unidirectional [61]. Unfolding such trajectories will be a challenge for research in years to come.

5. Conclusions

Overall, the findings of the present study suggest that part of the youths exposed to natural disasters is in especially high need as not only the child but also parents are affected. Therefore, it is of primary importance to screen parents on psychopathology, providing a broader clinical assessment. As the development of PTSD in offspring appears to be significantly influenced by parental depression, anxiety and somatization, post-disaster psychological screenings should include a range of internalizing problems.

Moreover, early interventions should be offered to prevent psychopathological outcomes, giving priority to subjects living in areas most affected by earthquakes. Parents and youths should be supported as a family, not only in the aftermath of a disaster but also in the long run, and should receive treatment programs to regain hope, challenging negative cognitions and feelings that might prevent them from adaptively processing their trauma [92].

These results should be carefully considered when developing mental health interventions for children and families in areas affected by earthquakes.

Author Contributions: Formal analysis, S.S.; Methodology, S.S. and E.R.; Supervision, E.C. and G.A.; Writing—original draft, B.F., M.C. and S.S.; Writing—review & editing, B.F., M.C. and E.R. All authors have read and agreed to the published version of the manuscript.

Funding: This research received no external funding. The open access publication was funded by the University of Modena and Reggio Emilia.

Institutional Review Board Statement: The study was conducted according to the guidelines of the Declaration of Helsinki and approved by the Ethical Committee of the Province of Modena (Protocol No. 268/12).

Informed Consent Statement: Informed consent was obtained from all subjects involved in the study.

Data Availability Statement: Due to ethical concerns, supporting data cannot be made openly available.

Acknowledgments: E. Botosso; E. Carluccio; O. Daolio; D. Gueraldi; L. Giamboni; R. La Torre; I. Maini; S. Leonardi; F. Soncini; E. Di Pietro; and G. Scarpini.

Conflicts of Interest: No conflict of interest was declared by the authors. All persons provided their informed consent prior to their inclusion in the study. Details that might disclose the identity of the subjects under study have been omitted.

References

1. Blanc, J.; Eugene, D.; Louis, E.F.; Cadichon, J.M.; Joseph, J.; Pierre, A.; Laine, R.; Alexandre, M.; Huang, K.Y. Mental health among children older than 10 years exposed to the Haiti 2010 earthquake: A critical review. *Curr. Psychiatry Rep.* **2020**, *22*, 1–13. [CrossRef] [PubMed]
2. Caffo, E.; Forresi, B.; Strik Lievers, L. Impact, psychological sequelae and management of trauma affecting children and adolescents. *Curr. Opin. Psychiatry* **2005**, *18*, 422–428. [CrossRef] [PubMed]
3. Dube, A.; Moffatt, M.; Davison, C.; Bartels, S. Health outcomes for children in Haiti since the 2010 earthquake: A systematic review. *Prehosp. Disaster Med.* **2018**, *33*, 77–88. [CrossRef] [PubMed]
4. Farooqui, M.; Quadri, S.A.; Suriya, S.S.; Khan, M.A.; Ovais, M.; Sohail, Z.; Shoaib, S.; Tohid, H.; Hassan, M. Posttraumatic stress disorder: A serious post-earthquake complication. *Trends Psychiatry Psychother.* **2017**, *39*, 135–143. [CrossRef] [PubMed]
5. Norris, F.H.; Friedman, M.J.; Watson, P.J. 60,000 disaster victims speak: Part II. Summary and implications of the disaster mental health research. *Psychiatry* **2002**, *65*, 240–260. [CrossRef] [PubMed]
6. Şalcıoğlu, E.; Başoğlu, M. Psychological effects of earthquakes in children: Prospects for brief behavioral treatment. *World J. Pediatr.* **2008**, *4*, 165–172. [CrossRef]
7. Wang, Y.; Xu, J.; Lu, Y. Associations among trauma exposure, post-traumatic stress disorder, and depression symptoms in adolescent survivors of the 2013 Lushan earthquake. *J. Affect. Disord.* **2020**, *264*, 407–413. [CrossRef]
8. Dai, W.; Chen, L.; Lai, Z.; Li, Y.; Wang, J.; Liu, A. The incidence of post-traumatic stress disorder among survivors after earthquakes: A systematic review and meta-analysis. *BMC Psychiatry* **2016**, *16*, 1–11. [CrossRef]
9. Ying, L.H.; Wu, X.C.; Chen, C. Prevalence and predictors of posttraumatic stress disorder and depressive symptoms among child survivors 1 year following the Wenchuan earthquake in China. *Eur. Child. Adolesc. Psychiatry* **2013**, *22*, 567–575. [CrossRef]
10. Ayub, M.; Poongan, I.; Masood, K.; Gul, H.; Ali, M.; Farrukh, A.; Shaheen, A.; Chaudhry, H.R.; Naeem, F. Psychological morbidity in children 18 months after Kashmir Earthquake of 2005. *Child. Psychiatry Hum. Dev.* **2012**, *43*, 323–336. [CrossRef]
11. Blanc, J.; Bui, E.; Mouchenik, Y.; Derivois, D.; Birmes, P. Prevalence of post-traumatic stress disorder and depression in two groups of children one year after the January 2010 earthquake in Haiti. *J. Affect. Disord.* **2015**, *1*, 121–126. [CrossRef]
12. Feo, P.; Di Gioia, S.; Carloni, E.; Vitiello, B.; Tozzi, A.E.; Vicari, S. Prevalence of psychiatric symptoms in children and adolescents one year after the 2009 L'Aquila earthquake. *BMC Psychiatry* **2014**, *14*, 1–12. [CrossRef]
13. Hong, C.; Efferth, T. Systematic review on post-traumatic stress disorder among survivors of the Wenchuan earthquake. *Trauma Violence Abuse* **2016**, *17*, 542–561. [CrossRef]
14. Laor, N.; Wolmer, L.; Kora, M.; Yucel, D.; Spirman, S.; Yazgan, Y. Posttraumatic, dissociative and grief symptoms in Turkish children exposed to the 1999 earthquakes. *J. Nerv. Ment. Dis.* **2002**, *190*, 824–832. [CrossRef]
15. Tang, B.; Deng, Q.; Glik, D.; Dong, J.; Zhang, L. A meta-analysis of risk factors for post-traumatic stress disorder (PTSD) in adults and children after earthquakes. *Int. J. Environ. Res. Public Health* **2017**, *14*, 1537. [CrossRef]
16. Forresi, B.; Soncini, F.; Bottosso, E.; Di Pietro, E.; Scarpini, G.; Scaini, S.; Aggazzotti, G.; Caffo, E.; Righi, E. Post-traumatic stress disorder, emotional and behavioral difficulties in children and adolescents 2 years after the 2012 earthquake in Italy: An epidemiological cross-sectional study. *Eur. Child. Adolesc. Psychiatry* **2020**, *29*, 227–238. [CrossRef] [PubMed]
17. Xu, J.; Wang, Y.; Zhang, J.; Tang, W.; Lu, Y. Influence of earthquake exposure and left-behind status on severity of post-traumatic stress disorder and depression in Chinese adolescents. *Psychiatry Res.* **2019**, *275*, 253–260. [CrossRef]
18. Jin, Y.; Deng, H.; An, J.; Xu, J. The prevalence of PTSD symptoms and depressive symptoms and related predictors in children and adolescents 3 years after the Ya'an earthquake. *Child. Psychiatry Hum. Dev.* **2019**, *50*, 300–307. [CrossRef]
19. Fan, F.; Long, K.; Zhou, Y.; Zheng, Y.; Liu, X. Longitudinal trajectories of post-traumatic stress disorder symptoms among adolescents after the Wenchuan earthquake in China. *Psychol. Med.* **2015**, *45*, 2885–2896. [CrossRef] [PubMed]
20. Terasaka, A.; Tachibana, Y.; Okuyama, M.; Igarashi, T. Post-traumatic stress disorder in children following natural disasters: A systematic review of the long-term follow-up studies. *J. Child. Fam. Stud.* **2015**, *6*, 111–133. [CrossRef]
21. Tian, Y.; Wong, T.K.; Li, J.; Jiang, X. Posttraumatic stress disorder and its risk factors among adolescent survivors three years after an 8.0 magnitude earthquake in China. *BMC Public Health* **2014**, *15*, 1073. [CrossRef] [PubMed]

22. Jia, Z.; Shi, L.; Duan, G.; Liu, W.; Pan, X.; Chen, Y.; Tian, W. Traumatic experiences and mental health consequences among child survivors of the 2008 Sichuan earthquake: A community-based follow-up study. *BMC Public Health* **2013**, *13*, 1–9. [CrossRef] [PubMed]
23. Zhang, Z.; Ran, M.S.; Li, Y.H.; Ou, G.J.; Gong, R.R.; Li, R.H.; Fan, M.; Jiang, Z.; Fang, D.Z. Prevalence of post-traumatic stress disorder among adolescents after the Wenchuan earthquake in China. *Psychol. Med.* **2012**, *42*, 1687–1693. [CrossRef]
24. Goenjian, A.K.; Pynoos, R.S.; Steinberg, A.M.; Najarian, L.M.; Asarnow, J.R.; Karayan, I.; Ghurabi, M.; Fairbanks, L.A. Psychiatric comorbidity in children after the 1988 earthquake in Armenia. *J. Am. Acad. Child. Adolesc. Psychiatry* **1995**, *34*, 1174–1184. [CrossRef]
25. Goenjian, A.K.; Walling, D.; Steinberg, A.M.; Roussos, A.; Goenjian, H.A.; Pynoos, R.S. Depression and PTSD symptoms among bereaved adolescents $6\frac{1}{2}$ years after the 1988 Spitak earthquake. *J. Affect. Disord.* **2009**, *112*, 81–84. [CrossRef]
26. Goenjian, A.K.; Roussos, A.; Steinberg, A.M.; Sotiropoulou, C.; Walling, D.; Kakaki, M.; Karagianni, S. Longitudinal study of PTSD, depression, and quality of life among adolescents after the Parnitha earthquake. *J. Affect. Disord.* **2011**, *133*, 509–515. [CrossRef]
27. Yule, W.; Bolton, D.; Udwin, O.; Boyle, S.; O'Ryan, D.; Nurrish, J. The long-term psychological effects of a disaster experienced in adolescence: I: The incidence and course of PTSD. *J. Child. Psychol. Psychiatry* **2000**, *41*, 503–511. [CrossRef]
28. Rezayat, A.A.; Sahebdel, S.; Jafari, S.; Kabirian, A.; Rahnejat, A.M.; Farahani, R.H.; Mosaed, R.; Nour, M.G. Evaluating the prevalence of PTSD among children and adolescents after earthquakes and floods: A systematic review and meta-analysis. *Psychiatr. Q* **2020**, *91*, 1265–1290. [CrossRef] [PubMed]
29. Trickey, D.; Siddaway, A.P.; Meiser-Stedman, R.; Serpell, L.; Field, A.P. A meta-analysis of risk factors for post-traumatic stress disorder in children and adolescents. *Clin. Psychol. Rev.* **2012**, *32*, 122–138. [CrossRef]
30. Furr, J.M.; Comer, J.S.; Edmunds, J.M.; Kendall, P.C. Disasters and youth: A meta-analytic examination of posttraumatic stress. *J. Consult. Clin. Psychol.* **2010**, *78*, 765–780. [CrossRef]
31. Lambert, J.E.; Holzer, J.; Hasbun, A. Association between parents' PTSD severity and children's psychological distress: A meta-analysis. *J. Trauma Stress* **2014**, *27*, 9–17. [CrossRef]
32. Kerns, C.E.; Elkins, R.M.; Carpenter, A.L.; Chou, T.; Green, J.G.; Comer, J.S. Caregiver distress, shared traumatic exposure, and child adjustment among area youth following the 2013 Boston Marathon bombing. *J. Affect. Disord.* **2014**, *167*, 50–55. [CrossRef]
33. Bonanno, G.A.; Brewin, C.R.; Kaniasty, K.; Greca, A.M.L. Weighing the costs of disaster: Consequences, risks, and resilience in individuals, families, and communities. *Psychol. Sci. Public Interest* **2010**, *11*, 1–49. [CrossRef]
34. Pfefferbaum, B.; Jacobs, A.K.; Houston, J.B.; Griffin, N. Children's disaster reactions: The influence of family and social factors. *Curr. Psychiatry Rep.* **2015**, *17*, 57. [CrossRef] [PubMed]
35. Bountress, K.E.; Gilmore, A.K.; Metzger, I.W.; Aggen, S.H.; Tomko, R.L.; Danielson, C.K.; Williamson, V.; Vladmirov, V.; Ruggiero, K.; Amstadter, A.B. Impact of disaster exposure severity: Cascading effects across parental distress, adolescent PTSD symptoms, as well as parent-child conflict and communication. *Soc. Sci. Med.* **2020**, *264*, 113293. [CrossRef] [PubMed]
36. Pynoos, R.S.; Steinberg, A.M.; Piacentini, J.C. A developmental psychopathology model of childhood traumatic stress and intersection with anxiety disorders. *Biol. Psychiatry* **1999**, *46*, 1542–1554. [CrossRef]
37. Bronfenbrenner, U. *The Ecology of Human Development: Experiments by Nature and Design*; Harvard University Press: Cambridge, MA, USA, 1979.
38. Kelley, M.L.; Self-Brown, S.; Le, B.; Bosson, J.V.; Hernandez, B.C.; Gordon, A.T. Predicting posttraumatic stress symptoms in children following Hurricane Katrina: A prospective analysis of the effect of parental distress and parenting practices. *J. Trauma Stress* **2010**, *23*, 582–590. [CrossRef] [PubMed]
39. Morris, A.; Gabert-Quillen, C.; Delahanty, D. The association between parent PTSD/depression symptoms and child PTSD symptoms: A meta-analysis. *J. Pediatr. Psychol.* **2012**, *37*, 1076–1088. [CrossRef] [PubMed]
40. Salmon, K.; Bryant, R.A. Posttraumatic stress disorder in children: The influence of developmental factors. *Clin. Psychol. Rev.* **2002**, *22*, 163–188. [CrossRef]
41. Spell, A.W.; Kelley, M.L.; Wang, J.; Self-Brown, S.; Davidson, K.L.; Pellegrin, A.; Palcic, J.L.; Meyer, K.; Paasch, V.; Baumeister, A. The moderating effects of maternal psychopathology on children's adjustment post–Hurricane Katrina. *J. Clin. Child. Psychol.* **2008**, *37*, 553–563. [CrossRef]
42. De Young, A.C.; Hendrikz, J.; Kenardy, J.A.; Cobham, V.E.; Kimble, R.M. Prospective evaluation of parent distress following pediatric burns and identification of risk factors for young child and parent posttraumatic stress disorder. *J. Child. Adolesc. Psychopharmacol.* **2014**, *24*, 9–17. [CrossRef]
43. Daviss, W.B.; Mooney, D.; Racusin, R.; Ford, J.D.; Fleischer, A.; McHugo, G.J. Predicting posttraumatic stress after hospitalization for pediatric injury. *J. Am. Acad Child. Adolesc. Psychiatry* **2000**, *39*, 576–583. [CrossRef]
44. Landolt, M.A.; Vollrath, M.; Ribi, K.; Gnehm, H.E.; Sennhauser, F.H. Incidence and associations of parental and child posttraumatic stress symptoms in pediatric patients. *J. Child. Psychol. Psychiatry* **2003**, *44*, 1199–1207. [CrossRef]
45. Landolt, M.A.; Ystrom, E.; Sennhauser, F.H.; Gnehm, H.E.; Vollrath, M.E. The mutual prospective influence of child and parental post-traumatic stress symptoms in pediatric patients. *J. Child. Psychol. Psychiatry* **2012**, *53*, 767–774. [CrossRef]
46. Nugent, N.R.; Ostrowski, S.; Christopher, N.C.; Delahanty, D.L. Parental posttraumatic stress symptoms as a moderator of child's acute biological response and subsequent posttraumatic stress symptoms in pediatric injury patients. *J. Pediatr. Psychol.* **2007**, *32*, 309–318. [CrossRef]

47. Scheeringa, M.S.; Myers, L.; Putnam, F.W.; Zeanah, C.H. Maternal factors as moderators or mediators of PTSD symptoms in very young children: A two-year prospective study. *J. Fam. Violence* **2015**, *30*, 633–642. [CrossRef]
48. Wise, A.E.; Delahanty, D.L. Parental factors associated with child post-traumatic stress following injury: A consideration of intervention targets. *Front. Psychol.* **2017**, *8*, 1412. [CrossRef]
49. Wong, S.S.; Kletter, H.; Wong, Y.; Carrion, V.G. A prospective study on the association between caregiver psychological symptomatology and symptom clusters of pediatric posttraumatic stress disorder. *J. Trauma Stress* **2013**, *26*, 385–391. [CrossRef] [PubMed]
50. Conway, A.; McDonough, S.C.; MacKenzie, M.J.; Follett, C.; Sameroff, A. Stress-related changes in toddlers and their mothers following the attack of September 11. *Am. J. Orthopsychiatry* **2013**, *83*, 536–544. [CrossRef] [PubMed]
51. de Vries, A.P.; Kassam-Adams, N.; Cnaan, A.; Sherman-Slate, E.; Gallagher, P.R.; Winston, F.K. Looking beyond the physical injury: Posttraumatic stress disorder in children and parents after pediatric traffic injury. *Pediatrics* **1999**, *104*, 1293–1299. [CrossRef] [PubMed]
52. Birmes, P.; Raynaud, J.P.; Daubisse, L.; Brunet, A.; Arbus, C.; Klein, R.; Cailhol, L.; Allenou, C.; Hazane, F.; Grandjean, H.; et al. Children's enduring PTSD symptoms are related to their family's adaptability and cohesion. *Community Ment. Health J.* **2009**, *45*, 290–299. [CrossRef]
53. Halevi, G.; Djalovski, A.; Vengrober, A.; Feldman, R. Risk and resilience trajectories in war-exposed children across the first decade of life. *J. Child. Psychol. Psychiatry* **2016**, *57*, 1183–1193. [CrossRef]
54. Koplewicz, H.S.; Vogel, J.M.; Solanto, M.V.; Morrissey, R.F.; Alonso, C.M.; Abikoff, H.; Gallagher, R.; Novick, R.M. Child and parent response to the 1993 World Trade Center bombing. *J. Trauma Stress* **2002**, *15*, 77–85. [CrossRef] [PubMed]
55. Samuelson, K.W.; Wilson, C.K.; Padrón, E.; Lee, S.; Gavron, L. Maternal PTSD and children's adjustment: Parenting stress and emotional availability as proposed mediators. *J. Clin. Psychol.* **2017**, *73*, 693–706. [CrossRef] [PubMed]
56. Pfefferbaum, B.; North, C.S.; Narayanan, P.; Dumont, C.E. The relationship between maternal psychopathology and parental perceptions of their children's reactions in survivors of the 1998 US Embassy bombing in Nairobi, Kenya. *Ann. Clin. Psychiatry* **2019**, *31*, 260–270. [PubMed]
57. Laor, N.; Wolmer, L.; Mayes, L.C.; Gershon, A.; Weizman, R.; Cohen, D.J. Israeli preschool children under Scuds: A 30-month follow-up. *J. Am. Acad. Child. Adolesc. Psychiatry* **1997**, *36*, 349–356. [CrossRef]
58. Laor, N.; Wolmer, L.; Cohen, D.J. Mothers' functioning and children's symptoms 5 years after a SCUD missile attack. *Am. J. Psychiatry* **2001**, *158*, 1020–1026. [CrossRef]
59. Endo, T.; Shioiri, T.; Someya, T.; Toyabe, S.; Akazawa, K. Parental mental health affects behavioral changes in children following a devastating disaster: A community survey after the 2004 Niigata-Chuetsu earthquake. *Gen. Hosp. Psychiatry* **2007**, *29*, 175–176. [CrossRef] [PubMed]
60. Honda, Y.; Fujiwara, T.; Yagi, J.; Homma, H.; Mashiko, H.; Nagao, K.; Okuyama, M.; Ono-Kihara, M.; Kihara, M. Long-term impact of parental post-traumatic stress disorder symptoms on mental health of their offspring after the great east Japan earthquake. *Front. Psychiatry* **2019**, *10*, 496. [CrossRef]
61. Juth, V.; Silver, R.C.; Seyle, D.C.; Widyatmoko, C.S.; Tan, E.T. Post-disaster mental health among parent–child dyads after a major earthquake in Indonesia. *J. Abnorm. Child. Psychol.* **2015**, *43*, 1309–1318. [CrossRef]
62. Kiliç, E.Z.; Özgüven, H.D.; Sayil, I. The psychological effects of parental mental health on children experiencing disaster: The experience of Bolu earthquake in Turkey. *Fam. Process.* **2003**, *42*, 485–495. [CrossRef]
63. Kiliç, C.; Kiliç, E.Z.; Aydin, I.O. Effect of relocation and parental psychopathology on earthquake survivor-children's mental health. *J. Nerv. Ment. Dis.* **2011**, *199*, 335–341. [CrossRef]
64. Shi, X.; Zhou, Y.; Geng, F.; Li, Y.; Zhou, J.; Lei, B.; Chen, S.; Chen, X.; Fan, F. Posttraumatic stress disorder symptoms in parents and adolescents after the Wenchuan earthquake: A longitudinal actor-partner interdependence model. *J. Affect. Disord.* **2018**, *226*, 301–306. [CrossRef]
65. Polusny, M.A.; Ries, B.J.; Meis, L.A.; DeGarmo, D.; McCormick-Deaton, C.M.; Thuras, P.; Erbes, C.R. Effects of parents' experiential avoidance and PTSD on adolescent disaster-related posttraumatic stress symptomatology. *J. Fam. Psychol.* **2011**, *25*, 220. [CrossRef]
66. Dyb, G.; Jensen, T.K.; Nygaard, E. Children's and parents' posttraumatic stress reactions after the 2004 tsunami. *Clin. Child. Psychol. Psychiatry* **2011**, *16*, 621–634. [CrossRef] [PubMed]
67. Li, Y.; Huang, X.; Tan, H.; Liu, A.; Zhou, J.; Yang, T. A study on the relationship between posttraumatic stress disorder in flood victim parents and children in Hunan, China. *Aust. N. Z. J. Psychiatry* **2010**, *44*, 543–550. [CrossRef] [PubMed]
68. Leen-Feldner, E.W.; Feldner, M.T.; Bunaciu, L.; Blumenthal, H. Associations between parental posttraumatic stress disorder and both offspring internalizing problems and parental aggression within the National Comorbidity Survey-Replication. *J. Anxiety Disorder* **2011**, *25*, 169–175. [CrossRef] [PubMed]
69. North, C.S.; Mendoza, S.; Simic, Z.; Pfefferbaum, B. Parent-reported behavioral and emotional responses of children to disaster and parental psychopathology. *J. Loss Trauma* **2018**, *23*, 303–316. [CrossRef] [PubMed]
70. Cobham, V.E.; McDermott, B.; Haslam, D.; Sanders, M.R. The role of parents, parenting and the family environment in children's post-disaster mental health. *Curr. Psychiatry Rep.* **2016**, *18*, 53. [CrossRef]
71. Self-Brown, S.; Lai, B.S.; Harbin, S.; Kelley, M.L. Maternal posttraumatic stress disorder symptom trajectories following Hurricane Katrina: An initial examination of the impact of maternal trajectories on the well-being of disaster-exposed youth. *Int J. Public Health* **2014**, *59*, 957–965. [CrossRef]

72. Pfefferbaum, B.; North, C.S. The association between parent-reported child disaster reactions and posttraumatic stress disorder in parent survivors of disasters and terrorism. *Ann. Clin. Psychiatry* **2020**, *32*, 256–265. [CrossRef] [PubMed]
73. Scheeringa, M.S.; Zeanah, C.H. Reconsideration of harm's way: Onsets and comorbidity patterns of disorders in preschool children and their caregivers following Hurricane Katrina. *J. Clin. Child. Adolesc. Psychol.* **2008**, *37*, 508–518. [CrossRef] [PubMed]
74. Beardselee, W.R.; Versage, E.M.; Giadstone, T.R. Children of affectively ill parents: A review of the past 10 years. *J. Am. Acad Child. Adolesc. Psychiatry* **1998**, *37*, 1134–1141. [CrossRef]
75. Rutter, M.; Quinton, D. Parental psychiatric disorder: Effects on children. *Psychol. Med.* **1984**, *14*, 853–880. [CrossRef]
76. Weissman, M.M.; Wickramaratne, P.; Nomura, Y.; Warner, V.; Pilowsky, D.; Verdeli, H. Offspring of depressed parents: 20 years later. *Am. J. Psychiatry* **2006**, *163*, 1001–1008. [CrossRef]
77. Pynoos, R.; Rodriguez, N.; Steinberg, A.; Stuber, M.; Frederick, C. *UCLA Posttraumatic Stress Disorder Reaction Index for DSM-IV*; UCLA Trauma Psychiatry Program; NCTSN: Los Angeles, CA, USA, 1998.
78. Derogatis, L.; Lipman, R.; Covi, L. The SCL-90: An outpatient psychiatric rating scale. *Psychopharmacol. Bull.* **1973**, *9*, 13–28.
79. Derogatis, L.R. *Symptom Checklist 90-R: Administration, Scoring, and Procedures Manual*, 3rd ed.; National Computer Systems: Eden Prairie, MI, USA, 1994.
80. Sarno, I.; Preti, E.; Prunas, A.; Madeddu, F. *SCL-90-R Symptom Checklist-90-R Adattamento Italiano*; Giunti Organizzazioni Speciali: Firenze, Italy, 2011.
81. Prunas, A.; Sarno, I.; Preti, E.; Madeddu, F.; Perugini, M. Psychometric properties of the Italian version of the SCL-90-R: A study on a large community sample. *Eur. Psychiatry* **2012**, *27*, 591–597. [CrossRef]
82. Panciroli, G.; Forresi, B.; Soncini, F.; Botosso, E.; Di Pietro, E.; Scarpini, G.; Scaini, S.; Aggazzotti, G.; Caffo, E.; Righi, E. Parental and offspring psychopathological disorders after the 2012 Italian earthquake. *Eur. J. Public Health* **2020**, *30*, 753. [CrossRef]
83. Hudson, J.L.; Doyle, A.M.; Gar, N. Child and maternal influence on parenting behavior in clinically anxious children. *J. Clin. Child. Adolesc. Psychol.* **2009**, *38*, 256–262. [CrossRef] [PubMed]
84. McLeod, B.D.; Wood, J.J.; Weisz, J.R. Examining the association between parenting and childhood anxiety: A meta-analysis. *Clin. Psychol. Rev.* **2007**, *27*, 155–172. [CrossRef] [PubMed]
85. Rork, K.E.; Morris, T.L. Influence of parenting factors on childhood social anxiety: Direct observation of parental warmth and control. *Child. Fam. Behav. Ther.* **2009**, *31*, 220–235. [CrossRef]
86. Rüstemli, A.; Karanci, A.N. Distress reactions and earthquake-related cognitions of parents and their adolescent children in a victimized population. *Soc. Behav. Pers.* **1996**, *11*, 767–780.
87. Ehlers, A.; Clark, D.M. A cognitive model of posttraumatic stress disorder. *Behav. Res. Ther.* **2000**, *38*, 319–345. [CrossRef]
88. Mirzamani, M.; Bolton, D. PTSD symptoms of mothers following occurrence of a disaster affecting their children. *Psychol. Rep.* **2002**, *90*, 431–438. [CrossRef] [PubMed]
89. Le Brocque, R.M.; Hendrikz, J.; Kenardy, J.A. Parental response to child injury: Examination of parental posttraumatic stress symptom trajectories following child accidental injury. *J. Pediatr. Psychol.* **2010**, *35*, 646–655. [CrossRef]
90. Hall, E.; Saxe, G.; Stoddard, F.; Kaplow, J.; Koenen, K.; Chawla, N.; Lopez, C.; King, L.; King, D. Posttraumatic stress symptoms in parents of children with acute burns. *J. Pediatr. Psychol.* **2006**, *31*, 403–412. [CrossRef]
91. Holt, T.; Cohen, J.; Mannarino, A.; Jensen, T.K. Parental Emotional Response to Children's Traumas. *J. Aggress Maltreat. Trauma* **2014**, *23*, 1057–1071. [CrossRef]
92. Cohen, J.A.; Deblinger, E.; Mannarino, A.P. Trauma-focused cognitive behavioral therapy for children and families. *Psychother. Res.* **2018**, *28*, 47–57. [CrossRef]

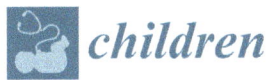

Article

Assessment of Psychological Distress and Peer Relations among Trans Adolescents—An Examination of the Use of Gender Norms and Parent–Child Congruence of the YSR-R/CBCL-R among a Treatment-Seeking Sample

Alexandra Brecht [1,*], Sascha Bos [1], Laura Ries [1], Sibylle M. Winter [1] and Claudia Calvano [1,2]

[1] Department of Child and Adolescent Psychiatry, Charité—Universitätsmedizin Berlin, Corporate Member of Freie Universität Berlin, Humboldt Universität zu Berlin and Berlin Insitute of Health, 13353 Berlin, Germany; sascha.bos@charite.de (S.B.); lauralenaries@gmail.com (L.R.); sibylle.winter@charite.de (S.M.W.); claudia.calvano@charite.de (C.C.)

[2] Department of Education and Psychology, Clinical Child and Adolescent Psychology and Psychotherapy, Freie Universität Berlin, 14195 Berlin, Germany

* Correspondence: alexandra.brecht@charite.de; Tel.: +49-30-450-566-653

Citation: Brecht, A.; Bos, S.; Ries, L.; Winter, S.M.; Calvano, C. Assessment of Psychological Distress and Peer Relations among Trans Adolescents—An Examination of the Use of Gender Norms and Parent–Child Congruence of the YSR-R/CBCL-R among a Treatment-Seeking Sample. *Children* **2021**, *8*, 864. https://doi.org/10.3390/children8100864

Academic Editor: Matteo Alessio Chiappedi

Received: 20 August 2021
Accepted: 23 September 2021
Published: 28 September 2021

Publisher's Note: MDPI stays neutral with regard to jurisdictional claims in published maps and institutional affiliations.

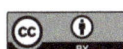

Copyright: © 2021 by the authors. Licensee MDPI, Basel, Switzerland. This article is an open access article distributed under the terms and conditions of the Creative Commons Attribution (CC BY) license (https://creativecommons.org/licenses/by/4.0/).

Abstract: Among trans adolescents, increased psychological distress is reported in the literature. The goal of this study was to examine psychological distress, associated peer relations and parent report congruence among the treatment-seeking sample of the Gender Identity Special Consultation (GISC) for youth at the Charité Berlin. Further, differences between the instruments' binary gender norms were investigated. Retrospectively, we analyzed clinical data derived from the GISC. By initial interviews and using the Youth Self-Report and Child Behavior Checklist, $n = 50$ trans adolescents aged 12–18 years ($M = 15.5$) were examined for psychological problems and peer relations. Congruence between self and parent report was analyzed by correlations. Half of the sample reported suicidality, self-harm and bullying. Trans adolescents showed significantly higher internalizing and total problems than the German norm population. The congruence between self and parent report proved to be moderate to high. The level of congruence and poor peer relations were identified as predictors of internalizing problems. Significant differences between the female vs. male gender norms emerged regarding mean scores and the number of clinically significant cases. Data provide valuable implications for intervention on a peer and family level. There are limitations to the suitability of questionnaires that use binary gender norms, and further research on adequate instruments and assessment is needed.

Keywords: trans adolescents; psychological distress; internalizing problems; YSR-R/CBCL-R; internalizing problems; parental congruence; peer relations; gender minority stress

1. Introduction

A topic that has been discussed, controversially, in medicine and psychology in recent years is the question of care for children and adolescents who do not identify with the gender they are assigned at birth [1]. While medicine calls this experience gender incongruence (GIC) or trans identity, affected people use various self-ascribed names to express their identity, such as transgender or genderqueer. A fluid perception between both female and male gender identity is, among others, described as gender variance. People who identify themselves neither as female nor male describe themselves, for example, as non-binary [2]. In this paper, we used the terms gender incongruence and trans as umbrella terms for people who do not identify with their at birth assigned sex (ABAS). This aims to acknowledge and include all variations of gender identity. It is noteworthy that the umbrella term used in this paper differs from the diagnosis of gender incongruence as defined in the ICD-11 classification system.

Prevalence rates for gender identity are provided by the large population-based Health Behaviour in School Aged Children study in Hamburg, Germany. Among 940 children and adolescents (10–16 years of age), 1.6% ($n = 15$) reported GIC, 1.1% gender variance and 1.5% identified themselves as non-binary [3].

Notably, treatment guidelines and legal frameworks vary across countries and even affirmative care has been of debate in several countries. In Germany, different, often interdisciplinary healthcare offers for trans adolescents, such as peer or psychological counseling, medical treatment options regarding a transition (social, judicial, medical) and endocrinological treatment, e.g., puberty-blockers, can provide time within the physical and sexual development and reduce gender dysphoria significantly [4]. In turn, a prerequisite for a medical transition is the utilization of psychological assessment and/or support.

While gender variety is a growing political and societal phenomenon—in Germany, for example, "diverse" was included as an official gender option for intersexual persons [5]—the relevance for child and adolescent psychiatry is increasing as well, as young people with GIC face several societal challenges and burdens that can lead to psychological distress. For example, in order to change their official surname, trans people have to undergo expensive psychological evaluation. Many suffer from being misgendered (being addressed as the wrong gender) and have to face discrimination, hostility and crimes [6]. Even though a tendency for increased healthcare-seeking among adolescents with GIC has been identified [7], specialized services and staff in the field of child and adolescent psychiatry are still lacking [8,9].

1.1. Mental Health Problems in Trans Adolescents

The prevalence of psychological distress in trans adolescents is alarmingly high. In their study among 218 adolescents aged 12–18 years with GIC and referred to the Gender Identity Development Service in London, Holt et al. [10] drew the conclusion that 49.7% suffered from depression, 23.7% from anxiety symptoms, 44% from self-harm and 39.5% from suicidal thoughts and intentions. Furthermore, 15.8% reported suicide attempts, 19.2% substance abuse, 16.4% had eating disorders, 6.8% ADHD and 5.7% psychoses. In a community-based non-clinical study on psychological distress among trans adolescents in Canada ($n = 923$) [11], 75% of the adolescents showed self-harming behavior and 65% suicidal thoughts and intentions, and 32% reported at least one suicide attempt in the past year. In Germany, too, high rates of suicidality and self-harm were found among adolescents with GIC who were referred to gender identity services [12,13]; although, thus far, surveys have been few in number and small in their sample sizes [14]. Looking at the most common psychological symptoms in adolescents with GIC, a strong tendency towards internalizing psychological problems is found [14,15]. In the area of child and adolescent psychiatry, a common way to assess mental health problems is using the questionnaires Youth Self-Report (YSR-R) and Child Behaviour Checklist (CBCL-R). There are several research groups who have used these instruments to evaluate the psychological distress of trans children and adolescents. Their findings can be summarized insofar as young trans people suffer significantly more frequently from mental health problems than their gender-conforming peer group, and especially from internalizing rather than from externalizing problems [14,16–18].

1.2. Bullying and Poor Peer Relationships

Bullying and poor peer relationships were identified as strong predictors of mental health problems in trans adolescents [10,16,19]. In the above mentioned study of Holt et al. [10], almost half of the trans adolescents (47%) experienced bullying in school and their social environment. Many young trans people suffer from social isolation and a lack of friendships and relationships [16,17]. In the literature, some research groups have investigated the association between mobbing and psychological distress using the Poor Peer Relation Scale (PPR Scale), which can be constructed out of the YSR-R. The findings showed a high level of poor peer relations among trans adolescents [16,17].

Since discrimination, mobbing and minority stress leads to mental health problems, it is important to investigate peer relations among trans adolescents who represent an often marginalized group in our society [6,19,20].

1.3. Gender-Related Distributions of Psychological Distress

In the general population, girls are more likely to show internalizing than externalizing problems, whereas boys are more likely to have externalizing problems [21–23]. The literature provides different findings regarding sex- or gender-based differences in mental health problems among trans adolescents, i.e., differences between the at birth assigned sex and the gender identity (GID). In a cross-national study of emotional and behavioral problems of trans adolescents in Toronto and Amsterdam [17], the data suggested that it was not the ABAS but the gender identity that was in line with the aforementioned general pattern. In their study, trans girls with a male at birth assigned sex (MABAS) suffered significantly more often from internalizing than externalizing problems, whereas trans boys with a female at birth assigned sex (FABAS) showed more externalizing than internalizing problems. In consequence, the authors postulated a "general pattern of reversal" [17] (p. 585) for trans adolescents since it was more common for girls to suffer from internalizing than externalizing problems and for boys vice versa. Other studies, however, found higher problem scores for trans boys [16] or no differences at all [24]. For the examination, the research group used the abovementioned YSR-R and CBCL-R. These established instruments, as well as others, evaluate the scores based on comparisons to the respective population's gender group (boys/girls). This process tends to be unclear when working with people who cannot identify with their ABAS. Most research groups used the ABAS for the evaluation [16–18], whereas some others mentioned uncertainty about which YSR/CBCL gender norm should be used with trans adolescents [14,16,25]. It is still unclear how to best use these instruments when working with trans and non-binary people [25]. Rider et al. [25] investigated the influence of the selection of the gender norm male/female of the CBCL-R on the scale scores of gender-nonconforming and trans children (n = 55) and adolescents (n = 53). Differences in somatic problems, oppositional behaviour and internalizing symptoms between the binary gender-normed scores were particularly evident. However, the choice of gender norm did not appear to have a significant impact on whether a score was considered clinically significant or not. Nevertheless, whether binary-normed instruments should be used with trans adolescents is still up for debate [26,27].

1.4. Congruence between Parent and Child Reports on Psychological Stress in Adolescents

Another relevant issue in the use of questionnaire measures for the assessment of psychological distress in children and adolescents is the role of parental perception of distress. Firstly, the use of counseling and treatment for mental health problems in adolescents is primarily related to parental perception of psychological distress [28–30]. Specifically for trans adolescents, parental perception and awareness of a child's distress play a central role with respect to their children's coming-out process, mental health and access to medical counseling and treatment [31–35]. In the general population, the congruence between adolescent and parent reports on adolescent psychopathology is low to moderate [36–39]. Furthermore, among population-based and clinical non-trans samples, the discordance between the child's and the parent's perception of mental health problems is associated with poorer outcomes [37,40,41]. Only a few studies have investigated the congruence between parent and child report among samples of trans adolescents. For example, Zucker et al. [42] found moderate correlations between the YSR and CBCL main scales (r = 0.44–0.48) for adolescents with a FABAS, whereas for adolescents with a MABAS, the correlations were low to moderate and only significant for the externalizing problems scale (r = 0.03–0.39). In a more recent study, De Graaf [43] compared a suicidality sum score, constructed by two items from YSR-R and CBCL-R asking for suicidal ideation and intentions, between parent and child report in cross-national samples. Interestingly, the correlations differed strongly from low to strong regarding ABAS and country. Since the discordance between parent and child report was identified as a predictor for poorer health outcomes among adolescents from general samples [36,37], it is important to obtain a firm analysis about parent–child congruence among trans adolescents, and investigate if the congruence can be identified as a predictor for psychological distress, too.

1.5. Aims and Hypotheses

Hence, the aims of this study are sixfold: (1) an analysis of mental health problems and gender differences among the treatment-seeking sample of trans youth, (2) the relationship between mental health problems and peer relations, (3) an evaluation of the congruence between parent and child report (4) its relation to trans adolescents' mental health problems, and (5) investigation as to whether the reports' congruence and poor peer relations predict psychological distress of trans adolescents. Further, we aim to (6) investigate the effect of the use of different genders norms of the YSR-/CBCL-R.

We hypothesized that (1) trans adolescents report significantly more mental health problems than the norm population, and that there are significant differences between the at birth assigned sexes (female/male) insofar as trans girls report higher internalizing problems than trans boys and trans boys report higher externalizing problems than trans girls; (2) trans adolescents' mental health problems are positively related to poor peer relations; (3) in the self report, trans adolescents report higher levels of psychological distress than their parents in the parent report, leading to a low report congruence/correlation; (4) higher levels of incongruence are significantly positively associated with higher scores of the trans adolescents' psychological problems; (5) the level of congruence and poor peer relations predict psychological distress significantly. We further hypothesize that (6) the results of the YSR and CBCL will be significantly different depending on the gender norm used: the gender norm for boys will lead to higher scores in internalizing problems than the norm for girls, whereas the gender norm for girls will result in higher scores in externalizing problems than the gender norm for boys.

2. Materials and Methods

2.1. Procedure

The present work investigated the psychological stress of adolescents with GIC who consulted the Gender Identity Special Consultation (GISC) at the Charité Universitätsmedizin Berlin, Germany. Affiliated with the Department of Child and Adolescent Psychiatry, the GISC is specialized in the care of children and adolescents with GIC, provided by an interdisciplinary team consisting of psychologists, endocrinologists, psychiatrists, pediatrics and speech therapists. The GISC offers interdisciplinary education and treatment services ranging from initial psychological counseling to endocrinological and phoniatric treatment. The patients seeking care are not restricted to the city of Berlin. The inclusion of caregivers as well as the recognition of the individual development stage of each person is of crucial importance.

The GISC includes concomitant research, covering interview and questionnaire measures on gender identity, sexual orientation and mental health. Parents are asked to provide data on socioeconomic background and also to report on their child's mental health. Further, in every initial consultation, suicidality, self-harm, other psychological symptoms or problems and bullying experiences are explored. This assessment includes the most common mental health problems in order to provide a thorough mental health screening; other parts of the psychiatric assessment such as the assessment of neurological symptoms were not included. However, in cases of a suspicion of other neurological problems, the GISC is able to refer to child psychiatrists at the clinic, which has, so far, not been the case. The diagnosis of gender incongruence according to ICD-11 is assigned and documented by the responsible psychologist according to the therapeutic assessment. This study was a retrospective analysis of the treatment-seeking sample based on the clinical documentation at time of first presentation of the GISC December 2018–November 2020. The concomitant research was approved by the Charité ethics committee (EA2/201/20, date 9 March 2020).

2.2. Material/Measures

2.2.1. Psychological Distress

Suicidality, the occurrence of self-injuries and the experience of bullying were evaluated and documented in the initial clinical assessment session by a licensed psychologists, specialized in gender identity and variety, at the GISC.

On a quantitative level, psychological distress was measured by the Youth Self-Report for 11–18 year olds (YSR-R) [44] and by the parent reported Child Behavior Checklist for 6–18 year olds (CBCL-R) [45]. Normative scores for the German populations are available [46]. All 120 items are answered on a 3-point scale (0 = does not apply, 1 = somewhat or sometimes applies, 2 = exactly or often applies). Both questionnaires provide eight problem scales (scales that intend to capture the construct of the respective problem area and its symptoms such as depressive/anxious), which in turn are assigned to three superordinate scales (main scales): Internalizing Problems, Externalizing Problems and Total Problems. For the assessment of clinical significance, a cut-off of a T-value > 69 was specified for the eight problem scales according to the manual [46]; the borderline range is from 65 to 69. For the superordinate problem scales of Internalizing and Externalizing Problems and the Total Problems scores, a $T > 63$ is clinically significant; the borderline range is defined by T-values from 60 to 63. The instruments' reliability is high, given an internal consistency for the main scales of $\alpha = 0.88$–0.94 for the YSR-R and $\alpha = 0.82$–0.93 for the CBCL. The convergent validity is proved by high correlations with validated syndrome scales for both instruments' scales [46].

Since uncertainty about the choice of gender norms when using the CBCL-R and YSR-R for young trans people had already been expressed in various studies [16,25,27], we used both female and male gender norms for each person's evaluation. This means that the raw scores of each questionnaire were compared with the values of both boys and girls from the standardization sample, which can result in different scale scores and corresponding T-values.

2.2.2. Peer Relations

The degree of problems in social interactions with peers is measured using three items from the YSR-R, defined as the Poor Peer Relations Scale (PPR Scale; [47]): Item 25 ("I don't get along with other children"), Item 38 ("I get teased a lot") and Item 48 ("I am not liked by other children"). The PPR Scale has already been used in various studies to examine adolescents with GIC [16–18]. In the present sample, the internal consistency of the scale is Cronbach's $\alpha = 0.75$. A higher number of points on the PPR Scale indicates a higher degree of peer problems (range 0–6).

2.3. Data Analysis

Data were analyzed using SPSS 25 [48]. For the first aim, comparisons with norm scores were conducted by one-sample t-tests. Additionally, differences in the psychological stress between the two groups MABAS and FABAS were calculated using t-tests for independent samples for the scales Internalizing, Externalizing and Total Problems.

Secondly, associations between psychological distress and peer relations were analyzed by Pearson correlations. Thirdly, congruence between parent and child report was also explored by Pearson's correlations. To calculate the difference between the self report and the parent's report, the mean value of the CBCL-R was subtracted from the mean value of the YSR-R for each scale (DIFF = M_YSR-R − M_CBCL-R). These differences were added up to form an aggregated total difference variable (DIFF_Tot). The sign of these difference values can already provide information for each case as to whether the scale scores of the YSR-R are greater than those of the CBCL-R (positive sign) or vice versa (negative sign). In order to determine a relationship between psychological distress and parental agreement, a Pearson correlation was performed between the total difference variables and the three main scales of the YSR-R.

For the fourth aim, we conducted a multiple linear regression analysis using the Internalizing Problem scores evaluated both by male gender norm and female gender norm as outcome variables. The predictors were entered blockwise into the regression model by entry in three steps. In the first step, the covariates age and ABAS were included in order to control possible confounding effects. In the second step, the PPR score was introduced to investigate whether poor peer relations can be identified as a predictor for psychological distress. In the third and last step, the reports' difference variable (DIFF_Tot) according to the respective gender norm evaluation was added. Since only T-scores and no raw scores were available, we used the Internalizing Problem score as an outcome variable because the items of the PPR Scale could not be extracted from the Total Problems score, which otherwise would have led to a confounding. Based on 1000 bootstrap samples, 95% bias-corrected and accelerated confidence intervals for the coefficient B and its standard errors were calculated, which makes the regression robust against violations of homoscedasticity that are often found in small sample sizes as ours. For our sample size of $n = 50$ and four predictors, large effects were assumed ($f = 0.26$) which can be tested with a power of 94% (calculated by GPower).

For the fifth aim, in order to check whether the YSR-R/CBCL-R scores differ significantly depending on the use of the assigned at birth norm vs. the gender identity norm, a comparison of the mean scores of the main and problem scales of the YSR-R and CBCL-R between the male and female gender norms was carried out using the t-test for dependent samples. For this, only cases with the same GID (male or female) are selected. One person who identified as non-binary was excluded from these hypotheses.

Finally, it was investigated whether the number of cases with clinically increased levels of distress changed depending on the use of the assigned at birth norm versus the gender identity's norm. For this purpose, a comparison between the dichotomous variables (0 = not clinically significant, 1 = clinically significant) according to each gender norm (cut-off value main scales: $T > 63$, problem scales: $T > 69$) (Döpfner et al., 2014), was calculated using the McNemar test. As an additional effect measure, the odds ratio (OR) was used. OR = 1 indicates no change in clinically significant proportions between evaluation according to GID and ABAS; OR < 1 means that the clinically significant cases in the evaluation according to ABAS are higher than according to GID, and OR > 1 indicates that the clinically significant proportions in the evaluation according to GID are higher than according to ABAS. Every analysis was run through a bias-corrected and accelerated (BCa) bootstrapping ($\alpha = 5\%$).

2.4. Sample

The primary inclusion criterion for this study was the determination of gender incongruence according to ICD-11 (still unpublished), a minimum age of twelve years and the presence of a complete CBCL and YSR dyad. Initially, $n = 66$ trans adolescents were referred to the GISC; $n = 53$ adolescents resp. their parents had filled out at least one questionnaire, leading to a final sample size of $n = 50$ that had filled out both YSR-R and CBCL-R. The sample was on average 15.5 years old ($SD = 1.64$; range 12–18). It consisted of 11 trans girls (22.0%) (MABAS) and 38 (76.0%) trans boys (FABAS), and one person identified as non-binary (FABAS). At this point it should be noted that some gender-variant people also use other self-descriptions and identities (e.g., non-binary, agender, queer), which, however, could not be recorded in this work and were therefore subsumed under the term trans.

3. Results
3.1. Psychological Distress

In the initial assessment interview, 54.0% of the adolescents reported suicidality (suicidal thoughts, intentions, or attempted suicide), 48.0% stated that they had already harmed themselves at least once and 44.0% had experienced bullying now or in the past.

The descriptive evaluation of YSR-R and CBCL-R shows elevated scores for the three main scales and the eight problem scales. Mean values, standard deviations and the percentage of cases whose scores are above the cut-off of the respective scale (main scale: $T > 63$, problem scale: $T > 69$) can be found in Table 1 for YSR-R and Table 2 for CBCL-R.

Table 1. Descriptive evaluation of the main and problem scales of the YSR-R ($n = 50$).

YSR Scale	Male Norm				Female Norm			
	MABAS [12] ($n = 11$)		FABAS [13] ($n = 39$)		MABAS ($n = 11$)		FABAS ($n = 39$)	
	M [14] (SD) [15]	% cl. Sign. [16]	M (SD)	% cl. Sign.	M (SD)	% cl. Sign.	M (SD)	% cl. Sign.
Int [1]	62.55 (10.85)	54.5%	66.82 (12.73)	61.5%	58.27 (9.78)	54.5%	63.05 (11.78)	48.7%
Ext [2]	52 (5.39)	-	53.59 (8.10)	12.8%	52.91 (5.77)	-	55.15 (9.18)	25.6%
Tot [3]	59.64 (8.8)	45.5%	62.49 (10.60)	48.7%	58.55 (8.29)	45.5%	62.59 (10.30)	51.3%
AD [4]	60.91 (10.62)	18.2%	67.05 (10.50)	43.6%	58.91 (9.24)	9.1%	64.87 (10.13)	35.9%
WD [5]	64.18 (10.04)	18.2%	64.33 (10.39)	28.2%	62.73 (10.45)	18.2%	63.15 (10.55)	28.2%
SC [6]	59.55 (6.65)	-	61.74 (9.98)	25.6%	56.09 (4.91)	-	58.56 (8.88)	10.3%
SP [7]	60.82 (8.40)	18.2%	59.54 (8.33)	10.3%	60.82 (7.56)	27.3%	60.31 (8.77)	20.5%
TP [8]	62.55 (9.22)	27.3%	67.46 (11.43)	51.3%	60.64 (8.57)	18.2%	65.90 (10.51)	48.7%
AP [9]	59.36 (6.90)	9.1%	61.33 (11.58)	15.4%	60.18 (6.79)	18.2%	61.87 (11.40)	28.2%
RB [10]	54.27 (6.00)	-	55.79 (5.97)	2.6%	55.27 (6.60)	9.1%	57.49 (7.16)	7.7%
AB [11]	52.36 (2.34)	-	55.15 (5.73)	-	52.82 (2.71)	-	56.03 (6.37)	2.6%

[1] Internalizing Problems, [2] Externalizing Problems, [3] Total Problems, [4] Anxious/Depressed, [5] Withdrawn/Depressed, [6] Somatic Complaints, [7] Social Problems, [8] Thought Problems, [9] Attention Problems, [10] Rule-Breaking Behaviour, [11] Aggressive Behaviour, [12] Male at birth assigned sex, [13] Female at birth assigned sex; [14] Mean; [15] Standard deviation; [16] Clinically significant (T-score main scale > 63, T-score problem scale > 69).

Table 2. Descriptive evaluation of the main and problem scales of the CBCL-R ($n = 50$).

CBCL Scale	Male Norm				Female Norm			
	MABAS [12] ($n = 11$)		FABAS [13] ($n = 39$)		MABAS ($n = 11$)		FABAS ($n = 39$)	
	M [14] (SD) [15]	% cl. Sign. [16]	M (SD)	% cl. Sign.	M (SD)	% cl. Sign.	M (SD)	% cl. Sign.
Int [1]	66.91 (13.10)	54.5%	66.58 (11.66)	56.4%	64.36 (12.04)	45.5%	64.13 (11.46)	56.4%
Ext [2]	56.82 (5.81)	18.2%	54.08 (10.08)	28.2%	56.45 (6.92)	9.1%	53.59 (11.38)	25.6%
Tot [3]	63.09 (8.14)	54.5%	61.05 (10.30)	51.3%	64.09 (9.89)	54.5%	61.77 (10.56)	53.8%
AD [4]	63.00 (10.75)	27.3%	64.25 (10.51)	35.9%	61.82 (10.73)	27.3%	64.11 (10.70)	38.5%
WD [5]	69.64 (14.92)	45.5%	63.35 (8.48)	12.8%	70.91 (15.17)	45.5%	64.37 (8.36)	17.9%
SC [6]	60.55 (10.12)	27.3%	62.64 (10.30)	33.3%	58.91 (9.64)	27.3%	61.31 (10.13)	28.2%
SP [7]	59.27 (8.91)	18.2%	58.35 (6.85)	10.3%	60.18 (10.45)	18.2%	59.36 (7.83)	17.9%
TP [8]	60.45 (8.60)	27.3%	62.21 (8.33)	28.2%	61.00 (8.96)	27.3%	62.32 (8.38)	25.6%
AP [9]	65.55 (11.30)	36.4%	58.30 (8.26)	10.3%	67.82 (11.14)	36.4%	59.94 (8.55)	10.3%
RB [10]	55.45 (5.22)	-	56.05 (6.42)	5.1%	57.18 (6.42)	18.2%	57.97 (7.56)	15.4%
AB [11]	55.73 (5.01)	-	55.02 (6.81)	5.1%	57.00 (6.29)	9.1%	56.10 (8.66)	12.8%

[1] Internalizing Problems, [2] Externalizing Problems, [3] Total Problems, [4] Anxious/Depressed, [5] Withdrawn/Depressed, [6] Somatic Complaints, [7] Social Problems, [8] Thought Problems, [9] Attention Problems, [10] Rule-Breaking Behaviour, [11] Aggressive Behaviour, [12] Male at birth assigned sex, [13] Female at birth assigned sex; [14] Mean; [15] Standard deviation; [16] Clinically significant (T-score main scale > 63, T-score problem scale > 69).

3.2. Psychological Distress of Trans Adolescents Compared to the Normative Sample

In the self-report YSR-R and in the parent report CBCL-R, the internalizing problems and total problems scales for both gender norms were significantly higher than the comparison samples, with large effect sizes ($p < 0.001$; $d = 0.87$–1.37). In contrast, no significant difference between the samples could be found for the Externalizing Problems scale in both child and parent report ($p > 0.05$) (see Table 3).

The mean values of the groups MABAS and FABAS for the main scales of the YSR-R were compared using a one-way ANOVA. No statistically significant main effect could be found between adolescents with FABAS and adolescents with MABAS with regard to their psychological distress ($p > 0.05$) (Table S1).

Table 3. Results of the one-sample *t*-test between the values of the sample and the mean values of the norm sample for the main scales of the YSR-R and CBCL-R.

Variable	M_GISC [6] (SD) [7]	M_Norm [8]	Statistics	Effect Size [9]	BCa 95% CI+ [10]	CI− [10]
YSR_Int [1]_m [2]	65.56 (12.03)	49	$t(53) = 10.12$	$d = 1.37$ *	13.45	20.31
YSR_Ext [3]_m	52.96 (7.44)	52	$t(53) = 0.95$	$d = 0.16$	−0.90	3.19
YSR_Tot [4]_m	61.69 (9.76)	51	$t(53) = 8.04$	$d = 1.08$ *	8.22	13.39
YSR_Int_f [5]	61.37 (11.47)	52	$t(53) = 6.01$	$d = 0.87$ *	6.88	12.94
YSR_Ext_f	54.09 (8.62)	52	$t(53) = 1.78$	$d = 0.31$	0.38	5.26
YSR_Tot_f	61.11 (10.01)	52	$t(53) = 6.70$	$d = 0.97$ *	7.19	12.07
CBCL_Int_m	66.82 (11.92)	54	$t(50) = 7.69$	$d = 1.07$ *	9.37	15.64
CBCL_Ext_m	54.98 (9.39)	54	$t(51) = 0.75$	$d = 0.07$	−0.21	0.35
CBCL_Tot_m	61.82 (9.87)	53	$t(50) = 6.39$	$d = 0.87$ *	5.84	11.13
CBCL_Int_f	64.11 (11.97)	53	$t(53) = 6.82$	$d = 0.96$ *	7.77	14.37
CBCL_Ext_f	54.31 (10.84)	52	$t(53) = 1.57$	$d = 0.21$	−0.79	5.10
CBCL_Tot_f	62.41 (10.52)	53	$t(53) = 6.57$	$d = 0.89$ *	6.52	11.90

[1] Internalizing Problems; [2] Male norm; [3] Externalizing Problems; [4] Total problems; [5] Female norm; [6] Mean of the GISC-sample; [7] Standard deviation; [8] Mean of the manual's norm sample; [9] Significance and effect; * $p < 0.001$; [10] 95% bias-corrected and accelerated confidence interval of mean differences. Each mean of the main scale's score in YSR-R and CBCL-R of the current sample was compared with the respective mean score of the manual's norm population score using both male and female gender norms.

3.3. Poor Peer Relations and Mental Health Problems

Both male and female norm evaluation showed a high, significantly positive Pearson correlation between the YSR-R Internalizing Problems scale and the PPR Scale ($M = 1.34$, $SD = 1.57$, Min = 0, Max = 5) (r PPR ~ YSR_Int_m = 0.52 (0.22, 0.75), $p < 0.001$ and r PPR ~ YSR_Int_w = 0.51 (0.20, 0.73), $p < 0.001$). Thus, a statistically significant, moderate association between poor peer relationships and internalizing problems of adolescents with GIC could be found.

3.4. Agreement between Self and Parent Report

For the main scales of both norm evaluations, there were strong correlations between self report and parent report ($p < 0.001$). The problem scales showed moderate to strong associations between YSR-R and CBCL-R for both norm evaluations ($p < 0.01$) (Table 4).

Table 4. Correlations between main and problem scales of the CBCL-R and YSR-R according to male norm evaluation.

Scale	r YSR_CBCL_m [12]	BCa 95% CI [14]	r YSR_CBCL_f [13]	BCa 95% CI [14]
Int [1]	0.59 **	(0.14, 0.58)	0.61 *	(0.42, 0.76)
Ext [2]	0.51 **	(0.19, 0.76)	0.61 *	(0.40, 0.76)
Tot [3]	0.57 **	(0.34, 0.74)	0.60 *	(0.39, 0.74)
AD [4]	0.47 **	(0.22, 0.70)	0.55 *	(0.31, 0.76)
WD [5]	0.47 **	(0.25, 0.70)	0.45 *	(0.21, 0.69)
SC [6]	0.56 **	(0.29, 0.74)	0.52 *	(0.27, 0.70)
SP [7]	0.44 **	(0.16, 0.66)	0.48 *	(0.23, 0.66)
TP [8]	0.53 **	(0.31, 0.71)	0.54 *	(0.35, 0.71)
AP [9]	0.40 **	(0.22, 0.61)	0.45 *	(0.25, 0.65)
RB [10]	0.53 **	(0.25, 0.72)	0.65 *	(0.43, 0.79)
AB [11]	0.41 **	(0.11, 0.67)	0.49 *	(0.21, 0.71)

[1] Internalizing Problems, [2] Externalizing Problems, [3] Total Problems, [4] Anxious/Depressed, [5] Withdrawn/Depressed, [6] Somatic Complaints, [7] Social Problems, [8] Thought Problems, [9] Attention Problems, [10] Rule-Breaking Behaviour, [11] Aggressive Behaviour, [12] Male norm, [13] Female norm; * $p < 0.01$, ** $p < 0.001$; [14] 95% bias-corrected and accelerated confidence interval of the correlation.

3.5. Association between Psychological Distress and Parental Perception

The mean values of the difference variables according to the male norm evaluation ($M = -1.38$, $SD = 24.81$, Max = 47, Min = −52) and the female norm evaluation ($M = -1.58$,

$SD = 24.34$, Max = 54, Min = −46) were both negative, i.e., the mean values of the CBCL-R were on average greater than those of the YSR-R. The relationships between the difference variables according to both norm evaluations and the Internalizing Problems and Total Problems scales turned out to be significantly positive ($p < 0.01$) with strong to moderate effects. No significant association could be found for the Externalizing Problems scale ($p > 0.05$) (Table 5). Thus, the results indicate that a larger incongruence between parental and self reports is related to a higher degree of internalizing and total problems. There were no significant differences found between the at birth assigned sexes male/female (MABAS/FABAS) regarding the level of parent–child congruence ($p < 0.05$; data not shown).

Table 5. Correlations and 95%-confidence intervals between the difference variable according to male and female norm evaluation with the corresponding scores of the main scales of the YSR-R.

	Int [5]_m/f	Ext [6]_m/f	Tot [2]_m/f
DIFF [1]_Tot [2]_m [3]	0.49 ** (0.24, 0.67)	0.23 (−0.04, 0.46)	0.43 ** (0.20, 0.62)
DIFF_Tot_f [4]	0.47 ** (0.25, 0.67)	0.26 (0.04, 0.47)	0.39 * (0.18, 0.58)

[1] Difference variable of the report's congruence; [2] Total Problems; [3] Male norm; [4] Female norm; [5] Internalizing Problems; [6] Externalizing Problems; * $p < 0.05$; ** $p < 0.01$.

3.6. Poor Peer Relations and Parental Congruence as Predictors of Internalizing Problems

Table 6 provides an overview of the multiple linear regression and the results of the final model with the YSR-R Internalizing Problem scale score by male and female gender norm functioning as an outcome variable. The results of the modeling steps were: first model with age and ABAS as predictors (male norm: adjusted $R^2 = -0.01$, $F(2) = 1.31$, $p = 0.28$; female norm: adjusted $R^2 = 0.03$, $F(2) = 0.1.7$, $p = 0.19$) second model added the PPR score (male norm: adjusted $R^2 = 0.27$; $F(3) = 7.14$, $p < 0.001$; female norm: adjusted $R^2 = 0.28$ $F(3) = 7.22$, $p < 0.001$) ending with the final model introducing the reports' difference variable (male norm: adjusted $R^2 = 0.39$, $F(4) = 8.75$, $p < 0.01$; female norm: adjusted $R^2 = 0.36$, $F(4) = 0.7.84$, $p < 0.001$). The overall male norm model fit was satisfactory, explaining 43.7% of the variance for the Internalizing Problem score, the female norm model was also satisfactory, explaining 41.1% of the outcome variable's variance. The average variance of inflation (male norm: VIF = 1.11; female norm: VIF = 1.16) was not substantially greater than 1. The Durbin–Watson statistics testing the independence of errors was 2.60 (male norm) and 2.48 (female norm) and therefore within the acceptable range (1.0–3.0).

Table 6. Final linear model of predictors of the YSR-R Internalizing Problem score evaluated by male and female gender norm, with 95% bias-corrected and accelerated confidence intervals reported in square brackets. Confidence intervals and standard errors based on 1000 bootstrap samples.

	Male Norm				Female Norm			
	Unstandardized Coefficients		Standardized Coefficents		Unstandardized Coefficients		Standardized Coefficents	
	B [5]	SE [6] B	β	p	B	SE B	β	p
Constant	53.33 (30.07, 79.94)	13.18		$p < 0.01$	49.69 (24.08, 77.16)	12.43		$p < 0.01$
ABAS [1]	1.62 (−4.88, 7.19)	3.18	0.06	$p = 0.64$	2.01 (−4.83, 7.44)	3.06	0.07	$p = 0.55$
Age [2]	0.44 (−1.29, 2.08)	0.82	0.06	$p = 0.62$	0.43 (−1.05, 1.88)	0.78	0.06	$p = 0.62$
PPR score [3]	3.54 (1.96, 5.17)	0.78	0.45	$p < 0.001$	3.19 (1.70, 4.86)	0.75	0.44	$p < 0.01$
DIFF score [4]	0.19 (0.08, 0.30)	0.06	0.38	$p < 0.01$	0.16 (0.05, 2.7)	0.06	0.35	$p < 0.05$

[1] At birth assigned sex; [2] Age at initial session; [3] Poor Peer Relations Scale score; [4] Difference between parent and child report; [5] Regression coefficient; [6] Standard error.

For both male and female gender norm evaluation, the PPR score and the reports' difference variable proved to be significant predictors in the final model, whereas neither age nor ABAS turned out to be significant. Looking at the bootstrapped confidence intervals, zero lay within the intervals for the non-significant but not the significant predictors. Therefore, poor peer relations and the congruence between parent and child report could be identified as predictors for internalizing problems.

3.7. Differences in Assessment Results According to Gender Norm

The differences between the mean scores according to male and female norm evaluation of the main scales of the YSR-R and CBCL-R for trans boys can be seen in Table 7. For higher readability, the results for the eight problem scales of the YSR-R and CBCL-R are summarized in the Supplementary Material (Tables S1 and S2).

Table 7. Differences between the gender norms for the main scales of YSR-R and CBCL-R.

	Trans Boys ($n = 38$)					
	Male Norm	Female Norm			BCa 95%	
Scale	M_GID [4] (SD) [5]	M_ABAS [6] (SD)	Statistics	Effect Size	CI+ [7]	CI− [7]
YSR_Int [1]	66.21 (12.31)	62.45 (11.30)	$t(37) = -6.42$	$d = 1.04$ *	2.20	4.63
YSR_Ex [2]	53.76 (8.14)	55.34 (9.23)	$t(37) = -3.89$	$d = -0.63$	−2.57	−0.97
YSR_Tot [3]	62.24 (10.62)	62.39 (10.36)	$t(37) = -0.18$	$d = -0.03$	−2.38	1.25
CBCL_Int	66.55 (11.81)	64.08 (11.61)	$t(37) = -5.54$	$d = 1.04$ *	−3.32	−1.62
CBCL_Ext	54.40 (10.02)	53.87 (11.39)	$t(37) = -0.49$	$d = -0.63$	−2.76	1.31
CBCL_Tot	61.08 (10.43)	61.79 (10.70)	$t(37) = 1.27$	$d = -0.03$	−0.40	1.68

[1] Internalizing Problems; [2] Externalizing Problems; [3] Total Problems; [4] Mean according gender identity norm; [5] Standard deviation; [6] Mean according at birth assigned sex norm; [7] 95% bias-corrected and accelerated confidence interval for mean differences; * $p < 0.01$.

For trans boys, the mean values of the YSR-R main scale Internalizing Problems and the associated problem scale Physical Complaints (PC) were found to be significantly higher according to male norm evaluation than according to female norm evaluation ($p < 0.01$), with large effect sizes of $d = 1.70$ and 1.04, respectively (Table S2). Similarly, the mean score of the problem scale Rule-Breaking Behaviour (RB), proved to be significantly lower according to the male norm than according to the female norm evaluation ($p < 0.01$), with a likewise large effect size of $d = -0.86$. The mean score of the scale Thinking Problems (TP) was significantly higher according to the male norm than according to the female norm ($p < 0.01$, $d = -0.86$). No significant differences were found for the other scales ($p > 0.05$).

The CBCL-R also showed significantly higher mean values for the scale Internalizing Problems ($p < 0.01$), with a high effect size of $d = 1.04$. The mean values of the problem scale RB proved to be significantly lower according to the male norm than according to the female norm ($p < 0.01$, $d = -0.86$; Table S3). For the problem scales AP and SP, the mean score was significantly higher according to the female norm than according to the male norm ($p < 0.05$, $d = -0.25$−−0.86). No significant difference in means could be determined for the other scales. Summing up, there were significant differences between the mean values of four out of the eleven scales of the YSR-R and the CBCL-R for the evaluations according to the GID and ABAS norms for trans boys.

For trans girls, the results of the *t*-test for dependent samples between the mean scores of the main scales of the YSR-R and CBCL-R according to female and male norm evaluation are presented below (Table 8) and for the problem scales in the Supplementary Material (Tables S4 and S5). The mean scores of the YSR-R Internalizing Problems and associated problems scales (AD, WD, SC) were found to be significantly lower according to the female norm than according to the male norm ($p < 0.01$), with large effect sizes ($d = 1.70$ to -0.46); the same was found for the TP scale ($p < 0.01$, $d = 0.69$). Again, the mean values of the main and problem scales of the Externalizing Problems (RB, AB) were significantly higher according to female than male norm evaluation ($p < 0.05$, $d = -0.35$−−0.86). The mean value of the Total Problem scale proved to be significantly higher according to the male than the female norm ($p < 0.01$) and the effect size was large ($d = 1.31$). Thus, there were significant mean differences for nine scales of the YSR-R between the evaluation according to the GID and ABAS norms for trans girls.

Table 8. Differences between the gender norms for the main scales of YSR-R and CBCL-R for trans girls.

Variable	Trans Girls ($n = 11$)						
	Female Norm	Male Norm				BCa 95%	
	M_GID (SD) [4]	M_ABAS (SD) [5]	Statistics	Effect Size		CI+ [6]	CI− [6]
YSR_Int [1]	58.27 (9.78)	62.55 (10.85)	$t(10) = 12.84$	$d = 1.04$ *		3.60	4.90
YSR_Ext [2]	52.91 (5.77)	52.00 (5.39)	$t(10) = -4.30$	$d = -0.63$ *		−1.30	−0.42
YSR_Tot [3]	58.55 (8.29)	59.64 (8.08)	$t(10) = 4.35$	$d = 1.31$ *		0.57	1.56
CBCL_Int	64.36 (12.04)	66.91 (13.10)	$t(10) = 12.84$	$d = -1.99$ *		−3.37	−1.76
CBCL_Ext	56.45 (6.92)	56.82 (5.81)	$t(10) = -4.30$	$d = -0.05$		−6.11	2.86
CBCL_Tot	64.09 (8.89)	63.09 (8.14)	$t(10) = 4.35$	$d = -0.03$		0.22	1.75

[1] Internalizing Problems; [2] Externalizing Problems; [3] Total Problems; [4] Mean according gender identity norm; [5] Mean according at birth assigned sex norm; [6] 95% bias-corrected and accelerated confidence interval for mean differences; * $p < 0.01$.

Considering the CBCL-R, a similar pattern emerged: significantly lower mean values were found for scales of Internalizing Problems, AD, SC according to the female norm than according to the male norm ($p < 0.05$), with a large effect size ($d = 0.67$–-1.99). For the main scale Externalizing Problems, there was no significant difference ($p > 0.05$), but the mean values of the scales RB and AB as well as AP were significantly higher according to the female norm than according to the male norm ($p < 0.05$, $d = 0.86$–1.91). No significant difference in means was found for the Total Problems scale. Accordingly, significant mean differences can be found for seven scales of the CBCL-R between the evaluation according to the GID and ABAS norms for trans girls.

The results of the McNemar test between the number of clinically significant cases of YSR-R and CBCL-R are presented in each case for trans boys (Tables S5 and S6) and trans girls (Tables S7 and S8) in the Supplementary Material. Trans boys showed a significantly higher clinically significant number of cases when evaluated according to GID than according to ABAS for the Somatic Complaints (SC) scale only ($p < 0.05$); the number of significant cases of the SC scale increased by an odds ratio of 3.04 according to the male norm than according to the female norm.

Thus, in the YSR-R, a significant change in the number of clinically significant cases between the GID and ABAS norm could only be observed for trans boys for one scale. For trans girls, there was no significant change in the clinically significant number of cases between the gender norms.

Looking at the CBCL-R, there were no significant changes in the number of clinically significant cases between the norm evaluation according to GID or ABAS ($p > 0.05$), either for trans boys or for trans girls.

4. Discussion

This study aimed to analyze psychological distress, peer relations and the role of parental perception and norm evaluation among a healthcare-seeking sample of trans adolescents.

Regarding the first research question, our sample reported above-average scores on the Internalizing and Total Problems scale of the YSR-R and CBCL-R, with clinically significant scores of 41.3% for Internalizing and 39.7% for the Total Problems score. These high prevalence rates are in line with the findings from other studies on the accompanying psychological symptoms of adolescents with GIC [10–13]. The 44–52% rates for suicidality, self-injuries and bullying are comparable with the literature [10].

We found no differences or interactions between the male/female at birth assigned sexes in symptom scores and, therefore, no "general pattern of inversion" [17] (p. 585) with regard to a gender-related distribution of the psychological distress, which is in line with recent findings, for example, of de Graaf et al. [43]. Moreover, other studies postulated contrary results, which indicated a higher degree of internalizing and associated problems in trans boys [49–51]. As significantly higher levels of exposure were found in non-binary than in binary-identified trans young people [52,53], non-binary identities should also be taken into account, in addition to a binary comparison. Since only one person in the sample identified as non-binary, such a comparison could not be carried out.

Second, greater levels of poor peer relations were associated with higher levels of psychological distress and poor peer relations could be identified as a predictor for internalizing problems of trans adolescents. This is also in line with previously confirmed findings on the mental health of young trans people [10,16,17]. In terms of the Minority Stress Model [20], adolescents with GIC represent a marginalized group in heteronormative societies, which, apparently, already experiences problems with peers, a lack of friendships, exclusion and teasing in adolescence. Since trans people can also have a non-heteronormative sexual orientation, some of the young people could belong to another socially marginalized group, which could increase minority stress and the associated experience of discrimination [54,55]. Future studies with larger sample sizes are needed to obtain a deeper insight into the experiences of these subgroups.

Third, we observed moderate to high agreement between the parental and adolescent's perception of their mental health. The data from our study showed a higher level of congruence than reported for population-based samples using the YSR and CBCL [39,56]. Additionally, the average difference between the reports was negative, implying that some parents rated psychological problems higher than their children themselves. These finding are plausible insofar as the adolescents and their parents had attended the GIF, the parents, thus, were already showing a form of support and recognition of the possible problems and the need for counseling for their child [26].

Fourth, a greater incongruity between self and parent report was associated with higher psychological stress of the adolescents, and the level of congruence could be identified as a predictor for internalizing problems. This finding is consistent with the literature on the role of parental awareness of psychological distress and supportiveness for the mental health of young trans people [32,57–59]. In the present study, we found no differences between the female and male at birth assigned sexes regarding the report discrepancy, which contradicts the literature on both population-based and trans samples [36,38,39,42].

Finally, following Rider et al. [25], this study examined differences in trans youth's mental health scores between evaluation by GID and ABAS norms. This paper showed that in the YSR-R, the mean scores in the main and problem scales differed significantly on four out of eleven scales among trans boys and on nine scales among trans girls between the binary gender norms. In the CBCL-R, mean scores differed significantly on four scales for trans boys and on seven scales for trans girls. Comparable to the results by Rider et al. [25], we did not find differences between the assessment of clinical significance according to GID and ABAS, with the exception for the somatic complaints scale for trans boys in the YSR-R, which was higher after GID evaluation.

4.1. Limitations

With regard to our sample, it should be taken into account that the adolescents already came to our counseling with their parents and can therefore not be representative of all young trans people in Germany, nor can their parents be representative of all parents. In addition, it should be noted that in the present work, as well as in the studies described, the group of trans girls with MABAS was much smaller ($n = 11$) than that of trans boys ($n = 48$), including one non-binary person with FABAS, and mean differences and interaction effects should therefore be interpreted with caution. With regard to the comparison sample used from the CBCL-R manual, it should be noted that the validation study took place in 2001 and that the standardization may have lost its representativeness and interpretability [60]. Further, it is unclear whether this norm sample also included adolescents who did not identify with their ABAS, as gender identity was not explicitly recorded in advance [27,46]. Additionally, we were only able to run analyses by using the T-scores of each case because raw scores were not available. Using raw scores for the multiple regression could have led to more precise results and Total Problems could also have been used as an outcome variable if it was possible to extract confounding items such as the PPR scale.

4.2. Implications and Prospects

Reducing the high psychological distress and vulnerability of trans youth should be one of the main future advances in child and adolescent psychiatry. This may contribute to improving trans-sensitive health care in the area of child psychiatry. Future research should explore the distress' causes. To ensure perspective, it is important to investigate in which contexts the experiences of bullying and poor peer relations are primarily reflected and to what extent it is possible for trans youth to create a supportive social network. Drawing on community-based knowledge presents as a valuable approach for professionals who offer counseling in the field of gender identity. Young trans people in particular are usually advised to network with the community, as peer counseling by other trans people or allies enables them to share experiences, to address uncertainties and victimization and to build up a social network with good peer relations. This approach is perceived as very empowering and helpful, and enables networking with other trans and genderqueer people [55]. Furthermore, awareness raising and educational measures on gender diversity should be implemented in schools to promote tolerance and openness, and to prevent discrimination in the form of bullying and bad peer relationships among both hetero- and gender-nonconforming people.

Due to the high congruence between the self and parent reports in the sample, as well as the central position of parents in the life and development of their gender-variant children, it would be relevant to explore how parents deal with their children's trans identity and whether there might have been determining factors that led them to attend the GISC. Further research should focus on the examination of parental support, which was not assessed in our study. However, further research is needed on family and social support for trans adolescents in the context of mental health in Germany, especially from families that are yet to seek healthcare assistance, which is in line with calls from other research groups [14,16].

In the area of clinical psychology, more research should be devoted to adequate assessment tools for gender-variant young people in consultation with their parents: "To assess discrepancies between what the child desires in terms of how they want to assert their gender identity versus what the parents perceive and feel is most appropriate" [26] (p. 118). In practice with trans youth, clinicians should be aware that the decision whether to evaluate a test according to GID or ABAS has an influence on the test score but not on its interpretation, except for the somatic problems scale. Since trans people do not identify with their ABAS, it is generally questionable when the ABAS and not the GID is used for the analysis [26]. For non-binary identifying adolescents, both gender norms should be considered, although a binary-gendered test format ultimately seems rather inappropriate for this group [26]. For example, having to choose a gender when filling out the questionnaire can already raise conflicts for trans youth and their parents, triggering experiences of discrimination and building mistrust towards the investigators [25].

The results of this study emphasize that against the background of the gender-affirmative paradigm, and the avoidance of experiences of discrimination and violation, it is necessary to reconsider whether binary-normed procedures should be avoided in future. We would like to join other research groups by proposing that at least both norms should be used in the evaluation, or if a binary identification is present, the GID should be used instead of the ABAS. There are no norms for trans clients yet and validity can be raised by using both templates and deciding case by case whether the score of the female or male norm represents the person the most [25–27]. Since trans youth belong to a marginalized group, and appropriate measures are not available, the development of specific instruments is needed. Participatory research designs are a promising approach, giving trans adolescents and their parents a voice and concretely including them in the research process.

In practice, culturally-sensitive and gender-affirmative test diagnostics therefore require sensitivity in test selection, implementation and interpretation [27]. Thus, the results from this study underline that adolescents with GIC represent a healthcare-seeking group that requires a reflective and thinking out of the box attitude throughout the health system, and especially from professionals working in the area of child psychiatry.

Supplementary Materials: The following are available online at https://www.mdpi.com/article/10.3390/children8100864/s1. Table S1. Results of the one-way ANOVA for testing the effect of the at birth assigned sex on the main problem scale scores of the YSR-R; Table S2. Results of the *t*-test for dependent samples between means according to gender norms of the main and problem scales of the YSR-R for trans boys; Table S3. Results of the *t*-test for dependent samples between means according to gender norms of the main and problem scales of the CBCL-R for trans boys; Table S4. Results of the *t*-test for dependent samples between means according to gender norms of the main and problem scales of the YSR-R for trans girls; Table S5. Results of the *t*-test for dependent samples between means according to gender norms of the main and problem scales of the CBCL-R for trans girls; Table S6. Results of the McNemar test indicating the change between the clinical significance of the evaluation norms from GID to ABAS from the YSR-R for trans boys; Table S7. Results of the McNemar test indicating the change between the clinical significance of the evaluation norms from GID to ABAS from the CBCL-R for trans girls; Table S8. Results of the McNemar test indicating the change between the clinical significance of the evaluation norms from GID to ABAS from the YSR-R for trans girls; Table S9. Results of the McNemar test indicating the change between the clinical significance of the evaluation norms from GID to ABAS from the CBCL-R for trans girls.

Author Contributions: Conceptualization, A.B., C.C., L.R., S.B. and S.M.W.; methodology, A.B. and C.C.; formal analysis, A.B.; writing—original draft preparation, A.B. and C.C.; writing—review and editing, A.B., C.C., L.R., S.B. and S.M.W.; supervision, C.C. All authors have read and agreed to the published version of the manuscript.

Funding: This research received no external funding.

Institutional Review Board Statement: The study was conducted according to the guidelines of the Declaration of Helsinki, and approved by the Institutional Ethics Committee of the Charité Universitätsmedizin Berlin (EA2/201/20, date 9 March 2020).

Informed Consent Statement: The retrospective study was carried out as part of the accompanying clinical research of the Charité Universitätsmedizin Berlin, which is why no separate consent was obtained for this study.

Data Availability Statement: The data presented in this study are available on appropriate request from the corresponding author. The data are not publicly available as the privacy of the human subjects must be ensured.

Conflicts of Interest: The authors declare no conflict of interest.

References

1. Pauli, D. Geschlechtsinkongruenz und Genderdysphorie bei Kindern und Jugendlichen. *PSYCH Up2date* **2017**, *11*, 529–543. [CrossRef]
2. Franzen, J.; Sauer, A. *Benachteiligung von Trans*Personen, insbesondere im Arbeitsleben*; Antidiskriminierungsstelle des Bundes: Berlin, Germany, 2010.
3. Becker, I.; Ravens-Sieberer, U.; Ottová-Jordan, V.; Schulte-Markwort, M. Prevalence of adolescent gender experiences and gender expression in Germany. *J. Adolesc. Health* **2017**, *61*, 83–90. [CrossRef] [PubMed]
4. Neyman, A.; Fuqua, J.S.; Eugster, E.A. Bicalutamide as an androgen blocker with secondary effect of promoting feminization in fale-to-female transgender adolescents. *J. Adolesc. Health* **2019**, *64*, 544–546. [CrossRef] [PubMed]

5. Antidiskriminierungsstelle des Bundes Mann—Frau—Divers: Die "Dritte Option" Und Das Allgemeine Gleichbehandlungsgesetz. Available online: https://www.antidiskriminierungsstelle.de/DE/ThemenUndForschung/Geschlecht/Dritte_Option/Dritte_Option_node.html (accessed on 23 December 2020).
6. Sterzing, P.R.; Ratliff, G.A.; Gartner, R.E.; McGeough, B.L.; Johnson, K.C. Social ecological correlates of polyvictimization among a national sample of transgender, genderqueer, and cisgender sexual minority adolescents. *Child Abuse Negl.* **2017**, *67*, 1–12. [CrossRef] [PubMed]
7. Möller, B.; Güldenring, A.; Wiesemann, C.; Romer, G. Geschlechtsdysphorie im Kindes- und Jugendalter. *Kinderanalyse* **2018**, *26*, 228–263. [CrossRef]
8. Eyssel, J.; Koehler, A.; Dekker, A.; Sehner, S.; Nieder, T.O. Needs and concerns of transgender individuals regarding interdisciplinary transgender healthcare: A non-clinical online survey. *PLoS ONE* **2017**, *12*, e0183014. [CrossRef]
9. Nieder, T.O.; Strauß, B. S3-Leitlinie zur Diagnostik, Beratung und Behandlung im Kontext von Geschlechtsinkongruenz, Geschlechtsdysphorie und Trans-Gesundheit: Hintergrund, Methode und zentrale Empfehlungen. *Zeitschr. Sex.* **2019**, *32*, 70–79. [CrossRef]
10. Holt, V.; Skagerberg, E.; Dunsford, M. Young people with features of gender dysphoria: Demographics and associated difficulties. *Clin. Child Psychol. Psychiatry* **2016**, *21*, 108–118. [CrossRef]
11. Veale, J.F.; Watson, R.J.; Peter, T.; Saewyc, E.M. Mental health disparities among Canadian transgender youth. *J. Adolesc. Health* **2017**, *60*, 44–49. [CrossRef]
12. Becker, I.; Gjergji-Lama, V.; Romer, G.; Möller, B. Merkmale von Kindern und Jugendlichen mit Geschlechtsdysphorie in der Hamburger Spezialsprechstunde. *Prax. Kinderpsychol. Kinderpsychiatr.* **2014**, *63*, 486–509. [CrossRef]
13. Meyenburg, B. Geschlechtsdysphorie im Jugendalter. Schwierige Behandlungsverläufe. *Prax. Kinderpsychol. Kinderpsychiatr.* **2014**, *63*, 510–522. [CrossRef]
14. Wiech, M.; Kutlar, C.; Günthard, M.; Schenker, T.; Pauli, D.; Möller, B. Psychische Auffälligkeiten und gesundheitsbezogene Lebensqualität bei Jugendlichen mit Geschlechtsdysphorie. *Prax. Kinderpsychol. Kinderpsychiatr.* **2020**, *69*, 554–569. [CrossRef]
15. Turban, J.L.; Shadianloo, S. *Transgender and Gender Nonconforming Youth*; International Association for Child and Adolescent Psychiatry and Allied Professions: Geneva, Switzerland, 2018.
16. Levitan, N.; Barkmann, C.; Richter-Appelt, H.; Schulte-Markwort, M.; Becker-Hebly, I. Risk factors for psychological functioning in German adolescents with gender dysphoria: Poor peer relations and general family functioning. *Eur. Child Adolesc. Psychiatry* **2019**, *28*, 1487–1498. [CrossRef]
17. de Vries, A.L.C.; Steensma, T.D.; Cohen-Kettenis, P.T.; VanderLaan, D.P.; Zucker, K.J. Poor peer relations predict parent- and self-reported behavioral and emotional problems of adolescents with gender dysphoria: A cross-national, cross-clinic comparative analysis. *Eur. Child Adolesc. Psychiatry* **2016**, *25*, 579–588. [CrossRef] [PubMed]
18. de Graaf, N.M.; Cohen-Kettenis, P.T.; Carmichael, P.; de Vries, A.L.C.; Dhondt, K.; Laridaen, J.; Pauli, D.; Ball, J.; Steensma, T.D. Psychological functioning in adolescents referred to specialist gender identity clinics across Europe: A clinical comparison study between four clinics. *Eur. Child Adolesc. Psychiatry* **2018**, *27*, 909–919. [CrossRef]
19. Proulx, C.N.; Coulter, R.W.S.; Egan, J.E.; Matthews, D.D.; Mair, C. Associations of lesbian, gay, bisexual, transgender, and questioning–inclusive sex education with mental health outcomes and school-based victimization in U.S. High School students. *J. Adolesc. Health* **2019**, *64*, 608–614. [CrossRef]
20. Meyer, I.H. Prejudice, social stress, and mental health in lesbian, gay, and bisexual populations: Conceptual issues and research evidence. *Psychol. Bull.* **2003**, *129*, 674–697. [CrossRef]
21. Oliva, A.; Parra, Á.; Reina, M.C. Personal and contextual factors related to internalizing problems during adolescence. *Child Youth Care Forum* **2014**, *43*, 505–520. [CrossRef]
22. Oswald, T.M.; Winter-Messiers, M.A.; Gibson, B.; Schmidt, A.M.; Herr, C.M.; Solomon, M. Sex differences in internalizing problems during adolescence in autism spectrum disorder. *J. Autism Dev. Disord.* **2016**, *46*, 624–636. [CrossRef]
23. Rönnlund, M.; Karlsson, E. The relation between dimensions of attachment and internalizing or externalizing problems during adolescence. *J. Genet. Psychol.* **2006**, *167*, 47–63. [CrossRef]
24. van der Miesen, A.I.R.; Steensma, T.D.; de Vries, A.L.C.; Bos, H.; Popma, A. Psychological functioning in transgender adolescents before and after gender-affirmative care compared with cisgender general population peers. *J. Adolesc. Health* **2020**, *66*, 699–704. [CrossRef] [PubMed]
25. Rider, G.N.; Berg, D.; Pardo, S.T.; Olson-Kennedy, J.; Sharp, C.; Tran, K.M.; Calvetti, S.; Keo-Meier, C.L. Using the Child Behavior Checklist (CBCL) with transgender/gender nonconforming children and adolescents. *Clin. Pract. Pediatr. Psychol.* **2019**, *7*, 291–301. [CrossRef]
26. Berg, D.; Edwards-Leeper, L. Child and family assessment. In *The Gender Affirmative Model: An Interdisciplinary Approach to Supporting Transgender and Gender Expansive Children*; Keo-Meier, C., Ehrensaft, D., Eds.; American Psychological Association: Washington, DC, USA, 2018; pp. 101–124. ISBN 978-1-4338-2912-3.
27. Keo-Meier, C.L.; Fitzgerald, K.M. Affirmative psychological testing and neurocognitive assessment with transgender adults. *Psychiatr. Clin. N. Am.* **2017**, *40*, 51–64. [CrossRef] [PubMed]
28. Bajeux, E.; Klemanski, D.H.; Husky, M.; Leray, E.; Chan Chee, C.; Shojaei, T.; Fermanian, C.; Kovess-Masfety, V. Factors associated with parent–child discrepancies in reports of mental health disorders in young children. *Child Psychiatry Hum. Dev.* **2018**, *49*, 1003–1010. [CrossRef]

29. Canino, G.; Shrout, P.E.; Rubio-Stipec, M.; Bird, H.R.; Bravo, M.; Ramírez, R.; Chavez, L.; Alegría, M.; Bauermeister, J.J.; Hohmann, A.; et al. The DSM-IV Rates of child and adolescent disorders in Puerto Rico: Prevalence, correlates, service use, and the effects of impairment. *Arch. Gen. Psychiatry* **2004**, *61*, 85–93. [CrossRef]
30. Ford, T. Practitioner review: How can epidemiology help us plan and deliver effective child and adolescent mental health services? *J. Child Psychol. Psychiatry* **2008**, *49*, 900–914. [CrossRef]
31. Riley, E.A.; Clemson, L.; Sitharthan, G.; Diamond, M. Surviving a gender-variant childhood: The vews of transgender adults on the needs of gender-variant children and their parents. *J. Sex Marital Ther.* **2013**, *39*, 241–263. [CrossRef]
32. Olson, K.R.; Durwood, L.; DeMeules, M.; McLaughlin, K.A. Mental health of transgender children who are supported in their identities. *Pediatrics* **2016**, *137*, e20153223. [CrossRef]
33. Ryan, C.; Russell, S.T.; Huebner, D.; Diaz, R.; Sanchez, J. Family acceptance in adolescence and the health of LGBT young adults: Family acceptance in adolescence and the health of LGBT young adults. *J. Child Adolesc. Psychiatr. Nurs.* **2010**, *23*, 205–213. [CrossRef]
34. Coolhart, D.; Ritenour, K.; Grodzinski, A. Experiences of ambiguous loss for parents of transgender male youth: A phenomenological exploration. *Contemp. Fam. Ther.* **2018**, *40*, 28–41. [CrossRef]
35. Clark, B.A.; Marshall, S.K.; Saewyc, E.M. Hormone Therapy Decision-Making Processes: Transgender Youth and Parents. *J. Adolesc.* **2020**, *79*, 136–147. [CrossRef]
36. Ferdinand, R.F.; van der Ende, J.; Verhulst, F.C. Parent-adolescent disagreement regarding psychopathology in adolescents from the general population as a risk factor for adverse outcome. *J. Abnorm. Psychol.* **2004**, *113*, 198–206. [CrossRef]
37. Ferdinand, R.F.; van der Ende, J.; Verhulst, F.C. Prognostic value of parent–adolescent disagreement in a referred sample. *Eur. Child Adolesc. Psychiatry* **2006**, *15*, 156–162. [CrossRef]
38. Grills, A.E.; Ollendick, T.H. Multiple informant agreement and the anxiety disorders interview schedule for parents and children. *J. Am. Acad. Child Adolesc. Psychiatry* **2003**, *42*, 30–40. [CrossRef]
39. Salbach-Andrae, H.; Klinkowski, N.; Lenz, K.; Lehmkuhl, U. Agreement between youth-reported and parent-reported psychopathology in a referred sample. *Eur. Child Adolesc. Psychiatry* **2009**, *18*, 136–143. [CrossRef]
40. Lewinsohn, P.M.; Rohde, P.; Seeley, J.R. Major depressive disorder in older adolescents: Prevalence, risk factors, and clinical implications. *Clin. Psychol. Rev.* **1998**, *18*, 765–794. [CrossRef]
41. Williams, C.D.; Lindsey, M.; Joe, S. Parent-adolescent concordance on perceived need for mental health services and its impact on service use. *Child. Youth Serv. Rev.* **2011**, *33*, 2253–2260. [CrossRef]
42. Zucker, K.J.; Bradley, S.J.; Owen-Anderson, A.; Kibblewhite, S.J.; Wood, H.; Singh, D.; Choi, K. Demographics, behavior problems, and psychosexual characteristics of adolescents with gender identity disorder or transvestic fetishism. *J. Sex Marital Ther.* **2012**, *38*, 151–189. [CrossRef]
43. De Graaf, N.; Steensma, T.; Carmichael, P.; Vanderlaan, D.; Aitken, M.; Cohen-Kettenis, P.; de Vries, A.L.; Kreukels, B.P.; Wasserman, L.; Wood, H.; et al. Suicidality in clinic-referred transgender adolescents. *Eur. Child Adolesc. Psychiatry* **2020**. [CrossRef]
44. Achenbach, T.M. *Manual for the Youth Self-Report and 1991 Profile*; Department of Psychiatry, University of Vermont: Burlington, VT, USA, 1991.
45. Achenbach, T.M.; Edelbrock, C.S. *Manual for the Child Behavior Checklist and Revised Child Behavior Profile*; Department of Psychiatry, University of Vermont: Burlington, VT, USA, 1983.
46. Döpfner, M.; Plück, J.; Kinnen, C. *Für die Arbeitsgruppe Deutsche Child Behavior Checklist: Manual Deutsche Schulalter-Formen der Child Behavior Checklist von Thomas, M. Achenbach. Elternfragebogen über das Verhalten von Kindern Und Jugendlichen (CBCL/6-18R), Lehrerfragebogen über das Verhalten von Kindern Und Jugendlichen (TRF/6-18R), Fragebogen für Jugendliche (YSR/11-18R)*; Hogrefe: Göttingen, Germany, 2014.
47. Zucker, K.; Bradley, S.; Sanikhani, M. Sex differences in referral rates of children with gender identity disorder: Some hypotheses. *J. Abnorm. Child Psychol.* **1997**, *25*, 217–227. [CrossRef]
48. IBM Corporation. *SPSS Statistics for Mac, Version 25*; IBM Corp.: Armonk, New York, USA, 2017.
49. Becerra-Culqui, T.A.; Liu, Y.; Nash, R.; Cromwell, L.; Flanders, W.D.; Getahun, D.; Giammattei, S.V.; Hunkeler, E.M.; Lash, T.L.; Millman, A.; et al. Mental health of transgender and gender nonconforming youth compared with their peers. *Pediatrics* **2018**, *141*, e20173845. [CrossRef]
50. Budge, S.L.; Adelson, J.L.; Howard, K.A.S. Anxiety and depression in transgender individuals: The roles of transition status, loss, social support, and coping. *J. Consult. Clin. Psychol.* **2013**, *81*, 545–557. [CrossRef]
51. Kaltiala-Heino, R.; Sumia, M.; Työläjärvi, M.; Lindberg, N. Two years of gender identity service for minors: Overrepresentation of natal girls with severe problems in adolescent development. *Child Adolesc. Psychiatry Ment. Health* **2015**, *9*, 9. [CrossRef]
52. Liszewski, W.; Peebles, J.K.; Yeung, H.; Arron, S. Persons of nonbinary gender—Awareness, visibility, and health disparities. *N. Engl. J. Med.* **2018**, *379*, 2391–2393. [CrossRef]
53. Rimes, K.A.; Goodship, N.; Ussher, G.; Baker, D.; West, E. Non-binary and binary transgender youth: Comparison of mental health, self-harm, suicidality, substance use and victimization experiences. *Int. J. Transgenderism* **2017**, *20*, 230–240. [CrossRef]
54. Winker, G.; Degele, N. *Intersektionalität: Zur Analyse sozialer Ungleichheiten*; Transcript Verlag: Bielefeld, Germany, 2015; ISBN 978-3-8394-1149-0.

55. Wolf, G.; Meyer, E. Sexuelle Orientierung und Geschlechtsidentität—(K)ein Thema in der Psychotherapie? *Psychotherapeutenjournal* **2017**, *16*, 130–139.
56. Achenbach, T.M.; Dumenci, L.; Rescorla, L.A. *Ratings of Relations between DSM-IV Diagnostic Categories and Items*; University of Vermont: Burlington, VT, USA, 2001.
57. Lev, A.I.; Gottlieb, A.R. *Families in Transition: Parenting Gender Diverse Children, Adolescents, and Young Adults*; Harrington Park Press: New York, NY, USA, 2019; ISBN 978-1-939594-31-0.
58. Olezeski, C.L.; Kamody, R.C. Parents matter: Considering evidence-based relationship variables within families when working with gender expansive youth. *Pract. Innov.* **2020**, *5*, 218–229. [CrossRef]
59. Pariseau, E.M.; Chevalier, L.; Long, K.A.; Clapham, R.; Edwards-Leeper, L.; Tishelman, A.C. The relationship between family acceptance-rejection and transgender youth psychosocial functioning. *Clin. Pract. Pediatr. Psychol.* **2019**, *7*, 267–277. [CrossRef]
60. Kersting, M. Wenn Tests in die Jahre kommen. Probleme des Einsatzes überalteter Testverfahren. In *Polizei und Psychologie*; Lorei, C., Ed.; Verlag für Polizeiwissenschaft: Frankfurt, Germany, 2007; pp. 565–577.

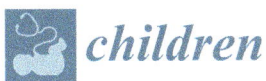

Article

Ten Years (2011–2021) of the Italian Lombardy ADHD Register for the Diagnosis and Treatment of Children and Adolescents with ADHD

Maurizio Bonati *[ ], Francesca Scarpellini [ ], Massimo Cartabia [ ], Michele Zanetti and on behalf of the Lombardy ADHD Group [†]

Laboratory for Mother and Child Health, Department of Public Health, Istituto di Ricerche Farmacologiche Mario Negri IRCCS, 20156 Milan, Italy; francesca.scarpellini@marionegri.it (F.S.); massimo.cartabia@marionegri.it (M.C.); michele.zanetti@marionegri.it (M.Z.)
* Correspondence: maurizio.bonati@marionegri.it
† Membership of the Lombardy ADHD Group is provided in the Acknowledgments.

Citation: Bonati, M.; Scarpellini, F.; Cartabia, M.; Zanetti, M.; on behalf of the Lombardy ADHD Group. Ten Years (2011–2021) of the Italian Lombardy ADHD Register for the Diagnosis and Treatment of Children and Adolescents with ADHD. *Children* **2021**, *8*, 598. https://doi.org/10.3390/children8070598

Academic Editor: Carl E. Stafstrom

Received: 3 June 2021
Accepted: 13 July 2021
Published: 15 July 2021

Publisher's Note: MDPI stays neutral with regard to jurisdictional claims in published maps and institutional affiliations.

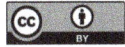

Copyright: © 2021 by the authors. Licensee MDPI, Basel, Switzerland. This article is an open access article distributed under the terms and conditions of the Creative Commons Attribution (CC BY) license (https://creativecommons.org/licenses/by/4.0/).

Abstract: Background: The purpose of this article is to update the diagnostic assessment, therapeutic approach, and 12–18 month follow-up of patients added to the Italian Lombardy Attention Deficit Hyperactivity Disorder (ADHD) Register. Methods: Medical records of patients added to the Registry from 2011 to 2021 were analysed. Results: 4091 of 5934 patients met the criteria for a diagnosis of ADHD, and 20.3% of them presented a familiarity with the disorder. A total of 2879 children (70.4%) had at least one comorbidity disorder, in prevalence a learning disorder (39%). Nearly all (95.9%) received at least one psychological prescription, 17.9% of them almost one pharmacological treatment, and 15.6% a combination of both. Values of ≥ 5 of the Clinical Global Impression—Severity scale (CGI-S) are more commonly presented by patients with a pharmacological prescription than with a psychological treatment ($p < 0.0001$). A significant improvement was reported in half of the patients followed after 1 year, with Clinical Global Impression—Improvement scale (CGI-I) ≤ 3. In all, 233 of 4091 are 18-year-old patients. Conclusions: A ten-year systematic monitoring of models of care was a fruitful shared and collaborative initiative in order to promote significant improvement in clinical practice, providing effective and continuous quality of care. The unique experience reported here should spread.

Keywords: attention deficit disorder with hyperactivity; child; adolescent; mental health; chronic disease; register; clinical protocol

1. Introduction

Attention deficit hyperactivity disorder (ADHD) is a neurodevelopmental disorder that affects 5.9% of children and persists into adulthood for two-thirds of them [1,2], with great impairments in academic achievement and work [3]. The core symptoms are inattention, restlessness, and impulsivity, which are more frequent in boys than girls (ratio 3:1). In Italy, the prevalence of the disorder ranges from 1.1 to 3.1% of the paediatric population, considering only subjects with a diagnosis confirmed by clinical evaluation [4].

The wide variability depends on the different diagnostic procedures adopted to assess children and the criteria used, and the period of time over which assessment is conducted [5]. The peak age of diagnosis of ADHD is in primary school children aged 5–10 years [6], and children born later in the school year are more likely to receive an ADHD diagnosis than their same school-year peers [7]. According to the national and international guidelines [8,9], the diagnosis of ADHD is based on a careful and systematic assessment of a lifetime history of symptoms, childhood onset, and impairment in some contexts (schools, relationships, home) [10]. Information about the medical history of psychiatric and neurological problems is also important. Psychiatric comorbidity is thus a clinically important factor that contributes to the persistence of ADHD in adulthood [11]. Oppositional defiant disorder (ODD), conduct disorder (CD) and autism spectrum disorder are the most common conditions associated with ADHD [12]. Concerning treatment, the guidelines suggest using a multimodal treatment combining psychosocial interventions with pharmacological therapies. Psychological therapies involve parents and teachers with training and a range of cognitive behavioural approaches to the patient. Medication includes stimulants, in particular methylphenidate, as a first choice and the most effective therapy. The stimulant medications for ADHD are more effective than non-stimulant medications but are also more likely to be diverted, misused, and abused [13,14]. Otherwise, non-medication treatments for ADHD are less effective than medication treatments for ADHD symptoms, but are frequently useful to help problems that remain after medication has been optimised [1]. A recent meta-analysis of the literature highlighted the positive effect of psychological interventions on ADHD cognitive symptomatology and supports the inclusion of non-pharmacological interventions in conjunction with the commonly used pharmacological treatments [15]. Despite the existence of clear and specific guidelines, access to services is limited [16,17], the waiting times for diagnosis are too long [18], and the treatment outcomes depend on many factors, such as the presence of comorbidities [19]. The Regional ADHD Registry was activated in June 2011 with the purpose of collecting data about the diagnosis and treatment of ADHD patients who had access to the 18 centres, with particular attention to the monitoring of pharmacological treatment. The Regional Registry was part of a more general project aiming to ensure appropriate ADHD management for children and adolescents once the disorder is suspected; the data recorded include common assessment processes as well as psychoeducational interventions for healthcare workers of the Lombardy region healthcare system [2]. After 10 years of the project, we aimed to update the diagnostic assessment and therapeutic approaches proposed to 5–17-year-old youths who had access to any of the 18 ADHD reference centres of the Lombardy region. In particular, we analysed the clinical characteristics of ADHD patients and the relation with the treatment prescription and the elevation in some scales of the test used for the diagnosis. We explored if there was an improvement on their Clinical Global Impression—Improvement scale (CGI-I) scores after 12–18 months of follow-up.

2. Materials and Methods

A retrospective study based on medical records was conducted. Data were identified from the Regional ADHD Registry. Formal ethical review board approval was not required for the present updating because it was previously approved by the Institutional Review Board of the Istituto di Ricerche Farmacologiche Mario Negri IRCCS, Milan, Italy. Written informed consent was obtained from all patients before data collection. We used the previously described methodology and reported data concerning the local health setting [7], the characteristics of the ADHD Registry activated in Lombardy in June 2011 [20,21], the systematic work carried out by the 18 ADHD centres [19], and the diagnostic assessment and the treatment conducted by all involved clinicians, according to the national and international guidelines [8,9]. Behavioural and emotional problems were highlighted with the most used and validated rating scales for parents and teachers, Conners' Parent Rating Scale (CPRS) [22], Conners' Teacher Rating Scale (CTRS) [23], and the Child Behaviour Checklist (CBCL) [24], while symptom severity and symptom improvement were quantified, respectively, with the use of the Clinical Global Impression—Severity scale and the Clinical Global Impressions—Improvement scale [25]. Results from the scales were analysed and compared with the perceptions of parents and teachers, as well as the perceptions of mothers and fathers. The Clinical Global Impressions—Improvement Scale scores were analysed after 12–18 months of follow-up. The percentages of completeness of the seven areas of the shared diagnostic assessment (Clinical Interview, Neurological Examination, IQ Evaluation, Diagnostic Interview, Parents and Teachers Assessment, Clinical Severity Evaluation) of all regional centres were analysed and displayed on radar chart axes with a range of 0 to 100%

Data were extracted from the database and analyses were updated on 1 April 2021, and data referred to patients added between 2011 and 2021.

Data Analyses

All data were entered in an SAS/STAT database (SAS Version 9, SAS Institute, Inc., Cary, NC, USA). Descriptive statistics were computed for the entire study population and for subgroups. The Wilcoxon test was used to compare continuous variables, whereas chi-square tests were used to compare categorical variables. V-Cramer and Wilcoxon effect sizes were calculated (Supplementary Materials). Both values vary from 0 to 1; the closer the value was to 1, the stronger the significant difference between the categorical and the continuous variables was. A multivariate logistic regression analysis with stepwise selection was also carried out to assess the determinants of disease and treatment. Moreover, interrater agreement (parents vs. teachers; mothers vs. fathers) on symptom scores for each diagnostic scale was established by Kappa coefficient of agreement (K). The results are presented as the number, frequency (%), and mean or median; $p < 0.05$ was considered to be significant.

3. Results

A total of 7053 children were added to the registry from June 2011 to December 2021, of whom 6188 were children and adolescents accessing the ADHD centres for the first time (range 89–1010 patients per centre, median = 248) for suspected ADHD diagnosis. Most of the patients (5934) had completed the diagnostic assessment (Table 1). Children had a median age of 9 years (range 7–11); most of them were males (4960 (83.6%)) and 974 (16.4%) were females. In all, 4091 patients received a diagnosis of ADHD based on the Diagnostic and Statistical Manual of Mental Disorders [26] criteria, 3484 (85.2%) of whom were males and 607 (14.8%) females. The cumulative incidence of ADHD in the 2011 and 2021 period was valued to be 0.26% (95% confidence interval (CI = [0.94–1.24]) of the resident population of the same age range, with a spike at 8 years of age (Figure 1).

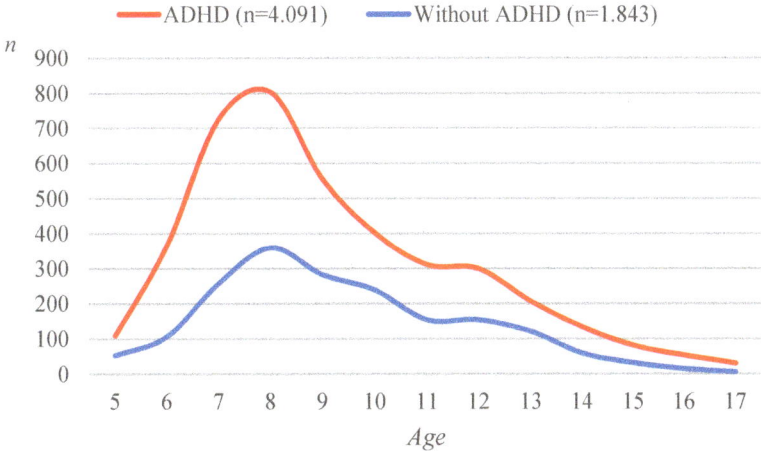

Figure 1. Age of the ADHD patients.

The characteristics strongly associated with ADHD were lower age, male gender, only child, not born in Italy, adopted, support teacher, lower educational level of parents, unemployed father, ADHD familiarity and psychiatric comorbidity (Table 1). According to both univariate and multivariate analysis, only child (odds ratio (OR) = 1.22, 95% CI = [1.07–1.41]), adopted (OR = 1.64, 95% CI = [1.07–2.52]), primary school (OR = 1.15, 95% CI = [1.00–1.31]), support teacher (OR = 2.82, 95% CI = [2.19–3.64]), employed mother

(OR = 1.14, 95% CI = [1.01–1.20]), unemployed father (OR = 1.31, 95% CI = [1.08–1.58]), and ADHD familiarity (OR = 2.21, 95% CI = [1.86–2.63]) were higher in ADHD patients. In all, 2879 of 3956 (70.4%) had at least one psychiatric disorder (1079 without ADHD), whereas 387 (6.5%) had another comorbidity chronic disease. Learning disorders (OR = 1.37, 95% CI = [1.21–1.55]), sleep disorders (OR = 1.83, 95% CI = [1.50–2.23]), oppositional defiant disorder (ODD) (OR = 2.87, 95% CI = [2.27–3.64]), language disorders (OR = 1.36, 95% CI = [1.05–1.77]), tics (OR = 1.87, 95% CI = [1.16–3.03]) and motor coordination disorders (OR = 1.68, 95% CI = [1.04–2.72]) were higher in ADHD patients. Anxiety (OR = 0.70, 95% CI = [0.56–0.87]) and conduct disorder (OR = 0.49, 95% CI = [0.32–0.76]) were higher in patients without ADHD. The presence of a neurological condition was more frequent (n = 121, 2%).

Table 1. Demographic characteristics of the ADHD patients.

		ADHD Yes	ADHD No	Total	p	OR (IC 95%)	Logistic
Children		4091	1843	5934			
Age at diagnosis	median (q1–q3)	9.0 (7.0–11.0)	9.0 (8.0–11.0)	9.0 (7.0–11.0)	<0.0001 *		
	media (ds)	9.2 (2.6)	9.4 (2.4)	9.2 (2.5)			
	(min–max)	(5.0–17.0)	(5.0–17.0)	(5.0–17.0)			
	Missing	30	14	44			
School age at diagnosis	5–11	3.264 (80.4)	1.447 (79.1)	4.711 (80.0)	0.2635	1.08 (0.94–1.24)	
	12–17	797 (19.6)	382 (20.9)	1.179 (20.0)		1.00 (Ref.)	
	Missing	30	14	44			
Gender	Female	607 (14.8)	367 (19.9)	974 (16.4)	<0.0001 *	1.00 (Ref.)	
	Male	3.484 (85.2)	1.476 (80.1)	4.960 (83.6)		1.43 (1.24–1.65) *	1.36 (1.17–1.58)
	Missing	-	-	-			
Only child	Yes	1.054 (25.8)	396 (21.5)	1.450 (24.5)	0.0004	1.27 (1.11–1.45)	1.22 (1.07–1.41)
	No	3.028 (74.2)	1.443 (78.5)	4.471 (75.5)		1.00 (Ref.)	
	Missing	9	4	13			
Born in Italy	Yes	3.869 (94.6)	1.774 (96.3)	5.643 (95.1)	0.0067	1.00 (Ref.)	
	No	220 (5.4)	69 (3.7)	289 (4.9)		1.46 (1.11–1.93)	
	Missing	2	-	2			
Adopted	Yes	149 (3.6)	34 (1.8)	183 (3.1)	0.0002	2.01 (1.38–2.93)	1.64 (1.07–2.52)
	No	3.938 (96.4)	1.807 (98.2)	5.745 (96.9)		1.00 (Ref.)	
	Missing	4	2	6			
School	Primary School	3.124 (76.4)	1.371 (74.5)	4.495 (75.8)	0.1124	1.11 (0.98–1.26)	1.15 (1.00–1.31)
	Middle/ High School	964 (23.6)	469 (25.5)	1.433 (24.2)		1.00 (Ref.)	
	Missing	3	3	6			
Support teacher	Yes	514 (12.6)	79 (4.3)	593 (10.0)	<0.0001	3.21 (2.51–4.09)	2.82 (2.19–3.64)
	No	3.577 (87.4)	1.764 (95.7)	5.341 (90.0)		1.00 (Ref.)	
	Missing	-	-	-			

Table 1. Cont.

		ADHD Yes	ADHD No	Total	p	OR (IC 95%)	Logistic
Educational level of mother	Yes	2.313 (56.5)	1.116 (60.6)	3.429 (57.8)	0.0038	0.85 (0.76–0.95)	
	No	1.778 (43.5)	727 (39.4)	2.505 (42.2)		1.00 (Ref.)	
	Missing	-	-	-			
Educational level of father	Yes	1.865 (45.6)	934 (50.7)	2.799 (47.2)	0.0003	1.00 (Ref.)	
	No	2.226 (54.4)	909 (49.3)	3.135 (52.8)		1.23 (1.10–1.37)	
	Missing	-	-	-			
Mother employed	Yes	2.729 (66.7)	1.227 (66.6)	3.956 (66.7)	0.9210	1.01 (0.90–1.13)	1.14 (1.01–1.30)
	No	1.362 (33.3)	616 (33.4)	1.978 (33.3)		1.00 (Ref.)	
	Missing	-	-	-			
Father employed	Yes	3.411 (83.4)	1.624 (88.1)	5.035 (84.9)	<0.0001	1.00 (Ref.)	
	No	680 (16.6)	219 (11.9)	899 (15.1)		1.48 (1.26–1.74)	1.31 (1.08–1.58)
	Missing	-	-	-			
ADHD familiarity	Yes	831 (20.3)	193 (10.5)	1.024 (17.3)	<0.0001	2.18 (1.84–2.58)	2.21 (1.86–2.63)
	No	3.260 (79.7)	1.650 (89.5)	4.910 (82.7)		1.00 (Ref.)	
	Missing	-	-	-			
Psychiatric comorbidity	Yes	2.879 (70.4)	1.079 (58.5)	3.958 (66.7)	<0.0001	1.68 (1.50–1.89)	
	No	1.212 (29.6)	764 (41.5)	1.976 (33.3)		1.00 (Ref.)	
	Missing	-	-	-			
Type of comorbidity (flag)	Learning disorder	1.594 (39.0)	613 (33.3)	2.207 (37.2)	<0.0001	1.28 (1.14–1.44)	1.37 (1.21–1.55)
	Sleeping disorder	582 (14.2)	145 (7.9)	727 (12.3)	<0.0001	1.94 (1.60–2.35)	1.83 (1.50–2.23)
	ODD	569 (13.9)	93 (5.0)	662 (11.2)	<0.0001	3.04 (2.42–3.81)	2.87 (2.27–3.64)
	Anxiety	280 (6.8)	162 (8.8)	442 (7.4)	0.0083	0.76 (0.62–0.93)	0.70 (0.56–0.87)
	Language disorder	287 (7.0)	88 (4.8)	375 (6.3)	0.0010	1.50 (1.18–1.92)	1.36 (1.05–1.77)
	Tic	95 (2.3)	22 (1.2)	117 (2.0)	0.0038	1.97 (1.23–3.14)	1.87 (1.16–3.03)
	Conduct disorder	69 (1.7)	41 (2.2)	110 (1.9)	0.1551	0.75 (0.51–1.11)	0.49 (0.32–0.76)
	Coordination disorder	95 (2.3)	23 (1.2)	118 (2.0)	0.0061	1.88 (1.19–2.98)	1.68 (1.04–2.72)
Chronic disease	Yes	265 (6.5)	122 (6.6)	387 (6.5)	0.8376	0.98 (0.78–1.22)	
	No	3.826 (93.5)	1.721 (93.4)	5.547 (93.5)		1.00 (Ref.)	
	Missing	-	-	-			

Table 1. Cont.

		ADHD Yes	ADHD No	Total	p	OR (IC 95%)	Logistic
Type of chronic disease (flag)	Neurological	91 (2.2)	30 (1.6)	121 (2.0)	0.1324	1.37 (0.91–2.08)	
	Breathing	60 (1.5)	32 (1.7)	92 (1.6)	0.4365	0.84 (0.55–1.30)	
	Gastrointestinal	18 (0.4)	11 (0.6)	29 (0.5)	0.4227	0.74 (0.35–1.56)	

ADHD = attention deficit hyperactivity disorder, ODD = oppositional defiant disorder, p = chi-squared test (categorical variables) or Wilcoxon test (continuous variables), OR = odds ratio, CI = confidence interval, Logistic = OR and CI from the multivariate logistic regression model with stepwise type selection. (*) = $p < 0.05$.

3.1. Prescription after Diagnosis

In all, 4016 ADHD patients (98.2%) received at least one prescription: 3282 (80.2%) received only psychological treatment, 94 (2.3%) only pharmacotherapy and 640 patients (15.6%) received both pharmacological and psychological treatment. A total of 734 patients received a drug prescription, 679 (16.6%) of them methylphenidate (0.5–80 mg daily), of those 21 (0.5%) together with another drug (i.e., risperidone, aripiprazole, haloperidol, lorazepam, sertraline, alprazolam, fluvoxamine, clomipramine, delorazepam), 23 (0.6%) atomoxetine (10–60 mg daily), and 53 (1.3%) other psychotropic drugs. Among the 3922 (95.9%) patients prescribed psychoeducational treatment, 2631 (64.3%) received at least one type of training intervention (parents, teacher or child), whereas 2820 (68.9%) received other psychological treatment. Parent training was the most frequently proposed psychological treatment (n = 2311, 56.5%), followed by child training (n = 1556, 38%) and teacher training (n = 870, 21.3%). All training types were proposed to 519 (12.7%) patients. In all, 2485 (61.9%) patients had an ADHD Combined subtype (ADHD-C), whereas 1218 (30.3%) were diagnosed with Inattentive Type (ADHD-I) and 313 (7.8%) Hyperactive Type (ADHD-HI) subtypes. Of all 4091 patients diagnosed with ADHD, 4016 patients received a prescription (Table 2).

Table 2. Clinical characteristics of the ADHD patients by treatment prescription.

		Pharmacological Treatment	Psychological Treatment	Total	p	OR (IC 95%)	Logistic
		734	3282	4016			
ADHD Subtype	Combined	586 (79.8)	1.899 (57.9)	2.485 (61.9)	<0.0001 *	3.41 (2.26–5.14)	* 3.48 (1.84–6.59)
	Inattentive	122 (16.6)	1.096 (33.4)	1.218 (30.3)		1.23 (0.79–1.91)	2.34 (1.19–4.62)
	Hyperactive	26 (3.5)	287 (8.7)	313 (7.8)		1.00 (Ref.)	
	Missing	-	-	-			
QI pathologic	Yes	82 (11.4)	79 (2.4)	161 (4.1)	<0.0001 *	5.18 (3.76–7.13)	
	No	635 (88.6)	3.166 (97.6)	3.801 (95.9)		1.00 (Ref.)	
	Missing	17	37	54			
CPRS-O	Pathological	384 (63.6)	1.305 (42.6)	1.689 (46.0)	<0.0001 *	2.36 (1.97–2.82)	
	Normal	220 (36.4)	1.761 (57.4)	1.981 (54.0)		1.00 (Ref.)	
	Missing	130	216	346			

Table 2. Cont.

		Pharmacological Treatment	Psychological Treatment	Total	p	OR (IC 95%)	Logistic
		734	3282	4016			
CTRS-O	Pathological	310 (59.0)	1.219 (41.7)	1.529 (44.3)	<0.0001 *	2.02 (1.67–2.44)	
	Normal	215 (41.0)	1.707 (58.3)	1.922 (55.7)		1.00 (Ref.)	
	Missing	209	356	565			
CPRS-I	Pathological	515 (85.3)	2.176 (70.9)	2.691 (73.3)	<0.0001 *	2.37 (1.87–3.01)	
	Normal	89 (14.7)	892 (29.1)	981 (26.7)		1.00 (Ref.)	
	Missing	130	214	344			
CTRS-I	Pathological	362 (69.0)	1.717 (58.6)	2.079 (60.2)	<0.0001 *	1.57 (1.28–1.91)	
	Normal	163 (31.0)	1.211 (41.4)	1.374 (39.8)		1.00 (Ref.)	
	Missing	209	354	563			
CPRS-H	Pathological	477 (79.0)	1.840 (60.0)	2.317 (63.1)	<0.0001 *	2.51 (2.03–3.09)	* 1.48 (1.10–1.99)
	Normal	127 (21.0)	1.228 (40.0)	1.355 (36.9)		1.00 (Ref.)	
	Missing	130	214	344			
CTRS-H	Pathological	403 (76.6)	1.893 (64.7)	2.296 (66.5)	<0.0001 *	1.79 (1.44–2.22)	
	Normal	123 (23.4)	1.035 (35.3)	1.158 (33.5)		1.00 (Ref.)	
	Missing	208	354	562			
CPRS-ADHD	Pathological	557 (92.2)	2.371 (77.3)	2.928 (79.7)	<0.0001 *	3.48 (2.56–4.75)	* 2.79 (1.82–4.28)
	Normal	47 (7.8)	697 (22.7)	744 (20.3)		1.00 (Ref.)	
	Missing	130	214	344			
CTRS-ADHD	Pathological	459 (87.3)	2.285 (78.1)	2.744 (79.5)	<0.0001 *	1.92 (1.47–2.52)	
	Normal	67 (12.7)	642 (21.9)	709 (20.5)		1.00 (Ref.)	
	Missing	208	355	563			
CGI-S	5–7	516 (71.9)	597 (18.8)	1.113 (28.6)	<0.0001 *	11.02 (9.15–13.26) *	8.04 (6.35–10.19)
	1–4	202 (28.1)	2.575 (81.2)	2.777 (71.4)		1.00 (Ref.)	
	Missing	16	110	126			
Psychiatric comorbidity	Yes	612 (83.4)	2.215 (67.5)	2.827 (70.4)	<0.0001 *	2.42 (1.96–2.97) *	
	No	122 (16.6)	1.067 (32.5)	1.189 (29.6)		1.00 (Ref.)	
	Missing	-	-	-			
Type of comorbidity (flag)	Learning disorder	265 (36.1)	1.296 (39.5)	1.561 (38.9)	0.0890	0.87 (0.73–1.02)	
	Sleeping disorder	130 (17.7)	443 (13.5)	573 (14.3)	0.0032 *	1.38 (1.11–1.71)	
	ODD	209 (28.5)	356 (10.8)	565 (14.1)	<0.0001 *	3.27 (2.69–3.97)	1.64 (1.25–2.15)

Table 2. Cont.

	Pharmacological Treatment	Psychological Treatment	Total	p	OR (IC 95%)	Logistic
	734	3282	4016			
Anxiety	70 (9.5)	208 (6.3)	278 (6.9)	0.0020 *	1.56 (1.17–2.07)	
Intellectual disability	94 (12.8)	150 (4.6)	244 (6.1)	<0.0001 *	3.07 (2.34–4.02)	2.47 (1.65–3.69)
Mood disorder	57 (7.8)	170 (5.2)	227 (5.7)	0.0061 *	1.54 (1.13–2.11)	
Language disorder	61 (8.3)	221 (6.7)	282 (7.0)	0.1307	1.26 (0.93–1.69)	
Tic	40 (5.4)	54 (1.6)	94 (2.3)	<0.0001 *	3.45 (2.27–5.23)	3.60 (2.02–6.43)
Conduct disorder	29 (4.0)	39 (1.2)	68 (1.7)	<0.0001 *	3.42 (2.10–5.57)	
Autism	60 (8.2)	65 (2.0)	125 (3.1)	<0.0001 *	4.41 (3.07–6.32)	
Coordination disorder	28 (3.8)	63 (1.9)	91 (2.3)	0.0018 *	2.03 (1.29–3.19)	3.67 (2.02–6.67)
Other	17 (2.3)	66 (2.0)	83 (2.1)	0.5994	1.16 (0.67–1.98)	

CPRS = Conners' Parent Rating Scale (CPRS-O = Oppositive Scale; CPRS-I = Inattention Scale; CPRS-H = Hyperactivity Scale; CPRS-ADHD = ADHD Index; CPRS-E = Emotion Lability Scale); CTRS = Conners' Teacher Rating Scale (CTRS-O = Oppositive Scale; CTRS-I = Inattention Scale; CTRS-H = Hyperactivity Scale; CTRS-ADHD = ADHD Index; CTRS-E = Emotion Lability Scale); CGI-S = Clinical Global Impression—Severity scale; p = Chi-squared test (categorical variables) or Wilcoxon test (continuous variables); OR = odds ratio; CI = confidence interval; Logistic = OR and CI from the multivariate logistic regression model with stepwise type selectio; (*) = $p < 0.05$.

Those with an ADHD-C diagnosis were treated more commonly with drug therapy (79.8%) than with psychological treatment (57.9%), $p < 0.0001$. Otherwise, ADHD-I patients were more often treated with psychological treatment (33.4%) than drug therapy (16.6%), $p < 0.0001$. Univariate analysis between patients treated with pharmacological and psychological treatment highlighted several significant differences, as reported in Table 2. Multivariate analysis highlighted a higher probability to receive both medication and psychological prescription for those children who received a diagnosis of the ADHD combination type (OR = 3.48, 95% CI = [1.84–6.59]), a pathological score on the Hyperactivity Scales of (OR = 1.48, 95% CI [1.10–1.99]) or on the ADHD Index of CPRS (OR = 2.79, 95% CI = [1.82–4.28]), a Clinical Global Impression—Severity scale (CGI-S) score of 5 or above (OR = 8.04, 95% CI = [6.35–10.19]), and a comorbidity condition, such as ODD (OR = 1.64, 95% CI = [1.25–2.15]), cognitive delay (OR = 2.47, 95% CI = [1.65–3.69]), tics (OR = 3.60, 95% CI = [2.02–6.43]) and coordination disorders (OR = 3.67, 95% CI = [2.02–6.67]).

3.2. Parents and Teachers Rating Scales

Results from the rating scales, filled out by the parents and teachers, were compared in order to highlight differences or similarities about how adults perceived the symptom severity and behavioural problems of the child. The same comparison was made between mothers' and fathers' perception (Table 3).

Table 3. Symptom severity perceptions by parents and teachers.

Conners' Rating Scales	Score	CPRS	CTRS	p	K (IC 95%)	Agreement %
Subscales		4909	4909			
O	Pathological	1.938 (39.5)	1.884 (38.4)	0.2637	0.32 (0.29–0.35)	68
	Normal	2.971 (60.5)	3.025 (61.6)			
I	Pathological	3.270 (66.6)	2.682 (54.6)	<0.0001 *	0.25 (0.22–0.28)	64
	Normal	1.639 (33.4)	2.227 (45.4)			
H	Pathological	2.646 (53.9)	2.846 (58.0)	<0.0001 *	0.31 (0.28–0.34)	66
	Normal	2.263 (46.1)	2.063 (42.0)			
ADHD Index	Pathological	3.530 (71.9)	3.478 (70.8)	0.2456	0.26 (0.23–0.29)	70
	Normal	1.379 (28.1)	1.431 (29.2)			
E	Pathological	1.645 (33.5)	1.942 (39.6)	<0.0001 *	0.26 (0.23–0.29)	65
	Normal	3.264 (66.5)	2.967 (60.4)			
CBCL	Score	Mother	Father	p	K (IC 95%)	Agreement %
		1082	1082			
I	Pathological	223 (20.6)	159 (14.7)	0.0003	0.64 (0.58–0.70)	89
	Normal	859 (79.4)	923 (85.3)			
E	Pathological	254 (23.5)	204 (18.9)	0.0085	0.69 (0.63–0.74)	89
	Normal	828 (76.5)	878 (81.1)			
T	Pathological	349 (32.3)	255 (23.6)	<0.0001	0.66 (0.61–0.71)	86
	Normal	733 (67.7)	827 (76.4)			

CPRS = Conners' Parent Rating Scale (CPRS-O = Oppositive Scale; CPRS-I = Inattention Scale; CPRS-H = Hyperactivity Scale; CPRS-ADHD = ADHD Index; CPRS-E = Emotion Lability Scale); CTRS = Conners' Teacher Rating Scale (CTRS-O = Oppositive Scale; CTRS-I = Inattention Scale; CTRS-H = Hyperactivity Scale; CTRS-ADHD = ADHD Index; CTRS-E = Emotion Lability Scale); CBCL = Child Behaviour Checklist (CBCL-I = Internalising problems; CBCL-E = Externalising problems; CBCL-T = Total); p = Chi-squared test; K = Cohen's Kappa Statistic; % = proportion of patients with the same results on tests; (*) = $p < 0.05$.

The results highlighted that parents tended to perceive more cognitive problems (CPRS-I = 3270, 66.6%; CTRS-I = 2682, 54.6%; $p < 0.0001$) than teachers, who reported more behavioural (CTRS-H = 2848, 58%; CPRS-H = 2646, 53.9%; $p < 0.0001$) and emotional problems (CTRS-E = 1942, 39.6%; CPRS-E = 1645, 33.5%; $p < 0.0001$). Mothers reported more child pathological problems than fathers did on both subscales (CBCL-I = 223, 20.6%; CBC-I father = 159, 14.7%; $p = 0.0003$) (CBCL-E = 254, 23.5%; CBCL-E father = 204, 18.9%; $p = 0.0085$) and on the CBCL-Total score (CBCL-T = 349, 32.3%; CBCL-T father = 255, 23.6%; $p < 0.0001$). Despite these differences, kappa values highlighted a "fair" agreement between parents and teachers (>60%) and "excellent" agreement between mothers and fathers (>85%).

3.3. Continuity of Care and Management

Throughout the regional database system, data on patient care from the first access to the diagnosis and data on treatment prescriptions and follow-up visits were systematically collected. As shown in Figure 2, the diagnostic evaluation was full and accurate: each axis has a range of 0 to 100% and represents one of the seven areas of the shared diagnostic assessment (Clinical Interview, Neurological Examination, IQ Evaluation, Diagnostic Interview, Parents and Teachers Assessment, Clinical Severity Evaluation), while the three datasets represent the performance scores of the most (average = 100%) and least compliant (average = 91.01%) ADHD centre, as well as the total completeness (average = 97.86%) estimated by the analysis of data recorded by all 18 ADHD centres. Overall, 320 of 4091 patients with a diagnosis of ADHD were discharged during the first 3 months; 1468 patients with ADHD had been monitored for more than 1 year after the diagnosis, half of whom had a significant improvement with CGI-I scores of 1–3, and the majority of these (89%) were in a stable condition with scores of 4 on the CGI-I. In all, 755 patients reached the legal age (range 18–27 years), 31.3% of whom just turned 18 years old.

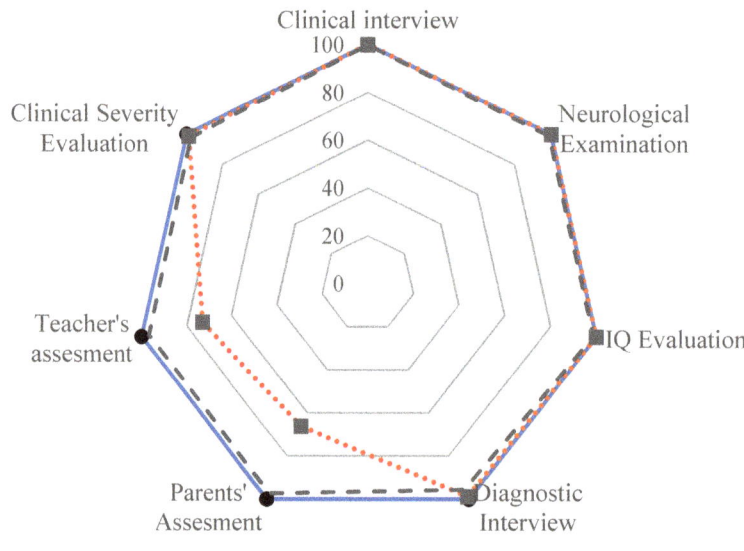

Figure 2. Rate of completeness levels based on data inputted in the registry.

4. Discussion

Ten years after the creation of the Lombardy Registry Project, clinical and service assessment data revealed the effectiveness and usefulness of this regional project in providing assistance and continuity of care to ADHD patients and their families. Over the years, the registry was monitored to achieve clinical improvement, using systematic activities and an interactive system evaluation to test the change, according to the main clinical quality improvement features [27]. The clinical characteristics of the ADHD patients of the Lombardy Registry Project were in line with the literature; the peak age of diagnosis was in primary school children aged 5–10 years [6], and LD was the main psychiatric comorbidity followed by ODD, anxiety, and sleeping disorders [1,12]. The most associated chronic disease was a neurological condition. Concerning treatment, data extracted from the registry highlighted a relation between some clinical characteristics and the type of prescription at diagnosis; according to the literature, the symptom severity increased the likelihood of being prescribed ADHD medication [28]. The higher the CGI-S score, the higher the probability of receiving a medical prescription, in particular for patients with ODD, an intellectual disability, tics or a coordination disorder. Differently from what we expected, learning problems were not associated with being prescribed medication, suggesting that learning problems may not be pertinent to pharmacological treatment decisions for children with ADHD. Pharmacological prescription was infrequent (18%), and nearly all of the patients (96%) received a psychological prescription such as child, parent or teacher training. Comparing data with higher rates reported in other countries [29], in Italy child psychiatrists' professional attitude leaned more toward behavioural treatments than to the use of drugs [30]. In general, half of the patients with a diagnosis of ADHD and in treatment for almost one year (follow-up between 12 and 18 months) reported an improvement in their level of symptom severity on the CGI-I score. These data were comforting, suggesting the clinical care utility of a continuously monitored, standardised system. The project represents a great opportunity to improve collaboration, share assessment approaches and promote the continuity of care of patients affected by ADHD, monitoring their treatments and healthcare pathway. This represented an important value for the project; continuously monitoring and sharing data is an important approach in order to ensure the quality of care. The ADHD project could represent an example of a healthcare system for other chronic conditions and psychiatric disorders in childhood in order to promote the continuity and improvement of childcare. Particular attention should be paid to a particular phase called transition—the passage between child care to adult care; after ten years of the project, many children became adolescents, and some of them are near the boundary age. The transition process not only concerns healthcare but also involves the transition to adulthood, finding employment or continuing the education process; therefore, it is important for the adolescent to be prepared to manage their medical condition and pharmacological treatment. Once reaching adulthood, the risk is being discharged by the services and not receiving prescribed medication. In order to avoid this situation, it is very important to promote the continuity and monitoring of childcare. A great deal has been done, but a lot of work is still necessary for the best management of ADHD across the lifespan. The limit of the project's approach is that it represents a national uniqueness. Moreover, the registry, due to its nature of being an observatory of healthcare provided by a service (even if public), does not contemplate the rate of patients who interrupted the care pathway or who did not start it, failing to show up from the start. Despite the remarkable improvements made in the last twenty years for providing appropriate diagnostic and treatment services for children with ADHD, also as a result of the landmark Multimodal Treatment Study of Children with Attention Deficit/Hyperactivity Disorder (MTA) trial [31], practice is still different between and within countries. Recommendations and guidelines for ADHD management in children and adolescents were produced by several parties and individual centres adapted their care. The findings reported here are not different from others reported in the literature where health services and care are different. However, the heart of the Italian Lombardy ADHD Registry lies in the approach: collaborative, shared between and within the participating centres, over time. It is an unusual approach in the interest of the patients and carers.

5. Conclusions

The Regional ADHD Registry represents a distinctive tool, a unique experience in the international context, to help guarantee a shared pathway of care in ADHD children. Continuous, systematic monitoring allows resources to be invested appropriately, such as in promoting progressive and significant improvement in clinical practice, ensuring a shared and efficient quality of care. Training initiatives involving clinicians, patients, parents and teachers may be useful in order to raise awareness about the disorder in clinical practice.

Supplementary Materials: The following are available online at https://www.mdpi.com/article/10.3390/children8070598/s1, Table S1: Demographic Characteristics of the ADHD patients. Table S2: Clinical Characteristics of the ADHD Patients by Treatment Prescription. Table S3: Symptoms severity perceptions by parents and teachers.

Author Contributions: M.B. had the idea for the study and designed it, F.S. drafted the initial version. M.C. and M.Z. managed and analysed the data. All collected data were analysed monthly, and the findings were reported and periodically discussed with all 18 ADHD centres belonging to the Lombardy ADHD Group. All authors participated in study design, contributed to the interpretation of data, critical review and revision of the report, and approved the final report as submitted. M.B. is the guarantor for the study. The views expressed are those of the authors and not necessarily those of the Regional Healthcare Directorate. All authors have read and agreed to the published version of the manuscript.

Funding: The authors disclosed receipt of the following financial support for the research, authorship, and publication of this article: The study is part of the "Sharing Diagnostic-Therapeutic Approaches for ADHD Lombardy" project partially funded by the Health Care Directorate of the Lombardy Region (D.G. sanità n.3798, 8/05/2014).

Institutional Review Board Statement: The study was approved by the ethics committee of the San Paolo hospital of Milan, Italy (2020/ST/106).

Informed Consent Statement: Informed consent was obtained from all subjects involved in the study.

Data Availability Statement: The datasets analyzed during the current study are available from the corresponding author upon reasonable request.

Acknowledgments: The study is part of the "Sharing diagnostic–therapeutic approaches for ADHD in Lombardy" project partially funded by the Healthcare Directorate of the Lombardy Region (D.G. sanità n.3798, 8 May 2014). The views expressed are those of the authors and not necessarily those of the regional Healthcare Directorate. We thank all the teams of the 18 participating ADHD centres who devoted significant time and energy to this project, joining and animating the Lombardy ADHD Group, in addition to the authors: Stoppa Patrizia, Stefano Conte, Valeria Renzetti (Bergamo); Massimo Molteni, Sara Trabattoni, Antonio Salandi, Valentina Mauri (Bosisio Parini, LC); Elisa Fazzi, Elena Filippini, Elisabetta Pedercini (Brescia); Patrizia Conti, Nadia Fteita, Elena Della Libera (Como); Maria Teresa Giarelli, Giacomo Piccini, Luciano Viola (Cremona); Federico Ravaglione, Simona Frassica, Stefania Villa (Garbagnate Milanese, MI); Daniela Alacqua, Ottaviano Martinelli, Davide Villani (Lecco); Emanuela Binaghi, Andrea Deriu, Gabriella Vasile, Matteo Caletti (Legnano, MI); Paola Morosini, Barbara Salvatore (Lodi); Maddalena Breviglieri, Giuseppe Capovilla (Mantova); Vera Valenti, Chiara Galantini, Gala Garden (FBF); Costantino De Giacomo, Fornaro Emiddio, Chiara Battaini, Alessandra Valentino (Niguarda); Costantino Antonella, Bissoli Claudio, Cropanese Isabella, Jessica Babboni, Eliana Antonacci (Policlinico); Maria Paola Canevini, Mauro Walder, Valentina Tessarollo, Ilaria Costantino (San Paolo); Renato Borgatti, Matteo Chiappedi, Elisa Baroffio (Pavia); Maria Luisa Carpanelli, Maria Grazia Palmieri, Gianpaolo Ruffoni, Connie Capici (Sondrio); Francesco Rinaldi, Federica Soardi, Sara Mometti (Vallecamonica–Sebino, BS); Giorgio Rossi, Cristiano Termine, Carla Sgrò (Varese). The authors would like to acknowledge Chiara Pandolfini and Daniela Miglio for manuscript language editing.

Conflicts of Interest: The authors declare the following potential conflict of interest with respect to the research, authorship, and/or publication of this article. All authors declare no financial relationships with any organisations that might have an interest in the submitted work; no other relationships or activities that could appear to have influenced the submitted work.

References

1. Faraone, S.V.; Banaschewski, T.; Coghill, D.; Zheng, Y.; Biederman, J.; Bellgrove, M.A.; Newcorn, J.H.; Gignac, M.; Al Saud, N.M.; Manor, I.; et al. The World Federation of ADHD International Consensus Statement: 208 Evidence-based conclusions about the disorder. *Neurosci. Biobehav. Rev.* **2021**. [CrossRef] [PubMed]
2. Bonati, M.; Reale, L.; Zanetti, M.; Cartabia, M.; Fortinguerra, F.; Capovilla, G.; Chiappedi, M.; Costantino, A.; Effedri, P.; Luoni, C.; et al. A Regional ADHD center-based network project for the diagnosis and treatment of children and adolescents with ADHD. *J. Atten. Disord.* **2018**, *22*, 1173–1184. [CrossRef] [PubMed]
3. Caye, A.; Rocha, T.B.-M.; Anselmi, L.; Murray, J.; Menezes, A.M.B.; Barros, F.C.; Gonçalves, H.; Wehrmeister, F.; Jensen, C.M.; Steinhausen, H.-C.; et al. Attention-Deficit/Hyperactivity Disorder trajectories from childhood to young adulthood: Evidence from a birth cohort supporting a late-onset syndrome. *JAMA Psychiatry* **2016**, *73*, 705–712. [CrossRef] [PubMed]
4. Reale, L.; Bonati, M. ADHD prevalence estimates in Italian children and adolescents: A methodological issue. *Ital. J. Pediatr.* **2018**, *44*, 108. [CrossRef]
5. Austerman, J. ADHD and behavioral disorders: Assessment, management, and an update from DSM-5. *Clevel. Clin. J. Med.* **2015**, *82*, S2–S7. [CrossRef] [PubMed]
6. Eysbouts, Y.; Poulton, A.; Salmelainen, P. Stimulant medication in pre-school children in New South Wales. *J. Paediatr. Child. Health* **2011**, *47*, 870–874. [CrossRef]
7. Bonati, M.; Cartabia, M.; Zanetti, M.; Reale, L.; Didoni, A.; Costantino, M.A.; the Lombardy ADHD Group. Age level vs grade level for the diagnosis of ADHD and neurodevelopmental disorders. *Eur. Child. Adolesc. Psychiatry* **2018**, *27*, 1171–1180. [CrossRef] [PubMed]
8. National Guideline Centre (UK). *Attention Deficit Hyperactivity Disorder: Diagnosis and Management*; National Institute for Health and Care Excellence (UK): London, UK, 2018.
9. Chiarenza, G.A.; Bianchi, E.; Marzocchi, M.M. Linee Guida del Trattamento Cognitivo Comportamentale Deidisturbi da Deficit Dell'attenzione con Iperattività (Adhd)—Linee Guida SINPIA 2003. Available online: https://www.sinpia.eu/wp-content/uploads/atom/allegato/147.pdf (accessed on 21 May 2021).

10. Harpin, V.; Mazzone, L.; Raynaud, J.P.; Kahle, J.; Hodgkins, P. Long-term outcomes of ADHD: A systematic review of self-esteem and social function. *J. Atten. Disord.* **2016**, *20*, 295–305. [CrossRef]
11. Faraone, S.V.; Asherson, P.; Banaschewski, T.; Biederman, J.; Buitelaar, J.K.; Ramos-Quiroga, J.A.; Rohde, L.A.; Sonuga-Barke, E.J.; Tannock, R.; Franke, B. Attention-deficit/hyperactivity disorder. *Nat. Rev. Dis. Primers* **2015**, *1*, 15020. [CrossRef]
12. Jensen, C.M.; Steinhausen, H.-C. Comorbid mental disorders in children and adolescents with attention-deficit/hyperactivity disorder in a large nationwide study. *Atten. Deficit Hyperact. Disord.* **2015**, *7*, 27–38. [CrossRef]
13. Wilens, T.E.; Adler, L.; Adams, J.; Sgambati, S.; Rotrosen, J.; Sawtelle, R.; Utzinger, L.; Fusillo, S. Misuse and diversion of stimulants prescribed for ADHD: A systematic review of the literature. *J. Am. Acad. Child. Adolesc. Psychiatry* **2008**, *47*, 21–31. [CrossRef]
14. Clemow, D.B.; Walker, D.J. The potential for misuse and abuse of medications in ADHD: A review. *Postgrad. Med.* **2014**, *126*, 64–81. [CrossRef]
15. Lambez, B.; Harwood-Gross, A.; Golumbic, E.Z.; Rassovsky, Y. Non-pharmacological interventions for cognitive difficulties in ADHD: A systematic review and meta-analysis. *J. Psychiatr. Res.* **2020**, *120*, 40–55. [CrossRef] [PubMed]
16. Clavenna, A.; Cartabia, M.; Sequi, M.; Costantino, M.A.; Bortolotti, A.; Fortino, I.; Merlino, L.; Bonati, M. Burden of psychiatric disorders in the pediatric population. *Eur. Neuropsychopharmacol.* **2013**, *23*, 98–106. [CrossRef] [PubMed]
17. Coghill, D.R. Organisation of services for managing ADHD. *Epidemiol. Psychiatr. Sci.* **2016**, *26*, 453–458. [CrossRef]
18. Bonati, M.; Cartabia, M.; Zanetti, M.; the Lombardy ADHD Group. Waiting times for diagnosis of attention-deficit hyperactivity disorder in children and adolescents referred to Italian ADHD centers must be reduced. *BMC Health Serv. Res.* **2019**, *19*, 1–10. [CrossRef]
19. Reale, L.; Bartoli, B.; Cartabia, M.; Zanetti, M.; Costantino, M.A.; Canevini, M.P.; Termine, C.; Bonati, M.; on behalf of Lombardy ADHD Group. Comorbidity prevalence and treatment outcome in children and adolescents with ADHD. *Eur. Child. Adolesc. Psychiatry* **2017**, *26*, 1443–1457. [CrossRef]
20. Didoni, A.; Sequi, M.; Panei, P.; Bonati, M.; Lombardy ADHD Registry Group. One-year prospective follow-up of pharmacological treatment in children with attention-deficit/hyperactivity disorder. *Eur. J. Clin. Pharmacol.* **2011**, *67*, 1061–1067. [CrossRef] [PubMed]
21. Zanetti, M.; Cartabia, M.; Didoni, A.; Fortinguerra, F.; Reale, L.; Mondini, M.; Bonati, M. The impact of a model-based clinical regional registry for attention-deficit hyperactivity disorder. *Health Inform. J.* **2016**, *23*, 159–169. [CrossRef]
22. Goyette, C.H.; Conners, C.K.; Ulrich, R.F. Normative data on revised conners parent and teacher rating scales. *J. Abnorm. Child. Psychol.* **1978**, *6*, 221–236. [CrossRef]
23. Conners, C.K.; Sitarenios, G.; Parker, J.D.A.; Epstein, J.N. The Revised Conners' Parent Rating Scale (CPRS-R): Factor structure, reliability, and criterion validity. *J. Abnorm. Child. Psychol.* **1998**, *26*, 257–268. [CrossRef]
24. Achenbach, T.M.; Edelbrock, C.S. *Manual for the Child. Behavior Checklist and Revised Child. Behavior Profile*; Univ Vermont/Dept Psychiatry: Burlington, VT, USA, 1983; pp. 85–121.
25. Guy, W. Clinical global impressions. In *ECDEU Assessment Manual for Psychopharmacology—Revised*; Scientific Research: Rockville, MD, USA, 1976; pp. 218–222.
26. American Psychiatric Association. *Diagnostic and Statistical Manual of Mental Disorders*, 5th ed.; American Psychiatric Publishing: Arlington, VA, USA, 2013.
27. Rubenstein, L.; Khodyakov, D.; Hempel, S.; Danz, M.; Salem-Schatz, S.; Foy, R.; O'Neill, S.; Dalal, S.; Shekelle, P. How can we recognize continuous quality improvement? *Int. J. Qual. Health Care* **2014**, *26*, 6–15. [CrossRef]
28. Mowlem, F.D.; Rosenqvist, M.A.; Martin, J.; Lichtenstein, P.; Asherson, P.; Larsson, H. Sex differences in predicting ADHD clinical diagnosis and pharmacological treatment. *Eur. Child. Adolesc. Psychiatry* **2019**, *28*, 481–489. [CrossRef] [PubMed]
29. Scheffler, R.M.; Hinshaw, S.P.; Modrek, S.; Levine, P. The global market for ADHD medications. *Health Aff.* **2007**, *26*, 450–457. [CrossRef]
30. Clavenna, A.; Rossi, E.; DeRosa, M.; Bonati, M. Use of psychotropic medications in Italian children and adolescents. *Eur. J. Pediatr.* **2006**, *166*, 339–347. [CrossRef] [PubMed]
31. Taylor, E. Development of clinical services for attention-deficit/hyperactivity disorder. *Arch. Gen. Psychiatry* **1999**, *56*, 1097–1099. [CrossRef] [PubMed]

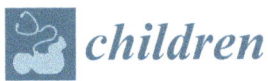

Article

Reading Skills of Children with Dyslexia Improved Less Than Expected during the COVID-19 Lockdown in Italy

Ilaria Maria Carlotta Baschenis [1,†], Laura Farinotti [1,†], Elena Zavani [2], Serena Grumi [1], Patrizia Bernasconi [1], Enrica Rosso [1], Livio Provenzi [1], Renato Borgatti [1,2], Cristiano Termine [3] and Matteo Chiappedi [1,*]

1. Child Neuropsychiatry Unit, IRCCS Mondino Foundation, 27100 Pavia, Italy; ilaria.baschenis@mondino.it (I.M.C.B.); laura.farinotti@mondino.it (L.F.); serena.grumi@mondino.it (S.G.); patrizia.bernasconi@mondino.it (P.B.); enrica.rosso@mondino.it (E.R.); livio.provenzi@mondino.it (L.P.); renato.borgatti@mondino.it (R.B.)
2. Department of Brain and Behavioral Sciences, University of Pavia, 27100 Pavia, Italy; elena.zavani01@universitadipavia.it
3. Department of Medicine and Surgery, University of Insubria, 21100 Varese, Italy; cristiano.termine@uninsubria.it
* Correspondence: matteo.chiappedi@mondino.it
† These authors contributed equally to this work.

Abstract: Following school closures due to the SARS-CoV-2 pandemic, for some months, children received only distance learning. The effects of this approach, however, are not clear for children with dyslexia. We conducted a cross-sectional comparison between children with and without dyslexia after the so-called "lockdown" and a comparison between pre- and post-lockdown parameters in children with dyslexia. We recruited sixty-five children with dyslexia (dyslexia group, DG) from an outpatient facility in Pavia (Lombardy, Italy) and fifty-two children without specific learning disabilities as the control group (CG) from summer camps in the same province. We performed neuropsychological tests to explore reading skills and an ad hoc questionnaire to explore how parents and children had experienced the measures taken to reduce spreading of SARS-CoV-2 infection. Between 59 to 63% of children with dyslexia did not reach the average expected increase of reading skills. According to their parents, they also showed greater social isolation and fewer worries about the pandemic and the school's closure. Our data indicate that children with dyslexia are at increased risk of consequences on their learning potential in case of school closure. They also seem to have a peculiar psychological experience of school closure. Specific interventions should therefore be provided to minimize the risk of negative effects on global development.

Keywords: COVID-19; dyslexia; reading skills; learning disability

1. Introduction

During the first months of 2020, Italy was rapidly and dramatically affected by the rapid outbreak of the SARS-CoV-2 pandemic [1]. Government attempts to mitigate and contain the virus spread required a massive reduction of physical contact and the lockdown that followed also included the suspension of school activities from February 24th to the end of the academic year in June 2020. Distance learning was recommended [2], but its implementation was not immediate for many institutes and the delivery modes varied during the lockdown months and among different schools [3].

In this scenario, a reduction of learning outcomes may be expected as reported in previous studies on partial or temporary interruptions of school attendance [4]. Nonetheless, more negative consequences may be expected for children who already presented special educational needs and learning disabilities [3]. According to the latest edition of the Diagnostic and Statistic Manual of Mental Disorders (DSM-5 [5]), specific learning disorder is a neurodevelopmental disorder with biological origin, characterized by persistent difficulties in learning and using academic skills. This diagnosis does not apply to

subjects with intellectual disabilities, uncorrected visual or auditory ability, other mental or neurological disorders, significant psychosocial adversities, inadequate language skills, or inadequate educational instruction. Dyslexia refers specifically to an impairment in word recognition, decoding, and spelling. Children with dyslexia require specific supports to reach adequate and satisfying learning goals. Besides rehabilitative attention [6], they need to receive specific teaching and to use compensative strategies and tools according to the specific needs of the single individual [7].

As such, as their educational needs require continuous dedicated and systematic care on a daily basis, children diagnosed with dyslexia may be at increased risk for detrimental learning consequences during the COVID-19 lockdown. The suspension of school in-presence activities may had impacted the continuity of educational care for children with dyslexia with the risk of increased emotional and psychological burden related to social distances, lack of dedicated specialist support, and isolation [3]. Moreover, during the lockdown, the engagement of parents in their children school activities dramatically increased as—in many case—they had to shift from working hours to a 24/7 care for their children's special educational needs at home [8]. Parents of children with special educational needs exhibited worries about the possibility for their children to fall even further behind in school because they did not feel adequate to meet their specific needs during the COVID-19 emergency [9]. Additionally, worries about the lack of supervised and specialist care for their children's disability condition and rehabilitation was the most significant predictor of parents' stress, depressive and anxious symptoms during the COVID-19 lockdown [10].

Although they should be considered as a specific vulnerable population during the COVID-19 emergency, to the best of our knowledge, no study to date has reported on the effects of school suspension and distance learning in children with dyslexia. In the present study, we compared the reading skills (i.e., accuracy and speed) of a sample of children with dyslexia before (T1) and after the COVID-19 lockdown (T2) with a control group at T2. A preliminary analysis was conducted to control for differences in the perception and experience of the lockdown and distance learning in the two groups. Then, we analyzed the presence of significant changes in reading skills between T1 and T2 within the group of children with dyslexia. In order to better explore the clinical relevance of significant changes in reading skills within dyslexic children, they were compared with two different parameters: the reading skills of typically developing counterparts and the expected one-year improvement in reading speed.

2. Materials and Methods

2.1. Participants

Sixty-five children ($n = 20$ females) with dyslexia (dyslexia group, DG) were enrolled consecutively at the Child Neuropsychiatry Unit of the IRCCS Mondino Foundation, Pavia, Italy. Children were included if they were students from the third to the eighth grade, if they had had a previous reading assessment in 2019, if they were monolingual, and in the absence of neurological and psychiatric comorbidities. Fifty-two ($n = 20$ females) children without specific learning disabilities as the control group (CG) were enrolled at a summer camp in Pavia from July to August 2020. Neither group physically attended the school from March to June 2020 due to the COVID-19 lockdown.

The mean age of children of the dyslexia group (DG) was 10.64 years (Standard Deviation (SD) = 1.60, range = 8–14), while that of the control group (CG) was 9.80 years (SD = 1.57, range = 7–13). The t-test showed that CG children were significantly younger compared to the DG counterparts ($t = 3.14$, $p < 0.01$), therefore in the subsequent comparison analyses on reading abilities, the age was controlled as the covariate.

2.2. Procedures

Both groups completed three tasks to assess their reading skills (see below) and they filled in a questionnaire about online school characteristics and challenges. DG children were evaluated for reading skills two times: before the lockdown in 2019 (T1) and after the lockdown (T2). CG children were evaluated only once at T2. In consideration of the reading difficulties of DG subjects, the questionnaire was administered by a nominated researcher to the children of both groups. Additionally, parents filled in a self-report questionnaire on online school management.

2.3. Measures

Reading assessment. The reading assessment was performed through three tasks. The first two tasks (i.e., reading aloud a list of words and a list of non-words) were derived from the Battery for the Assessment of Developmental Dyslexia and Dysorthography-2 (DDE-2 Battery by Sartori et al. [11]) to assess reading speed (syllables per second) and accuracy (number of errors). The third task was derived from the Assessment of Reading and Comprehension Skills for Elementary and Middle School (MT-3-Clinic tasks by Cornoldi and Carretti [12]) and it consists of reading a text aloud to assess reading speed (syllables per second) and accuracy (number of errors).

Ad hoc questionnaire. An ad hoc questionnaire provided a detailed characterization of the online school delivered during the lockdown period (March–June 2020), including which kinds of remote education were implemented (e.g., online vs. pre-recorded lessons), major challenges in managing online school (e.g., online platform, connection, family management), and parents' perception of their children learning trajectories. The questionnaire was filled in by parents as well as by children with the help of a dedicated researcher.

2.4. Plan of Analysis

Preliminary descriptive statistics were performed and the two groups of students were compared for demographic characteristics through an independent-sample t-test. Then, a set of χ^2 tests were performed in order to identify differences in the survey's results between the DG and CG subjects. In order to assess reading skills development of DG children, three different sets of analyses were used. First, T1-to-T2 differences in reading speed and accuracy (for words, non-words, and text) were tested in DG children through paired-sample t-tests. Second, two sets of analysis of covariance (ANCOVA) with age as the covariate were implemented to compare reading speed and accuracy between DG and CG children at T2. Third, a sub-group analysis was used to identify percentages of DG children that reached the expected one-year improvement in reading speed in Italian untreated dyslexic students, i.e., 0.30 syllables per second for words and 0.15 syllables per second for non-words (as reported by Tressoldi et al. [13]). IBM SPSS 25 was used for the statistical analyses and p was set at 0.05.

2.5. Ethics

All parents provided informed consent to participate and children accepted to take part in the study. All the procedures were consistent with the Declaration of Helsinki ethical principles for research involving human subjects and the study was approved by the Ethics Committee of the Policlinico San Matteo (Pavia) with number P-20200048574.

3. Results

3.1. Survey

As showed in Figure 1, the online school activities changed during the lockdown, with an increase of live classes: during the first months of the lockdown, the majority of the students attended online live classes only twice a week and received study sheets and/or pre-recorded video by teachers as integration, while from May to June, more than 80% of them attended daily online classes.

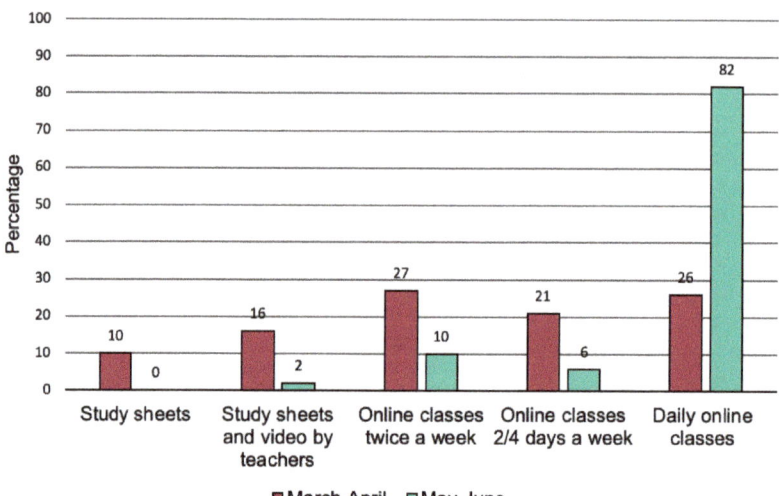

Figure 1. Remote school activities delivered during the first (March–April) and last (May–June) months of the lockdown period.

Table 1 reports significant differences between DG and CG subjects. As expected, a higher percentage of DG children reported difficulties in following online classes and managing homework during the lockdown. Moreover, more children with dyslexia compared to CG controls perceived a worsening in various tasks, including reading, comprehension, and mathematics. These main difficulties were confirmed also by the parents' point of view. Moreover, for DG children, greater social isolation and fewer worries about the pandemic and the school's closure emerged.

Table 1. Children and parents' comparison about online school management. Note: DG, dyslexia group; CG, control group.

Survey Items (Children)	DG, n = 65	CG, n = 52	χ^2	p
Difficulties following online classes	48%	23%	6.56	<0.05
Difficulties in doing homework	62%	13%	24.4	<0.001
Perceiving that learning abilities worsened during quarantine	19%	3%	14.86	<0.01
Perceiving that reading abilities remained the same during quarantine	64%	93%	11.35	<0.05
More difficulties in text comprehension without teacher's oral explanation	60%	33%	8.77	<0.05
Difficulties in mathematics	35%	10%	8.05	<0.01
More errors in mathematics	49%	18%	10.62	<0.01
Worsening in text comprehension	49%	18%	10.62	<0.01
More difficulties in studying	51%	13%	15.68	<0.01
Worsening in vocabulary	38%	8%	12.43	<0.01
More family conflicts	46%	20%	7.30	<0.05
Asking often when the school will reopen	19%	65%	22.36	<0.001
Missing friends	67%	93%	9.92	<0.01
Concerns about COVID-19	3%	25%	11.54	<0.01
Asking for information about COVID-19	30%	73%	32.66	<0.001
Survey Items (Parents)	**DG, n = 63**	**CG, n = 38**	χ^2	p
Difficulties following online classes	52%	0%	30.91	<0.001
Difficulties in doing homework	67%	11%	33.50	<0.001
Perceiving that reading worsened during quarantine	41%	16%	12.33	<0.05
Using more the keyboard	46%	76%	8.89	<0.01
More errors in mathematics	46%	13%	13.12	<0.05
Worsening in text comprehension	38%	5%	18.71	<0.001
Worsening in oral presentation	35%	3%	18.71	<0.001
Contac classmates for homework	11%	40%	14.81	<0.01
Teachers as emotional support	44%	82%	14.47	<0.01
Less contacts with friends	32%	11%	9.45	<0.01

3.2. Reading Skills Group Analysis

DG children improved their reading speed for all the three included tasks (see Figure 2A): words t(64)= −4.99, $p < 0.001$, non-words, t(64) = −3.51, $p = 0.001$, and text, t(64) = −6.25, $p < 0.001$. DG children also showed a significant reduction of the errors' occurrence for words, t(64) = 3.97, $p < 0.001$, non-words, t(64) = 2.25, $p = 0.028$, and text t(64) = 2.31, $p = 0.024$.

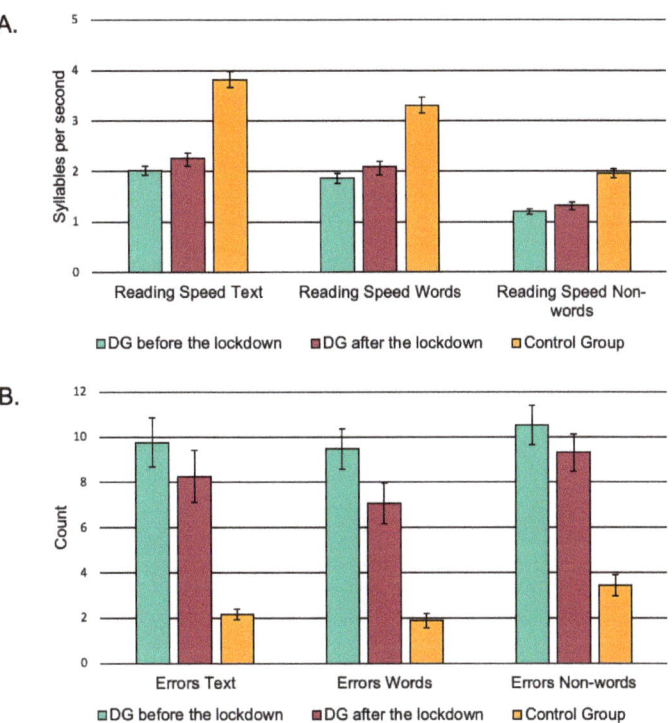

Figure 2. Dyslexia group (DG) and control group reading speed (**A**) and accuracy (**B**) for words, non-words, and text before and after the lockdown. Note: the control group was assessed only after the lockdown; bars represent standard errors.

At T2, DG subjects exhibited significantly worse performance than CG counterparts for what pertains to reading speed (words: $F(1,114) = 130.86$, $p < 0.001$; non-words, $F(1,114) = 89.32$, $p < 0.001$; text: $F(1,114) = 175.43$, $p < 0.001$) and accuracy (words: $F(1,114) = 46.16$, $p < 0.001$; non-words: $F(1,114) = 48.1$, $p < 0.001$; text: $F(1,114) = 22.82$, $p < 0.001$), as showed in Figure 2.

3.3. Expected Improvement in Reading Speed

As showed in Figure 3A, 70% to 85% of DG children exhibited an improvement with respect to zero, suggesting that there is a naturally occurring improvement in reading speed at this age. However, a percentage from 59% to 63% did not reach the expected improvement (0.30 syllables/second for words; 0.15 syllables/second for non-words) (Figure 3B). Notably, the availability of compensatory tools and the presence of a tutor during the lockdown did not significantly affect these percentages.

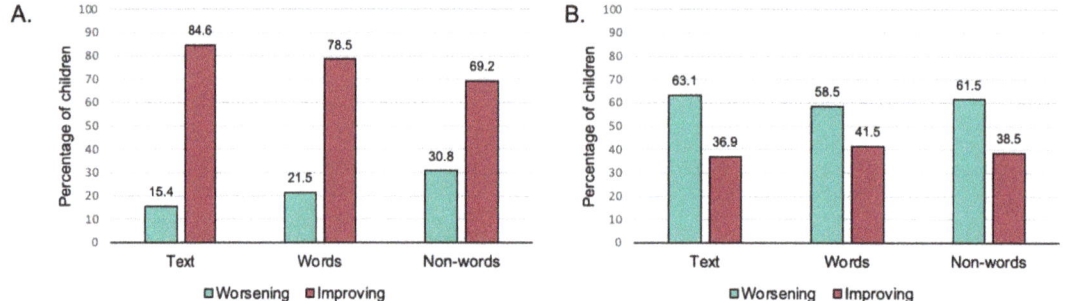

Figure 3. Percentages of DG children who improved after the lockdown with respect to improve-rate equal to zero (**A**) and equal to 0.30 for words and text and 0.15 for non-words (**B**). Note: DG, dyslexia group.

4. Discussion

The aim of this study was to investigate the evolution of reading speed and accuracy in children with dyslexia, following the closure of schools due to the spread of the SARS-CoV-2 infection.

The first relevant finding emerging from our data is that a high percentage of children did not receive daily online live classes for a prolonged period. As expected, children with dyslexia reported more difficulties in following online classes and managing homework compared to normally developing ("healthy") children. At the same time, however, children with dyslexia appeared to be less worried about the school closure: the school context implies the exposure to performance and social issues that usually trigger anxiety or feelings of inadequacy [14]; therefore, they may perceive the school closure as protective for them.

We also noted a failure to reach learning outcomes (in terms of expected increase of reading speed). Previous research evidenced that children with dyslexia tend to have a natural increase of reading skills, in terms both of accuracy and speed; this increase is not negligible, although significantly lower than that seen in normally developing children [13]. In keep with existing literature, we found a general significant improvement in reading speed and a reduction in the number of reading errors observed also in children with dyslexia, confirming that there is a naturally occurring improvement in reading speed at this age; however, a percentage from 59% to 63% of these children did not reach the improvement in reading skills expected in untreated children with the same diagnosis.

These data could be expected from existing literature, although the number of studies investigating the development of learning in contexts without education or with distance learning methods is low, except for those that refer to the summer break (whose duration was, however, lower than the period of school closure in Italy). Research conducted by Shynwell and Defeyter showed that during the seven-week summer vacation, children experienced a reduction of the physiological increase of learning skills, up to a total stop, but could start improving again after a similar amount of time of school frequency [15]. Alexander et al. showed that, during the summer months, the skills of children with higher socioeconomic status continued to advance (albeit, at a slower rate than the school year), whereas the skills of children with lower socioeconomic status mostly remained flat [16]. Cooper et al. suggested that skills requiring a procedural knowledge are more significantly influenced by the loss of the regular exercise provided by school frequency [17]. This could be especially relevant for children whose neuropsychological functioning towards reading is often characterized by a deficit of procedural learning [18].

The introduction of distance learning did not seem to reduce these risks. In Italy, despite regulatory prescriptions, it was realized in a way that was neither consistent nor sufficient (our findings suggest that after three months from the beginning of the lockdown, nearly one fifth of children were not receiving daily classes, despite the fact that children in our study were from Lombardy, usually considered to be one of the better organized parts of Italy). Moreover, recent data evidenced that distance learning in Italy increases educational deprivation and social inequalities, a fact more evident in children with developmental disabilities [19].

It should be also stressed that the feeling of being understood and supported by the teacher(s) is highly relevant in reducing the risk of anxiety symptoms in children with specific learning disabilities [14]. The lack of direct contact with teachers could reduce this feeling of receiving adequate attention and support, and therefore increase the risk of developing internalizing symptoms.

Our study has some limitations. First, the control group was not assessed before the so-called "lockdown"; this prevented us from knowing the increase in reading speed obtained in these subjects, which, however, had a reading speed and accuracy in line with what expected according to their grade. Second, the control group was tested after school ending; this could, however, have only reduced the difference in reading speed and accuracy [15,16]. Third, there was a difference in terms of age between the two groups, which we were, however, able to control through statistical analyses. To end with, we did not explore the possibility of a "catch up" in terms of reading speed and accuracy after returning to a normal school frequency; this could be, however, an interesting idea for future studies.

5. Practical Implications

Both existing literature and our findings support the idea that children with dyslexia appear to be a specific at-risk population that may deserve tailored support during a period of therapy and school suspension. School closures carry a heavy burden of risk to reduce children's health in a number of ways, including both biological (increased risk of overweight) and psychological (increased negative emotions and reduced discipline) aspects [20].

Moreover, our survey suggested that the school closure may impact also the social condition of children with learning difficulties: this could be in part a consequence of the internalizing comorbidities frequently seen in these children [21] but could also reflect an increased burden of distress caused by the feeling of an increased inadequacy coupled with a larger amount of time requested to fulfill school duties [3].

To end with, in the next years, these findings suggest increased caution in the interpretation of results of neuropsychological testing concerning reading skills, to avoid diagnostic errors which can have negative consequences in term of academic results [22] and of global well-being of the child [14].

Author Contributions: I.M.C.B., L.F. and E.Z. designed the study. E.Z., P.B., E.R., M.C. performed patients' evaluations. M.C. performed preliminary statistical analysis. S.G. and L.P. performed final statistical analysis and drafted the manuscript. R.B. and C.T. supervised study design and execution, and contributed to the final version of the manuscript. All authors have read and agreed to the published version of the manuscript.

Funding: The study was supported by the Italian Ministry of Health (Ricerca Corrente 2020).

Institutional Review Board Statement: The study was approved by the Ethics Committee of the Policlinico San Matteo (Pavia) with number P-20200048574.

Informed Consent Statement: All parents and/or legal guardians provided an informed consent.

Data Availability Statement: Raw data are available from Zenodo using DOI:10.5281/zenodo.4983550.

Conflicts of Interest: The authors declare no conflict of interest.

References

1. Remuzzi, A.; Remuzzi, G. COVID-19 and Italy: What next? *Lancet* **2020**, *395*, 1225–1228. [CrossRef]
2. Parodi, S.M.; Liu, V.X. From Containment to Mitigation of COVID-19 in the US. *JAMA* **2020**, *323*, 1441–1442. [CrossRef] [PubMed]
3. Petretto, D.R.; Masala, I.; Masala, C. School Closure and Children in the Outbreak of COVID-19. *Clin. Pract. Epidemiol. Ment. Health* **2020**, *16*, 189–191. [CrossRef] [PubMed]
4. Bonal, X.; González, S. The impact of lockdown on the learning gap: Family and school divisions in times of crisis. *Int. Rev. Educ.* **2020**. Epub ahead of print. [CrossRef] [PubMed]
5. American Psychiatric Association. *Diagnostic and Statistical Manual of Mental Disorders*, 5th ed.; APA Publisher: Washington, DC, USA, 2013.
6. Smirni, P.; Vetri, L.; Misuraca, E.; Cappadonna, M.; Operto, F.F.; Pastorino, G.M.G.; Marotta, R. Misunderstandings about developmental dyslexia: A historical overview. *Pediatr. Rep.* **2020**, *12*, 8505. [CrossRef] [PubMed]
7. Nadeau, M.F.; Massé, L.; Argumedes, M.; Verret, C. Education for students with neurodevelopmental disabilities-Resources and educational adjustments. *Handb. Clin. Neurol.* **2020**, *174*, 369–378. [PubMed]
8. Provenzi, L.; Grumi, S.; Borgatti, R. Alone with the Kids: Tele-Medicine for Children with Special Healthcare Needs during COVID-19 Emergency. *Front. Psychol.* **2020**, *11*, 2193. [CrossRef] [PubMed]
9. Asbury, K.; Fox, L.; Deniz, E.; Code, A.; Toseeb, U. How is COVID-19 Affecting the Mental Health of Children with Special Educational Needs and Disabilities and Their Families? *J. Autism Dev. Disord.* **2021**, *51*, 1772–1780. [CrossRef] [PubMed]
10. Grumi, S.; Provenzi, L.; Gardani, A.; Aramini, V.; Dargenio, E.; Naboni, C.; Vacchini, V.; Borgatti, R. Engaging with Families through On-line Rehabilitation for Children during the Emergency (EnFORCE) Group. Rehabilitation services lockdown during the COVID-19 emergency: The mental health response of caregivers of children with neurodevelopmental disabilities. *Disabil. Rehabil.* **2020**, *43*, 27–32. [PubMed]
11. Sartori, G.; Job, R.; Tressoldi, P.E. *DDE-2. Batteria per la Valutazione della Dislessia e della Disortografia Evolutiva (Battery for the Assessment of Developmental Dyslexia and Dysorthographia)*; Giunti OS: Firenze, Italy, 2007.
12. Cornoldi, C.; Carretti, B. *Prove MT-3-Clinica—La Valutazione delle Abilità di Lettura e Comprensione per la Scuola Primaria e Secondaria di I Grado (MT-3—Clinic Tasks. The Assessment of Reading and Comprehension Skills for Elementary and Middle School)*; Giunti EDU: Firenze, Italy, 2016.
13. Tressoldi, P.E.; Stella, G.; Faggella, M. The development of reading speed in Italians with dyslexia: A longitudinal study. *J. Learn. Disabil.* **2001**, *34*, 414–417. [CrossRef] [PubMed]
14. Chiappedi, M.; Baschenis, I.M. Specific learning disorders and anxiety: A matter of school experience? *Min. Pediatr.* **2016**, *68*, 51–55.
15. Shinwell, J.; Defeyter, M.A. Investigation of Summer Learning Loss in the UK-Implications for Holiday Club Provision. *Front. Public Health* **2017**, *5*, 270. [CrossRef] [PubMed]
16. Alexander, K.L.; Entwisle, D.R.; Olson, L.S. Summer learning and its implications: Insights from the Beginning School Study. *New Dir. Youth Dev.* **2007**, *114*, 11–32. [CrossRef] [PubMed]
17. Cooper, H.; Nye, B.; Charlton, K.; Lindsay, J.; Greathouse, S. The effects of summer vacation on achievement test scores: A narrative and meta-analytic review. *Rev. Educ. Res.* **1996**, *66*, 227–268. [CrossRef]
18. Nicolson, R.I.; Fawcett, A.J. Development of Dyslexia: The Delayed Neural Commitment Framework. *Front. Behav. Neurosci.* **2019**, *13*, 112. [CrossRef] [PubMed]
19. Chaabane, S.; Doraiswamy, S.; Chaabna, K.; Mamtani, R.; Cheema, S. The Impact of COVID-19 School Closure on Child and Adolescent Health: A Rapid Systematic Review. *Children* **2021**, *8*, 415. [CrossRef] [PubMed]
20. Scarpellini, F.; Segre, G.; Cartabia, M.; Zanetti, M.; Campi, R.; Clavenna, A.; Bonati, M. Distance learning in Italian primary and middle school children during the COVID-19 pandemic: A national survey. *BMC Public Health* **2021**, *21*, 1035. [CrossRef] [PubMed]
21. Giovagnoli, S.; Mandolesi, L.; Magri, S.; Gualtieri, L.; Fabbri, D.; Tossani, E.; Benassi, M. Internalizing Symptoms in Developmental Dyslexia: A Comparison Between Primary and Secondary School. *Front. Psychol.* **2020**, *11*, 461. [CrossRef] [PubMed]
22. Chiappedi, M.; Baschenis, I.M.; Dolci, R.; Bejor, M. Importance of a critical reading of neuropsychological testing. *Min. Pediatr.* **2011**, *63*, 239–245.

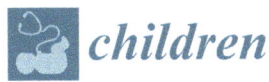

Article

The Child Behavior Checklist as a Screening Instrument for PTSD in Refugee Children

Ina Nehring [1,*], Heribert Sattel [2], Maesa Al-Hallak [1], Martin Sack [2], Peter Henningsen [2], Volker Mall [1] and Sigrid Aberl [2]

1 Department of Social Pediatrics, Technische Universität München, D-81377 Munich, Germany; Maesa.Al-Hallak@kbo.de (M.A.-H.); volker.mall@kbo.de (V.M.)
2 Department of Psychosomatic Medicine and Psychotherapy, Klinikum rechts der Isar, Technische Universität München, D-81377 Munich, Germany; h.sattel@tum.de (H.S.); martin.sack@mri.tum.de (M.S.); p.henningsen@tum.de (P.H.); sigrid.aberl@muenchen-klinik.de (S.A.)
* Correspondence: ina.nehring@kbo.de

Abstract: Thousands of refugees who have entered Europe experienced threatening conditions, potentially leading to post traumatic stress disorder (PTSD), which has to be detected and treated early to avoid chronic manifestation, especially in children. We aimed to evaluate and test suitable screening tools to detect PTSD in children. Syrian refugee children aged 4–14 years were examined using the PTSD-semi-structured interview, the Kinder-DIPS, and the Child Behavior Checklist (CBCL). The latter was evaluated as a potential screening tool for PTSD using (i) the CBCL-PTSD subscale and (ii) an alternative subscale consisting of a psychometrically guided selection of items with an appropriate correlation to PTSD and a sufficient prevalence (presence in more than 20% of the cases with PTSD). For both tools we calculated sensitivity, specificity, and a receiver operating characteristic (ROC) curve. Depending on the sum score of the items, the 20-item CBCL-PTSD subscale as used in previous studies yielded a maximal sensitivity of 85% and specificity of 76%. The psychometrically guided item selection resulted in a sensitivity of 85% and a specificity of 83%. The areas under the ROC curves were the same for both tools (0.9). Both subscales may be suitable as screening instrument for PTSD in refugee children, as they reveal a high sensitivity and specificity.

Keywords: child behavior checklist; post traumatic stress disorder; refugee; screening

1. Introduction

The number of refugees around the Middle East, Africa, and Afghanistan is increasing constantly, and disastrous conditions in their home countries as well as exhausting flights have an impact on the physical and psychological health of adults and children [1,2]. Hence, between 9% and 33% of adult refugees and 21–45% of children who experienced wars or armed conflicts suffer post traumatic stress disorder (PTSD) [3–6].

Psychological interventions, such as cognitive behavioral therapy, are shown to be highly effective in the treatment of traumatic symptoms [7,8] and thus may avoid chronic manifestation of the disorder. Therefore, detection of PTSD is necessary for appropriate treatment and the prevention of chronic courses; consequently, a routine screening is recommended [9]. A recent systematic review detected a lack of evidence in screening tools for PTSD in refugee children, especially below the age of six years [10]. Different self-report instruments are already in practice, such as the Child PTSD Symptom Scale, consisting of 20 items [11], the PTSD Reaction Index [12], or the Essener Trauma-Inventory for Children and Adolescents (ETI-KJ) [13]. These self-report measures, however, have been developed for children older than seven [12], eight [11], or twelve [13] years and are not appropriate for younger children. For this age group, parents or caregivers fill out the suitable checklists, such as the PTSD for Preschool Age Children [14], as well as a 15-item subscale of the Child Behavior Checklist (selection of suited items derived from the

Citation: Nehring, I.; Sattel, H.; Al-Hallak, M.; Sack, M.; Henningsen, P.; Mall, V.; Aberl, S. The Child Behavior Checklist as a Screening Instrument for PTSD in Refugee Children. *Children* 2021, *8*, 521. https://doi.org/10.3390/children8060521

Academic Editor: Matteo Alessio Chiappedi

Received: 31 May 2021
Accepted: 16 June 2021
Published: 18 June 2021

Publisher's Note: MDPI stays neutral with regard to jurisdictional claims in published maps and institutional affiliations.

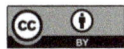

Copyright: © 2021 by the authors. Licensee MDPI, Basel, Switzerland. This article is an open access article distributed under the terms and conditions of the Creative Commons Attribution (CC BY) license (https://creativecommons.org/licenses/by/4.0/).

longer form [15]). Most of these instruments are specific tools for the detection of trauma induced disorders. The Child Behavior Checklist (CBCL), however, is a well-established, widely used instrument assessing not only trauma induced disorders but also the general behavioral problems of children of all age groups [15]. It is therefore an instrument that comprises a broad range of childhood psychological problems without additional strain for the patients. The CBCL, which has to be completed by parents or caregivers, is easily applicable in practice and available in more than 100 languages. A 20-item subscale of the CBCL selected by Wolfe et al. [16] covers PTSD relevant questions and might therefore be a suitable screening tool for PTSD. Previous studies already examined the use of this CBCL-PTSD subscale as a screening tool in children with traumatic experiences of various origin, such as domestic violence, sexual abuse, and unfavorable medical procedures, which may explain the different findings concerning sensitivity and specificity [15,17]. However, refugee children, according to the definition of the UNHCR (www.unhcr.org/refugees), have not yet been examined with this tool.

We therefore analyzed the data of refugee children from Syria who were hosted in a German reception camp to find out if the above mentioned CBCL-PTSD subscale might be an appropriate screening tool in this population. We further aimed to find out if a psychometrically guided item selection might be more appropriate and better tailored for the target population. Hence, we hypothesized that (i) the CBCL-PTSD subscale, as used in previous studies, would be a sensitive screening tool for PTSD in refugee children, and (ii) a psychometrically guided item selection would yield higher sensitivity and specificity in this particular population.

2. Methods

A cross sectional study was conducted between January and June 2014 in a former military barracks called "Bayernkaserne", which is used as reception camp for refugees in Munich, Germany. Data were directly collected in the barracks in separate examination rooms. The study included children with Syrian origin, aged 0 to 14 years, who were hosted in the Bayernkaserne reception camp and who were attended by at least one parent or legal guardian. Each newcomer who was listed by the agency and eligible for our study was contacted and received information about the study. They were asked to take part and invited to the first appointment.

Informed consent was given by the parents, and children were asked if they were willing to participate. The study protocol was approved by the ethics committee of the Technical University of Munich and adheres to the Helsinki Declaration.

The parents were interviewed and general information on age, sex, and religion, as well as subjective social status and socioeconomic status (according to MacArthur scale [18], which ranges from 1 to 10 points for low to high subjective socioeconomic status and has already been applied in immigrants) was collected. Because siblings were also included, there were less interview partners than analyzed children. For the purpose of our analyses, we extracted only children with completed psychological data who were older than 4 years.

2.1. Assessment

Clinical Examination and Interview: Parents were comprehensively interviewed and children were psychologically and physically examined. Details are described elsewhere [19]. In brief, trained study personnel interviewed the parents (i.e., one parent per family) and collected general data, information on former and current medical conditions of the parents, and information on their flight. For the single parents (mother or father) who voluntarily participated, the interviewer used open questions. A pediatrician of Syrian origin performed a comprehensive physical examination of the children. To diagnose psychiatric disorders (DSM-IV) like PTSD, the children were observed and interviewed by trained child and adolescent psychiatrists who collected the case histories and applied a psychometric assessment. A psychologist monitored the developmental, behavioral, and emotional problems of the children. Further, the investigators focused on the social interaction and specific PTSD-symptoms and established a psychopathological report. Depending on the child's age, information was received from the children or their parents. For children ≥ 6 years, the comprehensive structured Diagnostic Interview for Mental Disorders for Children and Adolescents, the Kinder-DIPS [20], was applied to establish a PTSD diagnosis according to DSM-IV. Children younger than 6 years received a clinical diagnosis from the psychologists and psychiatrists based on the German version [21] of the post-traumatic stress disorder semi-structured interview (PTSDSSI) for babies and toddlers developed by Scheeringa and Zeanah [22]. This instrument allows the diagnosis of PTSD in children older than 9 months by interviewing the main caregiver.

Interviews were accompanied by professional translators and native speaking doctors in order to minimize language restrictions. The duration of all examinations lasted 1–2 days for one family.

2.2. Psychometric Testing and Statistical Analyses

The Child Behavior Checklist (CBCL), developed by T.M. Achenbach [23], is a comprehensive questionnaire that comprises 113 items on child behavior, exploring the eight problem scales describing dimensions of problematic behavior: anxiety/depression, anti-social behavior, social problems, thought problems, somatic complaints, withdrawal/depression, attention problems, and aggressive behavior. The scale allows one to draw a conclusion on the internalizing, externalizing, and overall (total) problems of the child. Answers are given on a three-point Likert-scale (0—not true, 1—somewhat or sometimes true, 2—very true or often true). The CBCL was developed to identify problems by a respondent who knows the child well, such as a parent or caregiver. We applied the full German version of the CBCL for children of 4–18 years [24]. The checklist was completed by the parents. The instrument shows high 1-week test–retest reliability ($r > 0.8$) [25].

2.3. Statistical Analysis

As selected by Wolfe et al. [16] and applied in previous studies [15,17], firstly, we likewise examined the 20-item subscale of the CBCL (CBCL-PTSD subscale), which was developed to screen for potential PTSD in children older than four years. The computation of this subscale requires a recoding of each item by pooling the "somewhat/sometimes true" and "very true/often" replies, resulting in a statement on whether a problem is present or not (i.e., bivariate data). Then, the frequencies of the condensed problematic behaviors were determined, as well as the correlation of each item with the total score (item-total correlation), as well as with the diagnostic criterion "PTSD-present" (addressing reliability and validity issues, respectively).

In the second step, we replicated these analyses with all items of the CBCL. As criteria for potentially suitable items for the prediction of possible PTSD, a significant correlation with the presence of a PTSD diagnosis (Pearson correlation $r \geq 0.2$, $p < 0.05$, two-tailed) and a considerable prevalence of each particular behavior (present in at least 20% of the cases, rounded to nearest value) were chosen, resulting in a selection of 18 items from which an psychometrically guided item selection was derived [26–28].

To describe the sensitivity (ability to detect caseness) and specificity (precision of this detection) of this alternative and to determine possible cut-offs of both screening measures, we calculated receiver operating characteristic (ROC) curves, displaying the corresponding areas under the curve (AUC). The ROC curve graphically illustrates the suitability of a screening tool by plotting different sensitivity against specificity. An optimal cut-off considering a compromise of high sensitivity and high specificity would be chosen where the slope of the ROC-curve approaches 1, resulting in a maximum AUC of close to 1.0 [29].

Additionally, we calculated internal consistency (Cronbach's alpha) as a measure for internal reliability and the positive predictive value (PPV). The latter is defined as the quotient of the true positive test results divided by all positive test results. A low PPV would indicate that most of the positive test results are "false positive", suggesting a reduced test accuracy.

3. Results

3.1. Participants

Of initially 77 eligible children, 16 (20.8%) had either no complete CBCL or no complete clinical examination and were therefore excluded. Hence, the complete data of 61 children from 38 families could be analyzed. The mean age of the children was 8.9 years (SD: 2.8); 36 (59.0%) were boys (Table 1). PTSD was diagnosed in 20 of those children (32.8%) in the clinical examination. Parents were mostly of Syrian origin, Islamic religion, and had Arabic mother tongue (Table 2).

Table 1. General characteristics of the study population.

	PTSD (n = 20)	No PTSD (n = 41)
Children 4–14 years		
Age (years (SD))	8.2 (2.5)	9.3 (2.9)
Boys (n)	12	24
Religion (n)		
Islam	19	39
Other	1	2
In Germany since, months (SD)	1.1 (1.1)	1.1 (1.0)

SD: standard deviation.

Table 2. General characteristics of the parent who was interviewed.

	n (%)
Interview partner (n = 38)	
mother	27 (71.1)
father	11 (28.9)
Country of birth	
Syria	35 (92.1)
other (Iraq, Jordan, Libya)	3 (7.9)
Religion	
Islam	36 (94.7)
other	2 (5.3)
Mother tongue	
Arabic	30 (78.9)
Kurdish	5 (13.2)
other	3 (7.9)
Communication (language) problems in Germany [1]	29 (76.3)
Feels socially isolated [2]	17 (44.7)
Community-based subjective sociodemographic status in Germany above the median [3]	19 (51.3)
Society-based subjective sociodemographic status in Germany above the median [3]	12 (35.3)

[1] Interview partner was asked directly if he/she had any problems to communicate in Germany. [2] Interview partner was directly asked if he/she feels socially isolated in the camp. [3] Subjective sociodemographic status according to MacArthur Scale, "above the median"—at least 5 out of 10 points on the Scale, "community-based"—in the reception camp, "society-based"—Germany in general.

3.2. Test Results

Table 3 summarizes the results for both item selections. The CBCL-PTSD subscale comprises 20 items, whereas our psychometrically guided selection comprises 18 items. Of these, eleven CBCL items overlap in the two item selections.

Table 3. Selections of CBCL items used for analyses: CBCL-PTSD subscale as developed by Wolfe et al. [16] and psychometrically guided item selection. Eleven items (marked with [a]) are frequent behaviors, well associated with a PTSD-diagnosis and identical in both tested item selections.

CBCL Item Selections	Coincidence of Item with PTSD Diagnosis [1]	Occurrence/Frequency [2] [%]	Item—Total Correlation [1] (CBCL-PTSD-Scale)	Item—Total Correlation [1] (Psycho-Metrically Guided Item Selection)
Frequent Behaviors, Well Associated with a PTSD-Diagnosis **Overlapping Items of both Item Selections**				
Unhappy, sad, or depressed [a]	0.60	47.5	0.762	0.766
Nightmares [a]	0.48	41.0	0.597	0.702
Cannot concentrate, cannot pay attention for long [a]	0.45	23.0	0.483	0.552
Sudden changes in mood or feelings [a]	0.45	19.7	0.537	0.554
Trouble sleeping [a]	0.42	36.1	0.522	0.588
Too fearful, anxious [a]	0.39	37.7	0.451	0.507
Stubborn, sullen/irritable [a]	0.38	34.4	0.451	0.468
Fears certain places, animals, situations other than school [a]	0.37	35.0	0.467	0.412
Nervous, high-strung, or tense [a]	0.33	25.0	0.455	0.480
Clings to adults or too dependent [a]	0.22	35.0	0.381	0.394
Argues a lot [a]	0.20	45.9	0.257	0.274
Rare/Unassociated Behaviors **Additional Items of CBCL-PTSD Subscale**				
Withdrawn, does not get involved with others	0.36	9.8	0.337	–
Stomachaches and cramps	0.25	13.1	0.203	–
Feels others are out to get him/her	0.25	13.1	0.305	–
Cannot get his/her mind off certain thoughts, obsessions	0.25	13.1	0.367	–
Feels too guilty	0.12	9.8	0.258	–
Vomiting and throwing up	0.07	3.3	0.061	–
Secretive and keeps things to self	0.03	27.9	0.249	–
Headaches	0.01	5.0	0.140	–
Nausea and feels sick	−0.04	6.7	0.000	–
Additional Psychometrically Suitable Items **(Psychometrically Guided Item Selection)**				
Disobedient at home	0.41	32.8	–	0.561
Impulsive or acts without thinking	0.32	21.3	–	0.590
Cries a lot	0.30	39.3	–	0.649
Too shy or timid	0.28	36.1	–	0.371
Does not get along with others	0.28	23.3	–	0.383
Worries	0.27	29.7	–	0.653

Table 3. Cont.

CBCL Item Selections	Coincidence of Item with PTSD Diagnosis [1]	Occurrence/Frequency [2] [%]	Item—Total Correlation [1] (CBCL-PTSD-Scale)	Item—Total Correlation [1] (Psycho-Metrically Guided Item Selection)
Can't sit still, restless, or hyperactive	0.22	26.2	–	0.373

[a] Items identical in both item selections. [1] correlation coefficient (Spearman rank correlations, rho). [2] "somewhat/sometimes true" or "very true/often".

3.2.1. Item-Frequencies and Item/Criterion-Item/Total Correlations

(a) CBCL-PTSD subscale: The frequency of the assessed behaviors varies considerably and is observed from 2 children (3.3%, "vomiting and throwing up") up to 29 children (47.5%, "unhappy, sad, or depressed"). Moreover, the correlation of each item with the gold standard "established PTSD-diagnosis" ranges between 0.60 ("unhappy, sad, or depressed") to −0.04 ("nausea, feels sick"), indicating that not all items are significantly related to the presence of this diagnosis. The item-total correlation displayed concordant indices.

(b) Psychometrically guided item selection: The item frequency varies between 19.7% ($n = 12$ children with "sudden changes in moods or feelings") and 47.5% ($n = 29$ children who were "unhappy, sad, or depressed"). The correlation between the individual items and the PTSD diagnosis ranges between 0.60 ("unhappy, sad, or depressed") and 0.20 ("argues a lot"). Again, the item-total correlation displayed similar indices.

3.2.2. Internal Consistency and Proposed Cut-Offs

(a) With a Cronbach's $\alpha = 0.79$ for the CBCL-PTSD subscale, an acceptable internal consistency of the CBCL-PTSD subscale could be observed. The maximum AUC reached 0.88. A cut-off value of 5 (representing at least five symptoms present) was associated with a sensitivity of 85% and a specificity of 76%, whilst a cut-off of 7 and more symptoms present yielded a sensitivity of 75% and a specificity of 85%. Applying the higher cut-off, 24 children were tested positive, from which 17 suffered actually from PTSD according to the diagnostic interview. Accordingly, a positive predictive value (PPV) of 71.4% was determined.

(b) The psychometrically guided item selection having 18 items with a prevalence of more than 20% of the cases (Table 3) partly overlaps with the above analyzed CBCL-PTSD subscale. A Cronbach's α of 0.89 for this selection shows a slightly improved internal consistency, as compared to the CBCL-PTSD subscale, and can be estimated to be good.

While applying this item selection, we detected an AUC of 0.86. Again, we considered two cut-offs: The optimal cut-off value of 7 (representing at least seven symptoms present) yielded a sensitivity of 85% and a specificity of 83% (Figure 1). At this cut-off we identified 17 out of 20 children with PTSD. A lower cut-off of 5 results in a sensitivity of 90% and a specificity of 73%. The positive predictive value (PPV) of 70.8% indicates that a comparable proportion of all PTSD positives were detected correctly.

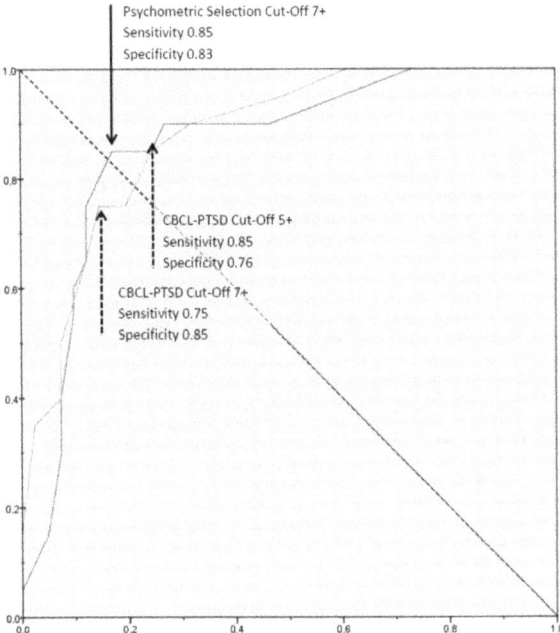

Figure 1. Receiver Operating Characteristic (ROC) Curve. The green line depicts the ROC curve of the PTSD-CBCL subscale (area under the curve (AUC) = 0.88), the blue line denotes the ROC curve of the psychometrically guided item selection (AUC = 0.86). "Cut-Off 7+"—at least 7 symptoms are present.

4. Discussion

Our study examined the suitability of two CBCL subscales in a population of Syrian refugee children and preadolescents. We were able to demonstrate that both the existing PTSD-subscale of the CBCL as well as a psychometrically guided selection of items show high sensitivity and specificity for this patient group. Although we cannot detect all PTSD cases with these measures, we are not aware of a PTSD screening tool with considerably higher sensitivity and specificity. However, it is important to consider the tools for screening purposes but not for diagnosis.

The principal aim of the detection of PTSD has already been studied by Dehon and Scheeringa and by Ruggerio and McLeer [15,17], who could demonstrate a high diagnostic accuracy of the CBCL-PTSD subscale in children with different traumatic experiences. In our analyses, the sensitivity and specificity of the CBCL-PTSD subscale were 85% and 76%, whereas the study of Ruggiero and McLeer [17] yielded a sensitivity of 87% and a specificity of 61.5% and the study of Dehon and Scheeringa [15] yielded 75% and 84.4%, respectively. Moreover, both previous studies defined the optimal sum score cut-off at 8 or more symptoms present, whilst our results revealed a lower cut-off of 5 or more symptoms. A cut-off of 8 or more would, in our sample, result in a sensitivity of 0.50 only, which cannot be considered appreciable for screening purposes. As possible explanations, differences in the observed study populations are likely: Ruggiero and McLeer examined 6–16-year-old children who had been sexually abused, Dehon and Scheeringa studied preschool aged children with different types of level I trauma (such as accidents, community, or domestic violence, medical procedures, sexual abuse), whereas our study consisted of a homogenous sample of 4–14-year-old Syrian refugee children who share different experiences in Syria and on their flight to Germany. Children who have been sexually abused frequently show psychiatric disorders that are not core symptoms of PTSD, e.g., attention deficits, anxiety-depression, and social withdrawal [30,31]. Accordingly, Ruggerio and McLeer described the examined children often as affected by additional related comorbidities such as dysthymic disorder, major depressive disorders, and specific phobia. The multimorbidity of these children is likely to lead to a high sum score as a statistically optimal cut-off, combined with a high sensitivity but relatively low specificity. In contrast, we have recently shown that our sample has a relatively low rate of comorbidities apart from PTSD [19], explaining the low optimal sum score with comparable sensitivity and higher specificity.

When considering an item selection for screening purposes for the detection of PTSD, it might be helpful to target a high sensitivity, combined with reasonable specificity. Therefore, we selected items according to their psychometric properties and determined sensitivity and specificity at the same population. Even in this context, maximum sensitivity remained at 85% with slightly higher specificity (83%). Comparing the ROC curves between the existing CBCL-PTSD subscale and the subscale optimized for our population, both provided comparable detection rates. However, at the cut-off in question, where there was an increment of 10 points in sensitivity while retaining a comparable specificity, one more child out of ten could be identified as "at risk for PTSD", with comparably small effort, when applying the psychometrically guided item selection. In general, sensitivity rates for both selections do not exceed 85% at reasonable expenses; this may point toward a ceiling effect of CBCL items concerning sensitivity for PTSD.

Regarding the individual items, those addressing sadness and depression, concentration deficits, sudden changes in mood, sleeping problems, and nightmares are strong indicators of a potential PTSD. However, some items of the CBCL-PTSD subscale, such as headaches or stomachaches, were not well correlated with the PTSD diagnosis in our population and showed a quite low item-total correlation. In particular, "physical problems without known medical cause", items 56b,c, and g in CBCL, (e.g., headaches, nausea/feels sick, vomiting/throwing up) were very low correlated with the PTSD diagnosis in our population. This finding is well in line with the new PTSD-criteria for children as proposed in ICD-11 [32], which consider the following clinical characteristics: disorganization, agitation, temper tantrums, clinging, excessive crying, social withdrawal, separation anxiety, distrust, trauma-specific re-enactments such as in repetitive play or drawings, frightening dreams without clear content or night terrors, sense of foreshortened future, and impulsivity. Although the majority of those criteria is covered by both item selections, a few of them are solely or more directly covered by the psychometrically guided selection (e.g., "crying a lot"). Furthermore, in contrast to the ICD-10, physical symptoms are no longer in use to specify a PTSD-diagnosis in the ICD-11. The elimination of these items from the CBCL-PTSD subscale may entail a better fit of the instrument to the forthcoming revision in ICD-11.

Strengths & Limitations

This is the first study that examines the CBCL-PTSD subscale in a population of refugee children and preadolescents. Substantial emphasis was put on the meticulous data collection and study conduct in this sensitive and strained population. The sample is homogenous concerning the cultural background and the kind of trauma experienced at their home countries and during the flight. Furthermore, all children were accompanied by at least one parent and therefore had partly intact family. Taken together, this may be a protective factor and a reason for the low rate of psychiatric disorders apart from PTSD. Although these are favorable conditions for the validation of a screening instrument for PTSD, it is likely to limit the transfer of the results to other populations. However, in general, refugee children have similar experiences such as home loss and flight [10], whereby the results might be generalizable, at least for refugee populations.

There are some limitations, most of them due to the situation in the field. The inclusion of siblings might have biased the results toward a specific direction. However, picking out only one child per family may lead to another selection bias. Hence, we decided to also include siblings, corresponding to a real field situation. The refugees may have been scared and may have tended not to report certain behaviors or to give more desirable answers in the interview. Because we included only children with Syrian origin we cannot exclude a cultural influence when considering a behavior as appropriate or problematic, which might systematically bias the results. Although children and parents were thoroughly examined, the discussed comorbidities could not be measured comprehensively. Additionally, working together with translators—although absolutely necessary for the study conduct—may have been imprecise or even error-prone. Moreover, children with pathological anxiety may be more likely to provide socially desirable responses on self-report measures. Finally, the limited number and the specific characteristics of the participants will not allow us to generalize our findings without rigorous examination.

5. Conclusions

It can be concluded that the existing CBCL-PTSD subscale developed by Wolfe et al. proved to be a suitable screening tool in refugee children with high sensitivity and specificity for the detection of PTSD. Psychometric data from our study and the revised classification of PTSD in the ICD-11, however, may suggest the elimination of items referring to somatoform symptoms.

Author Contributions: Conceptualization, I.N., H.S., V.M. and S.A.; formal analysis, I.N. and H.S.; funding acquisition, V.M.; investigation, M.A.-H., M.S., P.H. and S.A.; methodology, I.N., H.S., M.S., P.H., V.M. and S.A.; project administration, V.M.; software, H.S.; supervision, V.M. and S.A.; validation, S.A.; visualization, I.N.; writing—original draft, I.N. and H.S.; writing—review and editing, M.A.-H., M.S., P.H., V.M. and S.A. All authors have read and agreed to the published version of the manuscript.

Funding: This research was funded by "Kinder im Zentrum—Für Kinder e. V".

Institutional Review Board Statement: The study was conducted according to the guidelines of the Declaration of Helsinki and approved by the Ethics Committee of the Technical University of Munich (protocol code 5868/13, 2013).

Informed Consent Statement: Informed consent was obtained from all subjects involved in the study.

Data Availability Statement: Unfortunately, we cannot share the data because the approval by the ethics committee did not consider patient data publication. We are glad to be able to present the results of our analyses but are not allowed to share the original data.

Acknowledgments: We thank the professional team members, the assisting staff members, all professional translators, and the foundation "Kinder im Zentrum—Für Kinder e. V". We want to express our deep gratitude to all refugee families who participated and showed us their trust and support throughout the whole project. We wish only the best to all of them.

Conflicts of Interest: The authors declare no conflict of interest. The funders had no role in the design of the study; in the collection, analyses, or interpretation of data; in the writing of the manuscript, or in the decision to publish the results.

References

1. Alberer, M.; Wendeborn, M.; Löscher, T.; Seilmaier, M. Spectrum of diseases occurring in refugees and asylum seekers: Data from three different medical institutions in the Munich area from 2014 and 2015. *Dtsch. Med. Wochenschr.* **2016**, *141*, e8–e15. [PubMed]
2. van Berlaer, G.; Carbonell, F.B.; Manantsoa, S.; de Béthune, X.; Buyl, R.; Debacker, M.; Hubloue, I. A refugee camp in the centre of Europe: Clinical characteristics of asylum seekers arriving in Brussels. *BMJ Open* **2016**, *6*, e013963. [CrossRef]
3. Alpak, G.; Unal, A.; Bulbul, F.; Sagaltici, E.; Bez, Y.; Altindag, A.; Dalkilic, A.; Savas, H.A. Post-traumatic stress disorder among Syrian refugees in Turkey: A cross-sectional study. *Int. J. Psychiatry Clin. Pract.* **2015**, *19*, 45–50. [CrossRef] [PubMed]
4. Fazel, M.; Wheeler, J.; Danesh, J. Prevalence of serious mental disorder in 7000 refugees resettled in western countries: A systematic review. *Lancet* **2005**, *365*, 1309–1314. [CrossRef]
5. Slone, M.; Mann, S. Effects of War, Terrorism and Armed Conflict on Young Children: A Systematic Review. *Child Psychiatry Hum. Dev.* **2016**, *47*, 950–965. [CrossRef] [PubMed]
6. Soykoek, S.; Mall, V.; Nehring, I.; Henningsen, P.; Aberl, S. Post-traumatic stress disorder in Syrian children of a German refugee camp. *Lancet* **2017**, *389*, 903–904. [CrossRef]

7. Gutermann, J.; Schreiber, F.; Matulis, S.; Schwartzkopff, L.; Deppe, J.; Steil, R. Psychological Treatments for Symptoms of Posttraumatic Stress Disorder in Children, Adolescents, and Young Adults: A Meta-Analysis. *Clin. Child Fam. Psychol. Rev.* **2016**, *19*, 77–93. [CrossRef] [PubMed]
8. Morina, N.; Koerssen, R.; Pollet, T.V. Interventions for children and adolescents with posttraumatic stress disorder: A meta-analysis of comparative outcome studies. *Clin. Psychol. Rev.* **2016**, *47*, 41–54. [CrossRef] [PubMed]
9. AACAP. Practice Parameter for the Assessment and Treatment of Children and Adolescents with Posttraumatic Stress Disorder. *J. Am. Acad. Child Adolesc. Psychiatry* **2010**, *49*, 414–430.
10. Gadeberg, A.; Montgomery, E.; Frederiksen, H.; Norredam, M. Assessing trauma and mental health in refugee children and youth: A systematic review of validated screening and measurement tools. *Eur. J. Public Health* **2017**, *27*, 439–446. [CrossRef]
11. Foa, E.B.; Johnson, K.M.; Feeny, N.C.; Treadwell, K.R.H. The child PTSD Symptom Scale: A preliminary examination of its psychometric properties. *J. Clin. Child. Psychol.* **2001**, *30*, 376–384. [CrossRef] [PubMed]
12. Steinberg, A.M.; Brymer, M.J.; Decker, K.B.; Pynoos, R.S. The UCLA PTSD Reaction Index. *Curr. Psychiatry Rep.* **2004**, *6*, 96–100. [CrossRef]
13. Tagay, S.; Düllmann, S.; Hermans, E.; Repic, N.; Hiller, R.; Senf, W. Das Essener Trauma-Inventar für Kinder und Jugendliche (ETI-KJ). 2007. Available online: https://www.uni-due.de/rke-pp/essenertraumainventareti.php (accessed on 15 May 2017).
14. Levendosky, A.A.; Huth-Bocks, A.C.; Semel, M.A.; Shapiro, D.L. Trauma symptoms in preschool-age children exposed to domestic violence. *J. Interpers. Violence* **2002**, *17*, 150–164. [CrossRef]
15. Dehon, C.; Scheeringa, M.S. Screening for Preschool Posttraumatic Stress Disorder with the Child Behavior Checklist. *J. Pediatric. Psychol.* **2006**, *31*, 431–435. [CrossRef]
16. Wolfe, V.V.; Gentile, C.; Wolfe, D.A. The Impact of Sexual Abuse on Children: A PTSD Formulation. *Behav. Ther.* **1989**, *20*, 215–228. [CrossRef]
17. Ruggiero, K.J.; McLeer, S.V. PTSD scale of the Child Behavior Checklist: Concurrent and discriminant validity with non-clinic-referred sexually abused children. *J. Trauma. Stress* **2000**, *13*, 287–299. [CrossRef]
18. Adler, N.; Stewart, J. The MacArthur Scale of Subjective Social Status. 2007. Available online: http://www.macses.ucsf.edu/research/psychosocial/subjective.php (accessed on 15 May 2017).
19. Nehring, I.; Schlag, E.; Qirjako, E.; Büyükyaglioglu, C.; Mall, V.; Sattel, H.; Sack, M.; Henningsen, P.; Aberl, S. Health State of Syrian Children and Their Parents in a German Refugee Camp. *J. Refug. Stud.* **2019**, *29*. [CrossRef]
20. Unnewehr, S.; Schneider, S.; Margraf, J. *Kinder-DIPS: Diagnostisches Interview bei Psychischen Störungen im Kindes- und Jugendalter*; Springer: Berlin/Heidelberg, Germany, 2009.
21. Irblich, A.G.D.; Landhold, M.A. Posttraumatische Belastungsstörungen bei Säuglingen und Kleinkindern [Posttraumatic Stress Disorder in Infants and Toddlers]. *Praxis der Kinderpsychologie und Kinderpsychiatrie* **2008**, *57*, 247–263.
22. Scheeringa, M.S.; Zeanah, C.H. *PTSD Semi-Structured Interview and Observation Record for Infants and Young Children*; T.U.H.S.C. Department of Psychiatry and Neurology: New Orleans, LA, USA, 1994.
23. Achenbach, T.M. *Manual for the Child Behavior Checklist 4-18 and 1991 Profile*; University of Vermont, Department of Psychiatry: Burlington, VT, USA, 1991.
24. Döpfner, M.U.A. Elternfragebogen Über das Verhalten von Kindern und Jugendlichen: Deutsche Beabeitung der Child Behavior Checklist (CBCL/4-18). 1998. Available online: www.testzentrale.de (accessed on 1 June 2013).
25. Achenbach, T.M.; Rescorla, L.A. *Chapter 9 Reliability, Internal Consistency, Cross-Informant Agreement, and Stability in Manual for the ASEBA School-Age Forms and Profiles*; University of Vermont, Research Center for Children, Youth, & Families: Burlington, VT, USA, 2001.
26. Clark, L.A.; Watson, D. Constructing validity: Basic issues in objective scale development. *Psychol. Assess.* **1995**, *7*, 309–319. [CrossRef]
27. Lienert, G.A.; Raatz, U. *Testaufbau und Testanalyse*; Beltz PVU: Weinheim, Germany, 1998.
28. Moosbrugger, H.; Kelava, A. (Eds.) *Deskriptivstatistische Evaluation von Items (Itemanalyse) und Testwertverteilungen, in Testtheorie und Fragebogenkonstruktion*; Springer: Berlin/Heidelberg, Germany, 2007.
29. Fan, J.; Upadhye, S.; Worster, A. Understanding receiver operating characteristic (ROC) curves. *CJEM* **2006**, *8*, 19–20. [CrossRef] [PubMed]
30. McLeer, S.V.; Callaghan, M.; Henry, D.; Wallen, J. Psychiatric disorders in sexually abused children. *J. Am. Acad. Child Adolesc. Psychiatry* **1994**, *33*, 313–319. [CrossRef] [PubMed]
31. Ozbaran, B.; Erermis, S.; Bukusoglu, N.; Bildik, T.; Tamar, M.; Ercan, E.S.; Aydin, C.; Cetin, S.K. Social and emotional outcomes of child sexual abuse: A clinical sample in Turkey. *J. Interpers Violence* **2009**, *24*, 1478–1493. [CrossRef] [PubMed]
32. Hecker, T.; Maerker, A. Komplexe posttraumatische Belastungsstörung nach ICD-11. *Psychotherapeut* **2015**, *60*, 547. [CrossRef]

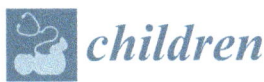

Article

Online Videogames Use and Anxiety in Children during the COVID-19 Pandemic

Concetta De Pasquale [1,†], Matteo Chiappedi [2,*,†], Federica Sciacca [1], Valentina Martinelli [3] and Zira Hichy [1]

1. Department of Education Science, University of Catania, 90100 Catania, Italy; depasqua@unict.it (C.D.P.); federica.sciacca@hotmail.com (F.S.); z.hichy@unict.it (Z.H.)
2. Developmental Psychopathology Research Unit, IRCCS Mondino Foundation, 27100 Pavia, Italy
3. Department of Brain and Behavioral Sciences, University of Pavia, 27100 Pavia, Italy; valentina.martinelli@unipv.it
* Correspondence: matteo.chiappedi@mondino.it
† These authors are to be considered as co-first authors.

Abstract: Videogames use has constantly increased among children and adolescents, with uncertain consequences on their health. This study aimed to assess the prevalence of videogames use and addiction in a sample of Italian children during the COVID-19 pandemic and their association with anxiety symptoms. One hundred and sixty-two children (M/F:78/84; age range: 8–10 years; average age 9.4 ± 0.7 years) completed the Videogame Addiction Scale for Children (VASC), the Test of Anxiety and Depression (TAD) and the Children's Anxiety Meter—State (CAM-S). Demographic variables and data on the access to electronic tools and games preferences were also collected. Overall, 96.3% of the study participants stated to have access to one or more device. They reported a low risk of videogame addiction (VASC score (mean ± SD): 46.7 ± 15.4), a moderate level of trait anxiety (TAD score (mean ± SD): 135 ± 16.8) and a low state anxiety (CAM-S score (mean ± SD): 2.2 ± 2.1). Males reported to spend more time on videogames, to perceive higher self-control and to be more influenced by reinforcement mechanisms; females described higher levels of trait anxiety. In the regression analysis, state anxiety was a predictor of videogame use and addiction ($p = 0.01$). Further research is needed to confirm these data and to maximize the developmentally positive effects of videogames and preventing the negative consequences.

Keywords: videogames; internet gaming disorder; anxiety

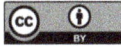

1. Introduction

Over the last decade, the amount of time that children and adolescents spend online playing videogames has constantly increased [1]. Lockdowns, quarantine measures and physical distancing imposed by the COVID-19 pandemic led to a further spread of indoor activities, including online gaming [2].

The consequences of online videogame use depend on frequency and duration. Previous studies found positive effects of online gaming in children, including distraction from pre-operative anxiety [3,4], motivational treatment of obesity [5], autism [6–8], amblyopia [9,10], psychiatric disorders [11], non-pharmacological treatment of cancer-related symptoms [12], improvement of intrinsic motivation [13], visual attention [14,15], visuospatial ability and speed of navigation [16] and physical activity [17].

By contrast, other studies found a correlation between excessive and compulsive use of videogames and retreat, social problems, attention difficulties and criminal and aggressive behaviors [18–20]. Recent studies showed that even a brief exposure to violent videogames can increase aggressive cognition and aggressive behaviors, especially in males [21]. According to the United Nations Children's Fund (UNICEF), millions of children are currently exposed to the growing risks associated with the virtual world [22].

Addictive behaviors towards playing online have been linked to a possible diagnosis of Internet Gaming Disorder (IGD) [1]. The Diagnostic and Statistical Manual of Mental

Disorders, Fifth Edition (DSM-5), includes IGD in Section 3, as a new condition warranting more clinical research. According to the current definition, IGD is characterized by a "persistent and recurrent use of the Internet to engage in games, often with other players, leading to clinically significant impairment or distress", as suggested by the presence of 5 (or more) diagnostic criteria within a 12-month period. The diagnostic criteria include preoccupation or obsession with gaming, withdrawal symptoms, tolerance, loss of control, loss of other interests, continued overuse despite negative consequences, deceptive behaviors in order to play, mood alterations and escape of negative feelings due to gaming, as well as work, relational and functional impairment [23]. More recently, the World Health Organization (WHO) included this gaming disorder in the International Statistical Classification of Diseases and Related Health Problems (ICD-11) [24].

Recent research documented the association between IGD and psychosocial variables in adolescents, including anxiety, depression, OCD, somatization and social difficulties [19,25,26]. Moreover, IGD was shown to be a significant contributor to the increase in sleep difficulties and impaired quality of life in adolescents during the COVID 19 outbreak, with anxiety being a strong mediator of the effects of IGD on sleep disturbances [2]. Parenting styles and family rules about videogaming were reported to be a significant factor in reducing the negative effects due to the use of videogames, in particular in terms of increased aggressivity and fighting behaviors [27].

A recent study [28] has provided data supporting the possibility of the existence of an optimal amount of time spent playing videogames that can at the same time maximize the possible benefits and be safe (i.e., not induce behavioral and emotional dyscontrol). However, this topic needs to be further studied, taking also into consideration variables related to psychopathological dysfunctions.

In this respect, anxiety can be defined as an alarm reaction to a stimulus perceived as dangerous, with the feeling that something bad is going to happen [23,29]. It represents a common reaction to stress. In 1961, Cattel and Scheier introduced the distinction between trait and state anxiety. Trait anxiety is a relatively stable individual personality characteristic, which refers to a general tendency to respond with anxiety and worry to perceived threats and dangers in the external environment. State anxiety reflects a transitory emotional state, characterized by feelings of tension and apprehension, with increased autonomic nervous system activity. When the subject experiences high state anxiety, he tries to limit these feelings through specific mechanisms, both psychological and behavioral [30].

According to the DSM 5, anxiety disorders include conditions that share features of excessive fear and anxiety and related behavioral disturbances, leading to an impairment in daily functioning [23]. A number of reports has shown that children were at risk of increased anxiety and anxiety-related behaviors during the COVID-19 pandemic, especially during the so-called "lockdown" [31]. To date, limited research specifically investigated the association between anxiety and videogames use in this age group [32]. Moreover, no epidemiological or quasi-epidemiological data have been published regarding the prevalence of videogames use and videogame addiction in Italy.

We conducted a cross-sectional study to assess the prevalence of videogames use and videogames addiction in a sample of Italian children during the COVID-19 pandemic. We also investigated the prevalence of trait and state anxiety symptoms, given their possible increase related to the COVID-19 pandemic, and their association to videogames use.

2. Materials and Methods

2.1. Recruitment

We recruited a sample of children in three primary schools in the province of Catania (Italy); all children were attending school in presence in the last three months (i.e., from September to November 2020). After discussing with the school heads and receiving their consent to the administration of the tests during school hours, we sent written information to all parents or legal guardians of children attending these primary schools, being available for face-to-face contacts but also to discuss the study and its characteristics by phone or messaging systems. After that, all parents or legal guardians signed an informed consent. In total, 162 children (78 males, 84 females), 8–10 years old (average; 9.4; SD: 0.7), were included in this study: 24.7% of them were an only child, while 75.3% had brothers or sisters.

2.2. Instruments

We administered an ad hoc questionnaire to explore the demographic variables (i.e., age, sex, having brothers or sisters), the access to electronic tools that could be used for playing and the games usually played.

Moreover, each child completed three questionnaires:

(1) the Videogame Addiction Scale for Children (VASC) [1]: specifically designed for children, this is a self-administered 21-item questionnaire investigating a possible addiction to videogames. All items are scored on a 5-point scale (from never to very often). The test provides a total score (range 21–105), and 4 sub-scores, related to four psychological dimensions (self-control, reinforcement, life-style and time-use problems and game involvement). A global score above 90 indicates the possibility of videogame addiction. The scale proved a Cronbach's alpha of 0.898 in our study sample;

(2) the Test of Anxiety and Depression (TAD) [33]: this is a self-report questionnaire investigating anxiety and depression. In the present study, we administered only the 11 items related to trait anxiety, in order to reduce the number of questions to be answered and improve children's collaboration and attention. The score obtained (range: 55–150) was classified as follows: anxiety symptoms below average (99 or lower), average non pathological (100–114), mildly pathological (115–129), moderately pathological (130–144) and highly pathological (145 or higher). The Cronbach's alpha in our study sample was 0.822;

(3) the Children's Anxiety Meter—State (CAM-S) [34]: this is a validated visual analogue scale, drawn to resemble a thermometer with ten levels. To measure state anxiety (CAM-S), children are asked to mark how they feel "right now". The Cronbach's alpha was 0.867 in our study sample.

2.3. Data Analysis

Statistical analysis was performed using IBM SPSS Statistics 26 for Windows.

2.4. Ethical Approval

Ethical approval for the study was granted by the Ethic committee of the Department of Education Science, University of Catania.

3. Results

Overall, 96.3% of the 162 children recruited reported access to one or more devices used to play videogames (console (65.4%), smartphone (56.2%), tablet (48.1%) or personal computer (36.4%)). Their favorite games were Fortnite (21.6%), FIFA (10.5%), Minecraft (7.4%), SuperMario (6.2%) and Just Dance (4.3%).

We found an average score at the VASC of 46.7 (SD: 15.4), indicating a low risk of videogame addiction; the average score at the TAD was 135 (SD 16.8), indicating a moderate level of pathological trait anxiety; as for the CAM-S, a low level of state anxiety was reported (average 2.2, SD 2.1).

There were significant differences comparing males and females (Table 1). Despite not being in general at risk for videogame addiction (VASC global score below 90), males used videogames more than females (t = 4.06; $p < 0.001$), declared higher self-control (t = 3.63, $p < 0.001$) and had a higher level of reinforcement mechanisms (t = 4.36; $p < 0.001$), but also of trait anxiety (TAD score; t = -5.18, $p < 0.001$).

Table 1. Differences comparing males and females in the Videogame Addiction Scale for Children (VASC), the Children's Anxiety Meter—State (CAM-S) and the Test of Anxiety and Depression (TAD).

	Male		Female			
	M	SD	M	SD	T	p
Self-control	7.95	2.43	6.59	2.31	3.637	<0.001
Reinforcement mechanisms	11.90	4.63	9.11	3.46	4.363	<0.001
Problems	9.68	3.72	8.30	3.51	2.435	0.016
Involvement in videogames	2.17	1.36	1.89	1.13	1.396	0.165
VASC	51.63	16.58	42.20	12.79	4.068	<0.001
CAM-S	2.24	2.40	2.23	1.71	0.053	0.957
TAD	14.77	3.88	18.81	5.76	−5.183	<0.001

The correlation analysis showed in the whole sample that state anxiety was positively related to videogames use ($r = 0.19$; $p < 0.05$), reinforcement mechanisms ($r = 0.21$; $p < 0.01$) and involvement in videogames use ($r = 0.17$; $p < 0.05$), while we found no significant correlations between trait anxiety levels and the VASC score or sub-scores. Analyzing males, state anxiety had a positive correlation with videogame involvement ($r = 0.26$; $p < 0.05$), while trait anxiety correlated with more frequent use of videogames ($r = 0.34$; $p < 0.01$), problems with life-style and time-use ($r = 0.27$; $p < 0.05$) and self-control (0.26; $p < 0.05$). As for females, state anxiety was positively related to videogames use ($r = 0.22$; $p < 0.05$) and with reinforcement mechanisms ($r = 0.35$; $p < 0.01$), while trait anxiety correlated with videogames use ($r = 0.31$; $p < 0.01$), reinforcement mechanisms (0.27; $p < 0.05$) and involvement in videogames ($r = 0.28$; $p < 0.05$).

We also conducted two linear regression analyses with the enter method between a dependent variable (VASC) and two independent variables (TAD and CAM) on the whole sample. They showed that state anxiety (standardized beta 0.152; t = 1.94; $p = 0.01$) was a possible predictor of videogame use and addiction, while trait anxiety was only "nearly significant" (standardized beta 0.192, t = 2.47; $p = 0.054$).

4. Discussion

Children in our sample showed on average a low risk of videogame addiction, a moderate level of trait anxiety and a low state anxiety. We found significant gender-related differences: males tend to spend more time on videogames, were perceived to have a higher self-control and to be more influenced by reinforcement mechanisms; females describe higher levels of trait anxiety. State anxiety emerged from the regression analysis as a risk factor for problematic videogame use in these children.

The mean VASC scores in our study were similar to those reported by Ylmaz et al. (2017), in a sample of 780 school children before the COVID-19 pandemic [1]. Moreover, in line with previous research, boys reported higher scores compared to girls [1,25].

To date, there is still an ongoing debate about the proper conceptualization of IGD [35,36]. Videogame playing has become one of children's favorite leisure activities. Previous research emphasized that the classification of videogaming behavior as an addiction or mental disorder can be problematic since excessive use of videogames concerns mainly adolescents and young adults, with a high rate of spontaneous remission [25]. The positive or negative consequences of videogames for child development have been widely debated in the scientific literature [5,36]. Videogames can have a number of positive effects, being well-accepted methods to stimulate motor, attentive and perceptual skills, but also motivation towards a goal and social skills [4,37].

The existing literature has focused on five aspects to be considered to assess the effect of videogames on children: the amount of time spent playing (especially if without pauses and with a complete immersion in the videogame), the content of the videogame, the game context, the game structure and the game mechanics [5,35]. Videogames can lead to unhealthy behaviors, including a sedentary lifestyle (with the consequent risk of developing over-weight), a reduction of time dedicated to academic learning (or a lack of concentration in performing school duties) and the substitution of all other forms of social relations with the videogame (favoring a state of isolation and a tendency towards introversion) [32,38–40].

Moreover, a large body of research clearly documented the association between IGD and anxiety symptoms in adolescents. In this regard, previous studies showed how videogames may be used as a treatment tool for internalized anxiety [41–43] while others highlighted that anxiety could be the reason for excessive videogames use, or vice versa [29,32]. According to the comorbidity hypothesis, IGD shares common psychological and neurobiological features (including craving) with other addictive behaviors and psychiatric problems. The experience of persistent high levels of anxiety could lead to problematic videogaming in order to avoid negative affective states, and this behavior could be maintained through reinforcement mechanisms [25,44].

Regarding gender differences, previous studies found that an increased amount of time spent playing with videogames was associated with higher anxiety symptoms in female adolescents. By contrast, it was associated with decreased anxiety levels in males [42,43]. Social support may represent a probable explanation, given the important differences in terms of the "social connection" that videogames seem to provide to boys compared to girls. Of note, male adolescents, while playing, seem to interact and create new friends much more frequently than females [45]. In our sample, male children perceived to have a higher self-control and to be more influenced by reinforcement mechanisms.

5. Conclusions

Our data are relevant to help children and caregivers to be aware of the risk of developing addiction to videogames [41]. Of note, males tend to perceive themselves as more "in control" of videogames use. Caregivers should define rules for videogaming, in terms of duration and of access to the devices [46]. Finally, given the role of state anxiety as a risk factor for problematic videogame use, it is important to monitor anxiety symptoms and their intensity in children as a preventive strategy.

Our study has some limitations. First, its cross-sectional design does not allow to understand the evolution of the relationship between anxiety and videogaming. Second, children were recruited during the so-called "second wave" of the SARS-CoV-2 diffusion in Italy, a fact that could have increased the reported levels of anxiety. Third, we used only self-administered questionnaires, a fact that could limit the interpretation of our results. Specifically, we assessed IGD and anxiety symptoms. Only a detailed clinical assessment can identify IGD and anxiety disorders. Fourth, the sample size was relatively small; therefore, our data should be replicated on larger samples. In fact, the number of children recruited is limited and could therefore be insufficient to represent the population of subjects of the same age range.

Notwithstanding these limitations, this study provides information about an emergent important issue in children in the context of a highly stressful and unique situation, such as the COVID-19 pandemic. Recently, a possible use of active video games for improving mental health and physical fitness during isolation periods was reported [47]; however, more studies are needed to define the most adequate interventions to be activated by caregivers to prevent the negative consequences and maximize the developmentally positive effects of videogames [14,48].

Author Contributions: Conceptualization, C.D.P., F.S. and Z.H.; methodology, C.D.P., F.S. and Z.H.; software, C.D.P. and M.C.; validation, C.D.P., F.S. and Z.H.; formal analysis, C.D.P., F.S. and Z.H.; investigation, C.D.P.; resources, C.D.P. and M.C.; data curation, C.D.P., F.S. and Z.H.; writing—original draft preparation, C.D.P., F.S. and Z.H.; writing—review and editing, V.M. and M.C.; supervision, M.C.; funding acquisition, C.D.P. and M.C. All authors have read and agreed to the published version of the manuscript.

Funding: This research was partially funded by the Italian Health Ministry (Ricerca Corrente 2020).

Institutional Review Board Statement: The study was conducted according to the guidelines of the Declaration of Helsinki, and approved by the Ethics Committee of the Department of Education Science, University of Catania.

Informed Consent Statement: Informed consent was obtained from legal guardians of all subjects involved in the study.

Data Availability Statement: Raw data are available from the corresponding author upon reasonable request.

Conflicts of Interest: The authors declare no conflict of interest.

References

1. Yılmaz, E.; Griffiths, M.D.; Kan, A. Development and Validation of Videogame Addiction Scale for Children (VASC). *Int. J. Ment. Health Addict.* **2017**, *15*, 869–882. [CrossRef]
2. Fazeli, S.; Mohammadi Zeidi, I.; Lin, C.Y.; Namdar, P.; Griffiths, M.D.; Ahorsu, D.K.; Pakpour, A.H. Depression, anxiety, and stress mediate the associations between internet gaming disorder, insomnia, and quality of life during the COVID-19 outbreak. *Addict. Behav. Rep.* **2020**, *12*, 100307. [CrossRef]
3. Dwairej, D.A.; Obeidat, H.M.; Aloweidi, A.S. Video game distraction and anesthesia mask practice reduces children's preoperative anxiety: A randomized clinical trial. *J. Spec. Pediatr. Nurs.* **2020**, *25*, e12272. [CrossRef]
4. Jurdi, S.; Montaner, J.; Garcia-Sanjuan, F.; Jaen, J.; Nacher, V. A systematic review of game technologies for pediatric patients. *Comput. Biol. Med.* **2018**, *97*, 89–112. [CrossRef]
5. Del Río, N.G.; González-González, C.S.; Martín-González, R.; Navarro-Adelantado, V.; Toledo-Delgado, P.; García-Peñalvo, F. Effects of a Gamified Educational Program in the Nutrition of Children with Obesity. *J. Med. Syst.* **2019**, *43*, 198. [CrossRef] [PubMed]
6. Travers, B.G.; Mason, A.H.; Mrotek, L.A.; Ellertson, A.; Dean, D.C., 3rd; Engel, C.; Gomez, A.; Dadalko, O.I.; McLaughlin, K. Biofeedback-Based, Videogame Balance Training in Autism. *J. Autism Dev. Disord.* **2018**, *48*, 163–175. [CrossRef] [PubMed]
7. Wijnhoven, L.A.M.W.; Creemers, D.H.M.; Vermulst, A.A.; Lindauer, R.J.L.; Otten, R.; Engels, R.C.M.E.; Granic, I. Effects of the video game 'Mindlight' on anxiety of children with an autism spectrum disorder: A randomized controlled trial. *J. Behav. Ther. Exp. Psychiatry* **2020**, *68*, 101548. [CrossRef] [PubMed]
8. Ghanouni, P.; Jarus, T.; Zwicker, J.G.; Lucyshyn, J.; Fenn, B.; Stokley, E. Design Elements during development of Videogame Programs for Children with Autism Spectrum Disorder: Stakeholders' Viewpoints. *Games Health J.* **2020**, *9*, 137–145. [CrossRef]
9. Kelly, K.R.; Jost, R.M.; Dao, L.; Beauchamp, C.L.; Leffler, J.N.; Birch, E.E. Binocular iPad Game vs Patching for Treatment of Amblyopia in Children: A Randomized Clinical Trial. *JAMA Ophthalmol.* **2016**, *134*, 1402–1408. [CrossRef] [PubMed]
10. Gao, T.Y.; Guo, C.X.; Babu, R.J.; Black, J.M.; Bobier, W.R.; Chakraborty, A.; Dai, S.; Hess, R.F.; Jenkins, M.; Jiang, Y.; et al. Effectiveness of a Binocular Video Game vs Placebo Video Game for Improving Visual Functions in Older Children, Teenagers, and Adults With Amblyopia: A Randomized Clinical Trial. *JAMA Ophthalmol.* **2018**, *136*, 172–181. [CrossRef]
11. Bioulac, S.; de Sevin, E.; Sagaspe, P.; Claret, A.; Philip, P.; Micoulaud-Franchi, J.A.; Bouvard, M.P. Qu'apportent les outils de réalité virtuelle en psychiatrie de l'enfant et l'adolescent ? *Encephale* **2018**, *44*, 280–285. [CrossRef]
12. Lopez-Rodriguez, M.M.; Fernández-Millan, A.; Ruiz-Fernández, M.D.; Dobarrio-Sanz, I.; Fernández-Medina, I.M. New Technologies to Improve Pain, Anxiety and Depression in Children and Adolescents with Cancer: A Systematic Review. *Int. J. Environ. Res. Public Health* **2020**, *17*, 3563. [CrossRef]
13. Wan, C.S.; Chiou, W.B. The motivations of adolescents who are addicted to online games: A cognitive perspective. *Adolescence* **2007**, *42*, 179–197. [PubMed]
14. Bertoni, A.; Franceschini, S.; Puccio, G.; Mancarella, M.; Gori, S.; Facoetti, A. Action Video Games Enhance Attentional Control and Phonological Decoding in Children with Developmental Dyslexia. *Brain Sci.* **2021**, *11*, 171. [CrossRef] [PubMed]
15. García-Baos, A.; D'Amelio, T.; Oliveira, I.; Collins, P.; Echevarria, C.; Zapata, L.P.; Liddle, E.; Supèr, H. Novel Interactive Eye-Tracking Game for Training Attention in Children with Attention-Deficit/Hyperactivity Disorder. *Prim. Care Companion CNS Disord.* **2019**, *21*, 19m02428. [CrossRef] [PubMed]
16. Rodriguez-Andres, D.; Mendez-Lopez, M.; Juan, M.C.; Perez-Hernandez, E. A Virtual Object-Location Task for Children: Gender and Videogame Experience Influence Navigation; Age Impacts Memory and Completion Time. *Front. Psychol.* **2018**, *9*, 451. [CrossRef] [PubMed]
17. Schneider, K.L.; Carter, J.S.; Putnam, C.; Keeney, J.; DeCator, D.D.; Kern, D.; Aylward, L. Correlates of Active Videogame Use in Children. *Games Health J.* **2018**, *7*, 100–106. [CrossRef]
18. Yousef, S.; Eapen, V.; Zoubeidi, T.; Mabrouk, A. Behavioral correlation with television watching and videogame playing among children in the United Arab Emirates. *Int. J. Psychiatry Clin. Pract.* **2014**, *18*, 203–207. [CrossRef]
19. De Pasquale, C.; Sciacca, F.; Martinelli, V.; Chiappedi, M.; Dinaro, C.; Hichy, Z. Relationship of Internet Gaming Disorder with Psychopathology and Social Adaptation in Italian Young Adults. *J. Environ. Res. Public Health* **2020**, *17*, 8201. [CrossRef] [PubMed]
20. De Pasquale, C.; Dinaro, C.; Sciacca, F. Relationship of Internet gaming disorder with dissociative experience in Italian university students. *Ann. Gen. Psychiatry* **2018**, *17*, 28. [CrossRef]

21. Zhang, Q.; Cao, Y.; Tian, J.J. Effects of Violent Video Games on Aggressive Cognition and Aggressive Behavior. *Cyberpsychol. Behav. Soc. Netw.* **2021**, *24*, 5–10. [CrossRef] [PubMed]
22. Unicef. Office on Global Insight and Polices. Available online: https://www.unicef.org/globalinsight/stories/rethinking-screen-time-time-covid-19 (accessed on 13 December 2020).
23. American Psychiatric Association. *Diagnostic and Statistical Manual of Mental Disorders*, 5th ed.; American Psychiatric Association: Washington, DC, USA, 2013.
24. Jo, Y.S.; Bhang, S.Y.; Choi, J.S.; Lee, H.K.; Lee, S.Y.; Kweon, Y.S. Clinical Characteristics of Diagnosis for Internet Gaming Disorder: Comparison of DSM-5 IGD and ICD-11 GD Diagnosis. *J. Clin. Med.* **2019**, *8*, 945. [CrossRef]
25. Fumero, A.; Marrero, R.J.; Bethencourt, J.M.; Peñate, W. Risk factors of internet gaming disorder symptoms in Spanish adolescents. *Comput. Hum. Behav.* **2020**, *111*, 106416. [CrossRef]
26. Männikkö, N.; Ruotsalainen, H.; Miettunen, J.; Pontes, H.M.; Kääriäinen, M. Problematic gaming behaviour and health-related outcomes: A systematic review and meta-analysis. *J. Health Psychol.* **2020**, *25*, 67–81. [CrossRef]
27. Cote, A.C.; Coles, S.M.; Dal Cin, S. The interplay of parenting style and family rules about video games on subsequent fighting behavior. *Aggress. Behav.* **2021**, *47*, 135–147. [CrossRef]
28. Kovess-Masfety, V.; Keyes, K.; Hamilton, A.; Hanson, G.; Bitfoi, A.; Golitz, D.; Koç, C.; Kuijpers, R.; Lesinskiene, S.; Mihova, Z.; et al. Is time spent playing video games associated with mental health, cognitive and social skills in young children? *Soc. Psychiatry Psychiatr. Epidemiol.* **2016**, *51*, 349–357. [CrossRef] [PubMed]
29. Sullivan, H.S. The Meaning of Anxiety in Psychiatry and in Life. *Psychiatry* **1948**, *11*, 1–13. [CrossRef]
30. Cattell, R.B.; Scheier, I.H. *The Meaning and Measurement of Neuroticism and Anxiety*; Ronald: New York, NY, USA, 1961.
31. Conti, E.; Sgandurra, G.; De Nicola, G.; Biagioni, T.; Boldrini, S.; Bonaventura, E.; Buchignani, B.; DellVecchia, S.; Falcone, F.; Fedi, C.; et al. Behavioural and Emotional Changes during COVID-19 Lockdown in an Italian Paediatric Population with Neurologic and Psychiatric Disorders. *Brain Sci.* **2020**, *10*, 918. [CrossRef]
32. González-Bueso, V.; Santamaría, J.J.; Fernández, D.; Merino, L.; Montero, E.; Ribas, J. Association between Internet Gaming Disorder or Pathological Video-Game Use and Comorbid Psychopathology: A Comprehensive Review. *Int. J. Environ. Res. Public Health* **2018**, *15*, 668. [CrossRef] [PubMed]
33. Lachar, D. Test Reviews: Newcomer, P. L., Barenbaum, E. M., & Bryant, B. R. (1994). Depression and Anxiety in Youth Scale. Austin, TX: PRO-ED. *J. Psychoeduc. Assess.* **1999**, *17*, 58–61. [CrossRef]
34. Ersig, A.L.; Kleiber, C.; McCarthy, A.M.; Hanrahan, K. Validation of a clinically useful measure of children's state anxiety before medical procedures. *J. Spec. Pediatr. Nurs.* **2013**, *18*, 311–319. [CrossRef]
35. Van Rooij, A.J.; Schoenmakers, T.M.; van de Mheen, D. Clinical validation of the C-VAT 2.0 assessment tool for gaming disorder: A sensitivity analysis of the proposed DSM-5 criteria and the clinical characteristics of young patients with 'video game addiction'. *Addict. Behav.* **2017**, *64*, 269–274. [CrossRef] [PubMed]
36. van Rooij, A.J.; Ferguson, C.J.; Colder Carras, M.; Kardefelt-Winther, D.; Shi, J.; Aarseth, E.; Bean, A.M.; Bergmark, K.H.; Brus, A.; Coulson, M.; et al. A weak scientific basis for gaming disorder: Let us err on the side of caution. *J. Behav. Addict.* **2018**, *7*, 1–9. [CrossRef] [PubMed]
37. Kietglaiwansiri, T.; Chonchaiya, W. Pattern of video game use in children with attention-deficit-hyperactivity disorder and typical development. *Pediatrics Int.* **2018**, *60*, 523–528. [CrossRef] [PubMed]
38. Schuurmans, A.A.; Nijhof, K.S.; Vermaes, I.P.; Engels, R.C.; Granic, I. A Pilot Study Evaluating "Dojo," a Videogame Intervention for Youths with Externalizing and Anxiety Problems. *Games Health J.* **2015**, *4*, 401–408. [CrossRef]
39. Fish, M.T.; Russoniello, C.V.; O'Brien, K. The Efficacy of Prescribed Casual Videogame Play in Reducing Symptoms of Anxiety: A Randomized Controlled Study. *Games Health J.* **2014**, *3*, 291–295. [CrossRef]
40. Schuurmans, A.A.T.; Nijhof, K.S.; Engels, R.C.M.E.; Granic, I. Using a Videogame Intervention to Reduce Anxiety and Externalizing Problems among Youths in Residential Care: An Initial Randomized Controlled Trial. *J. Psychopathol. Behav. Assess.* **2018**, *40*, 344–354. [CrossRef]
41. Peracchia, S.; Presaghi, F.; Curcio, G. Pathologic Use of Video Games and Motivation: Can the Gaming Motivation Scale (GAMS) Predict Depression and Trait Anxiety? *Int. J. Environ. Res. Public Health* **2019**, *16*, 1008. [CrossRef]
42. Ohannessian, C.M. Media Use and Adolescent Psychological Adjustment: An Examination of Gender Differences. *J. Child. Fam. Stud.* **2009**, *18*, 582–593. [CrossRef]
43. Vannucci, A.; Flannery, K.M.; Ohannessian, C.M. Social media use and anxiety in emerging adults. *J. Affect. Disord.* **2017**, *207*, 163–166. [CrossRef]
44. Bargeron, A.H.; Hormes, J.M. Psychosocial correlates of internet gaming disorder: Psychopathology, life satisfaction, and impulsivity. *Comput. Hum. Behav.* **2017**, *68*, 388–394. [CrossRef]
45. Lenhart, A.; Smith, A.; Anderson, M.; Duggan, M.; Perrin, A. *Teens, Technology, and Friendships*; Pew Research Center: Washington, DC, USA, 2015. Available online: http://www.pewinternet.org/2015/08/06/teens-technology-and-friendships/ (accessed on 18 December 2020).
46. Hernandez, M.W.; Estrera, E.; Markovitz, C.E.; Muyskens, P.; Bartley, G.; Bollman, K.; Kelly, G.; Silberglitt, B. *Uses of Technology to Support Early Childhood Practice*; OPRE Report; OPRE: Washington, DC, USA, 2015. Available online: https://www.acf.hhs.gov/sites/default/files/opre/useoftechreport_execsummary.pdf (accessed on 18 December 2020).

47. Santos, I.K.D.; Medeiros, R.C.D.S.C.; Medeiros, J.A.; Almeida-Neto, P.F.; Sena, D.C.S.; Cobucci, R.N.; Oliveira, R.S.; Cabral, B.G.A.T.; Dantas, P.M.S. Active Video Games for Improving Mental Health and Physical Fitness—An Alternative for Children and Adolescents during Social Isolation: An Overview. *Int. J. Environ. Res. Public Health* **2021**, *18*, 1641. [CrossRef] [PubMed]
48. Levac, D.E.; Miller, P.A. Integrating virtual reality video games into practice: Clinicians' experiences. *Physiother. Theory Pract.* **2013**, *29*, 504–512. [CrossRef] [PubMed]

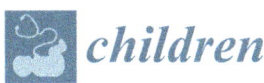

Article

The Role of Alexithymia in Social Withdrawal during Adolescence: A Case–Control Study

Sara Iannattone *, Marina Miscioscia, Alessia Raffagnato and Michela Gatta

Child and Adolescent Neuropsychiatry Unit, Department of Women's and Children's Health, Padua University Hospital, 35128 Padua, Italy; marina.miscioscia@unipd.it (M.M.); alessiaraffagnato@gmail.com (A.R.); michela.gatta@unipd.it (M.G.)
* Correspondence: sara.iannattone@studenti.unipd.it

Abstract: Although social withdrawal is becoming increasingly common among adolescents, there is still no consensus on its definition from the diagnostic and psychopathological standpoints. So far, research has focused mainly on social withdrawal as a symptom of specific diagnostic categories, such as depression, social phobia, or anxiety disorders, or in the setting of dependence or personality disorders. Few studies have dealt with social withdrawal in terms of its syndromic significance, also considering aspects of emotion control, such as alexithymia. The present case-control study aimed to further investigate the issue of social withdrawal, and try to clarify the part played by alexithymia in a sample of Italian adolescents diagnosed with psychological disorders ($n = 80$; Average Age$_g$ = 15.2 years, SD = 1.49). Our patients with social withdrawal (cases) scored significantly higher than those without this type of behavior (controls) in every domain of alexithymia investigated, using the Toronto Alexithymia Scale (TAS-20) and with the scales in the Youth Self-Report (YSR) regarding internalizing problems, anxiety–depression, social problems, and total problems. Internalizing problems and total levels of alexithymia also emerged as predictors of social withdrawal. These variables may therefore precede and predispose adolescents to social withdrawal, while social problems may develop as a consequence of the latter.

Keywords: social withdrawal; alexithymia; adolescence; psychological disorders; anxiety; depression; social problems

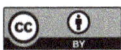

1. Introduction

Extreme social withdrawal, also known as "hikikomori syndrome", was first systematically conceptualized at the end of the 1990s by the Japanese psychiatrist Saito [1]. The term was used to refer to individuals who withdraw completely from society for at least six months, refusing to engage in any activities and social relationships. Their circadian rhythm is disrupted, and they may become violent with members of their own family. Such behavior cannot be attributed to other disorders [2].

Hikikomori was initially considered a culture-bound syndrome associated with the features of Japanese society [3,4]. However, when the experiences of these socially-withdrawn young people in Japan attracted more interest, similar cases emerged in other parts of the world too, and it became clear that the phenomenon is not only associated with eastern cultural factors. There are currently no precise data available on the prevalence of social withdrawal in the world's population.

In Italy, the topic of social withdrawal in adolescence is relatively new, and not enough studies have been conducted to ascertain its statistical prevalence. As reported by the Agenzia Nazionale Stampa Associata (ANSA), in 2018 it was estimated that approximately 100,000 young people in Italy between 13 and 20 years old were socially withdrawn [5]. A study conducted in the same year by the regional school board for Emilia-Romagna on 687 schools found that 21% of them reported cases of pupils who had stopped attending school. In all, 346 cases had been reported to the territorial services, and the majority (59%)

of them involved adolescents between 13 and 16 years old [6]. An epidemiological study conducted by a mental health service for children and adolescents run by a local public health unit in Arezzo, central Italy, found that—leaving aside those who were ill—the number of students failing to attend school for more than 40 days accounted for 1% of the school population, with a slight prevalence of males [7].

Generally speaking, several authors have emphasized how difficult it is to conduct cross-cultural studies on social withdrawal, because of the variety of ways in which it can become manifest and be interpreted in different cultures [8–10]. For this reason, it is hard to find an unequivocal and shared definition of it in the literature. Some consider it synonymous with hikikomori syndrome, while others use it as an umbrella term covering a vast array of emotions, motives, and behavior associated with the rejection of social interactions [11,12]. According to Asendorpf [13,14], social withdrawal is a multidimensional construct, since it can derive from three different motivations: shyness, peer avoidance, and unsociability. Shyness is a temperamental trait that prevents children and adolescents from interfacing with peers. Shy individuals experience an approach-avoidance conflict because their underlying desire for interaction is inhibited by fear and anxiety. Peer avoidance is the result of need of solitude and avoidance of all the social situations due to fear of judgment. Unsociability, instead, is a characteristic of children and adolescents who are happy alone and are not interested in interacting with peers.

1.1. Social Withdrawal in Adolescence: Risk Factor, Symptom, or Clinical Syndrome?

There is currently no consensus on how social withdrawal should be clinically diagnosed. Many psychologists and psychiatrists would agree that the condition of extreme social withdrawal represents a genuine syndrome [7], though it is hard to classify nosographically as a separate entity. In fact, the Diagnostic and Statistical Manual of Mental Disorders fourth edition (DSM-IV-TR) [15] included hikikomori among the cultural syndromes, but then the fifth edition of the Manual (DSM-5) [16] omitted it. The International Classification of Diseases eleventh edition (ICD-11) [17] includes social withdrawal among the "symptoms or signs involving appearance or behavior" in the category of "symptoms, signs or clinical findings not elsewhere classified", whereas this entity had not been envisaged in the ICD-10 [18].

In the literature on developmental age, social withdrawal has been alternately conceived as a risk factor for the onset of psychological disorders, or as a symptom thereof. Because social withdrawal is reportedly persistent during periods of transition, in the various stages of childhood and in the passage from childhood to adolescence [19], it has been interpreted as an early risk factor for the onset of full-blown psychopathological conditions. Some researchers have found that social withdrawal in developmental age often precedes the onset of various affective–relational problems, including rejection by peers, poor social competence, internalizing problems like anxiety and depression, and loneliness [20–23]. Rubin and Mills proposed a theoretical model that connects an individual's social withdrawal (intended as a tendency to remain on the margins of their group) with difficult experiences with their peers, as well as the onset of internalizing problems [24]. These authors suggest that withdrawal behavior at school exposes adolescents to a greater risk of problems with their classmates (rejection, exclusion, victimization). This in turn exacerbates their internalizing symptoms (anxiety, depression, loneliness), further increasing their propensity to become socially withdrawn, and generating a vicious circle. Nevertheless, the relationship between social withdrawal and social problems is still discussed in the literature, because it seems to be unclear whether the former represents a risk factor for the latter or vice versa. For example, according to a research by Oh et al. [25], negative peer relationships (including victimization and rejection) and friendlessness may exacerbate social withdrawal trajectories during childhood and adolescence. Moreover, Spiniello et al. [26] considered social problems as distinctive of the stage before social withdrawal in adolescence. In fact, relational difficulties and lack of interest in interacting with others are typical behaviors that anticipate social withdrawal itself.

Regarding social withdrawal as a symptom of psychiatric disorders, various studies have shown that the diagnoses most often presenting in comorbidity or confused with it are autism, selective mutism, psychotic disorders, personality disorders, mood disorders, anxiety, social phobia, and internet dependence [11,27–29]. That said, there have been reports of socially-withdrawn adolescents not meeting any of the criteria for these known psychopathological conditions [8]. Teo and Gaw have consequently recommended including severe social withdrawal as a mental disorder in the DSM [30]. They say it has particular clinical characteristics that distinguish it from the psychiatric problems with which it is often associated (i.e., internalizing disorders, internet dependence, psychotic disorders), but do not enable it to be unequivocally and conclusively defined as a separate disorder.

Suwa and Suzuki have offered a possible solution in the debate over whether social withdrawal is a symptom or a syndrome by distinguishing between primary and secondary social withdrawal [31]. In addition to the inability to be part of and adapt to society, primary social withdrawal also involves a weak self-image that adolescents try to protect with their avoidance behavior. Secondary social withdrawal would instead be one of the symptoms of a known psychopathological condition [32].

1.2. Social Withdrawal and Alexithymia in Adolescence

Alexithymia is characterized by the inability to identify and communicate one's own emotions [33]. Several studies have shown that it is not a condition secondary to situations of stress, but a personality trait that frequently lies behind the onset of psychiatric disorders [34–36]. Failure to develop an adequate capacity for emotion control in childhood prevents people from dealing adequately with difficult situations, prompting the emergence of negative feelings that can then impair their mental health.

Referring more specifically to psychological disorders in adolescence, alexithymia has been associated particularly with internalizing disorders [36–39], eating disorders [40,41], social problems [42], self-harming [43,44], internet dependence [45], borderline personality disorder [46], substance dependence [47], and primary headache [48,49]. In short, studies have placed alexithymia in relation to disorders frequently found in comorbidity with social withdrawal, such as internet dependence, internalizing disorders, and social problems. There is still a severe shortage of published research directly investigating the possible association between social withdrawal and alexithymia, however. One such study was conducted by Frankova, starting from an analysis of the various psychological and psychopathological characteristics of primary and secondary social withdrawal, including alexithymia, comparing groups with the two conditions, and with a healthy control group [29]. Although both the socially-withdrawn groups were less able to identify and verbalize their emotions than the controls, the group with primary social withdrawal showed higher levels of alexithymia than the group with secondary social withdrawal.

Hattori focused instead on the presence of general emotional problems in socially-withdrawn adolescents [2]. The author suggested that these individuals tend to repress their authentic emotions and personality in an effort to adapt to emotionally dysfunctional parents. They create a false identity to protect themselves against other people's negative opinions of them.

Honkalampi et al. [42] analyzed the correlations between scores obtained on the Toronto Alexithymia Scale-20 (TAS-20) [50] and the Youth Self-Report (YSR) 11–18 [51] scales in a sample of adolescents from the general population. They found the difficulty describing feelings (DDF) factor on the TAS-20 to be more strongly associated with the internalizing problems and withdrawal scales on the YSR. Nevertheless, this study was not specifically focused on the relationship between social withdrawal and emotional difficulties, since it aimed to underline the different psychopathological outcomes linked to alexithymia.

Difficulty describing feelings was also identified in socially-withdrawn adolescents in the clinical experience reported by Piotti, who found these patients unable to find the words to express their experiences of suffering [52].

Other published studies have not associated alexithymia directly with social withdrawal, but have investigated the possible link between difficulties with managing emotions and certain phenomena often encountered in situations of self-isolation, such as interpersonal problems [53], loneliness [54], and shyness [55]. It therefore seems interesting, from both the clinical and the research standpoints, to examine the potential direct association between adolescent social withdrawal and alexithymia, with a view to further clarifying their features, and thereby obtaining more information on the most appropriate types of intervention for the adolescents affected.

1.3. The Study: Aims and Hypotheses

Based on the above premises, the main aim of this work was to further analyze the role of alexithymia in adolescent social withdrawal, and the clinical characteristics of the latter. There is still not enough literature on this latter phenomenon, which is becoming increasingly common among teenagers. Despite its growing importance worldwide, there is still no consensus on how to define, diagnose, and manage social withdrawal in adolescence, partly because of the different ways in which it can become manifest and be interpreted in different cultures [8–10]. Research conducted to date has focused on social withdrawal mainly as a symptom of a specific diagnostic category, such as depression, social phobia, anxiety disorders, internet dependence, or personality disorders [20,28,29]. There is clearly still a shortage of studies on social withdrawal in its syndromic sense, also considering the issue of managing emotions, i.e., alexithymia. In fact, most studies have analyzed just the behavioral component of this phenomenon, without considering how socially-withdrawn teenagers feel their emotions and their suffering. Currently, due to the lack of research in this field, little is known about the characteristics of socially-withdrawn adolescents, especially from the emotional standpoint. Thus, we decided to better investigate the alexithymic traits of these youths, in order to contribute to the overall understanding of this phenomenon, considering not only its behavioral manifestations, but also the emotional experience.

The first objective of our study was therefore to analyze the link between alexithymia and social withdrawal, also seeking to identify which factor of alexithymia is most impaired in socially withdrawn adolescents. In a sample of adolescents with clinically-diagnosed psychological disorders, we expected to see higher levels of alexithymia in those who were socially withdrawn than in those who were not [29].

As a second objective, we wanted to further examine the adaptability and psycho-behavioral profile of socially-withdrawn adolescents. We predicted that they would be less able to adapt. In terms of the link between social withdrawal and psychopathology, we also expected them to be impaired not only in global functioning, but also and especially in terms of internalizing and social problems [21,22,25–27].

In conclusion, the innovative contribution of our work is that it was specifically focused on social withdrawal and its emotional aspects. In addition, it aimed to better investigate the clinical profile of socially-withdrawn adolescents, with the ultimate purpose of developing new trajectories for prevention and treatment programs.

2. Methods

2.1. Participants and Procedure

The individuals in our study included patients referred between January 2009 and March 2019 to a semi-residential service for psychopathological disorders in a territorial Neuropsychiatry for Children and Adolescents Unit provided by a local public health service in Padova, Italy. This service offers multidisciplinary intervention for adolescents in situations of psychological, behavioral, and environmental stress, in the form of pedagogical–educational activities, psychotherapy sessions, and pharmacological treatments. When patients first come to the service, the protocol requires that parents sign to give their informed consent to the administration of test materials, and to their use for clinical and research purposes. The present study was part of a broader research project on developmental psychopathologies, conducted in accordance with the Declaration of Helsinki and approved by the local ethical committee (CESC, May 2017, prot.95006).

Questionnaires were completed by the adolescent patients and the educators on the former's first visit to the semi-residential service. The data used in the present study were collected retrospectively from the patients' clinical records.

The sample as a whole consisted of 80 patients, including 39 males (48.8%) and 41 females (51.2%). At the time of their referral to the semi-residential service, these patients were from 12 to 17 years old (Average age = 15.2 years, SD = 1.49). As concerns their schooling, they had stopped going to school in 12.5% of cases, while 27.5% and 60% of them were attending lower and upper secondary schools, respectively. The reasons for their neuropsychiatric assessment prior to their referral to the semi-residential program included affective–relational problems (43.8%), behavioral problems (31.2%), and problems at school (25%). Taking the ICD-10 classification system for reference [18], 66.2% of the patients had been diagnosed with an affective–emotional disorder (F30–39, F40–48), while 33.8% had behavioral and personality disorders (F90–98, F60–69).

The power analysis, conducted by means of G*Power 3.1 software, showed that with a sample of 80 participants, we had a power of 0.90 in reliably detecting an odds ratio of 0.31, with a type I error of 0.05 [56].

A case–control study design was chosen to investigate patients' social withdrawal component. The whole sample was therefore divided into two groups: a group of 40 patients with social withdrawal (Average age = 15.3 years, SD = 1.62), and a group of 40 patients (Average age = 15.2 years, SD = 1.36) matched for age and psychiatric diagnoses with a group without any signs of social withdrawal. For the case group, we first selected all patients who had "withdrawal, isolation, refusal to make contact" among the symptoms recorded on their arrival at the semi-residential service ($n = 134$). This is the format used by the service, which records a patient's main clinical details and history, obtained from an information sheet completed by the clinician referring the patient to the service. Subsequently, from this initial sample of socially-withdrawn adolescents, we excluded those who did not complete the Toronto Alexithymia Scale-20 (TAS-20), Youth Self-Report 11–18 (YSR), and Global Assessment of Functioning (GAF) on their first visit to the service, or had not a borderline (65–69) or clinical (>69) score on the scale for withdrawal in the YSR ($n = 94$). According to these inclusion and exclusion criteria, the total number of socially withdrawn patients included in our study was 40. The patients excluded from this first step were not placed in the pool to select matched controls. Then, for the control group, we started selecting patients on the basis of their clinical records, in chronological order of their accessing the service. The first inclusion criterion were not having "withdrawal, isolation, refusal to make contact" among the symptoms recorded on their arrival at the semi-residential service, so we automatically excluded all patients who were previously included in the pool to select cases. After this first step, the total number of patients considered was 86. Subsequently, we excluded patients who did not complete TAS-20, YSR, and GAF at the arrival at the semi-residential service or had borderline or clinical scores on the scale for withdrawal in the YSR. The resulting number of patients was 71, of which we selected 40 patients matched for age and psychiatric diagnosis with socially-withdrawn adolescents. Table 1 shows the characteristics of the two groups.

Table 1. Frequencies of the characteristics of the case and control groups.

		Group	
		Cases n (%)	Controls n (%)
Sex	Males	23 (57.5%)	16 (40.0%)
	Females	17 (42.5%)	24 (60.0%)
Age	12–14 years old	11 (27.5%)	13 (32.5%)
	15–17 years old	29 (72.5%)	27 (67.5%)
Personality organization [1]	Neurotic	11 (27.5%)	9 (22.5%)
	Borderline	22 (55%)	25 (62.5%)
	Psychotic	7 (17.5%)	6 (15.0%)
Diagnosis [2]	F30–39, F40–48	25 (62.5%)	28 (70.0%)
	F90–98, F60–69	15 (37.5%)	12 (30.0%)
Traumas	Yes [3]	31 (77.5)	26 (65.0%)
	No	9 (22.5%)	14 (35.0%)
Attendance at the semi-residential service	Continuous	35 (87.5%)	31 (77.5%)
	Discontinuous	5 (12.5%)	9 (22.5%)
Hours per week of attendance at the semi-residential service	1–5	3 (7.5%)	2 (5.0%)
	5–10	12 (30.0%)	23 (57.5%)
	10–15	14 (35.0%)	10 (25.0%)
	>15	11 (27.5%)	5 (12.5%)
Parental couple	Single parent [4]	14 (35.0%)	16 (40.0%)
	Intact	26 (65.0%)	24 (60.0%)
Parents' education level [5]	High	11 (27.5%)	6 (15.0%)
	Average	20 (50.0%)	23 (57.5%)
	Low	9 (22.5%)	9 (22.5%)
	Not known	0	2 (5.0%)

Notes: [1] Personality organization as established from a structural interview based on Kernberg's criteria [57]. [2] F30–39, F40–48 = affective—emotional disorders; F90–98, F60–69 = behavioral and personality disorders. [3] In this category are included the following typologies of trauma, reported in the format used by the semi-residential service: conflict/domestic violence, separation/deaths, psychiatric disorders, changes/relocations. [4] Single parent due to separation or death of the other. [5] Parents' education level: high = both parents have a university degree, or one has a degree and the other a high school diploma; average = both parents have a high school diploma, or one has a degree and the other completed middle school; low = both parents completed middle school, or one has a high school diploma and the other completed middle school.

2.2. Tools

The validated Italian versions of the following standardized questionnaires were administered:

(a) Global Assessment of Functioning (GAF) [58]: this is a scale compiled by the operators to assess a patient's psychosocial functioning and activities (at school or at work, interpersonal relations, hobbies, and leisure activities). It considers functioning on a continuum from excellent (100) to severely impaired (1). Individuals are scored and assigned to one of 10 levels, assessing both symptom severity and functional impairment;

(b) Youth Self-Report 11–18 (YSR) [51,59]: this self-reported questionnaire consisting of 113 items that examine social competences and psychopathological behavior. The latter is classified on eight syndrome scales: anxiety–depression; social withdrawal; somatic complaints; social problems; thought disorders; attention disorders; deviant behavior; and aggressive behavior. These subscales are then grouped to obtain three global scales for internalizing problems, externalizing problems, and total problems. In our study, we considered the anxiety–depression, social withdrawal, social problems, internalizing problems, and total problems scales. Items of the anxiety–depression scale reflect symptoms of those syndromes (e.g., fears, worries, sleeping problems, sadness, crying a lot). The social withdrawal scale is made up of items referring to behaviors and individual characteristics (e.g., shyness, isolation, talking difficulties). The social problems scale identifies relational difficulties (e.g., teasing, loneliness, exclusion, clumsiness). The internalizing problems scale is composed of social withdrawal, somatic complaints, and anxiety–depression scales, while the total problems scale is the sum of all the YSR items, reflecting the global level of disease. The tool has a good reliability, with Cronbach's alpha ranging from 0.71 to 0.95. Specifically, in the present study, Cronbach's alpha coefficients for each scale ranged from 0.66 to 0.91;

(c) Toronto Alexithymia Scale (TAS-20) [50,60]: this is a self-administered questionnaire comprised of 20 items that respondents score on a five-point Likert scale from "strongly disagree" to "strongly agree". It consists of three subscales: difficulty describing feelings (DDF; i.e., difficulties in communicating feelings to other people), difficulty identifying feelings (DIF; i.e., problems in recognizing emotions and distinguishing them from bodily sensations), and externally-oriented thinking (EOT; i.e., concrete cognitive style oriented to external reality). Moreover, it has a total score that points out the global level of alexithymia. Respondents obtaining a total score of 61 or more are considered alexithymic, while those who score 50 or less are not alexithymic. A total score between 51 and 60 indicates the possible presence of alexithymia (borderline level). The Italian version of the tool has a good reliability, with Cronbach's alpha in the range of 0.52 to 0.75 for normal samples, and between 0.54 and 0.82 for clinical samples. In the present study, Cronbach's alpha coefficients for each scale ranged from 0.50 (for EOT) to 0.78 (for the total score).

2.3. Data Analysis

The data were analyzed using Jamovi statistical software, version 1.2 [61].

We first calculated the descriptive statistics and frequency tables to clarify the characteristics of the sample as a whole ($n = 80$) and of the two groups ($n = 40$ each).

Then the chi-square test (χ^2) for categorical variables was used to see whether the two groups were comparable in terms of gender (two levels), age (two levels: 12–14 years and 15–17 years), diagnosis (two levels), and personality organization (three levels).

The *t*-test for independent samples was used to identify any statistically significant differences between the two groups in relation to adaptability, level of alexithymia, and presence of psychopathological features. Social withdrawal (two levels) was input as an independent variable in the model, while the dependent variables were the total score on the GAF, the TAS-20 scales (i.e., DDF, DIF, EOT, and the total score), and several YSR scales, chosen on the basis of the psychopathological issues most often associated with social withdrawal in the literature [21,22,27,28], i.e., anxiety–depression, social problems, internalizing problems, and total problems.

Subsequently, two binomial logistic regressions were run after calculating Pearson's *r* correlations between the TAS-20 and YSR subscales used as predictors.

The first binomial logistic regression was run to identify the dimension of alexithymia most impaired in socially-withdrawn adolescents. In fact, considering that the presence of alexithymic traits is a characteristic of different psychopathological disorders [43,44,47], we wanted to better investigate which specific aspect of alexithymia (i.e., difficulty in recognizing emotions, difficulty in expressing them, or concrete and externally-oriented thinking) was the most influential on social withdrawal. The presence or absence of social withdrawal (two levels) was input in the model as the dependent variable, with the three subscales of the TAS-20—difficulty describing feelings (DDF), difficulty identifying feelings (DIF) and externally-oriented thinking (EOT)—as predictors.

As mentioned earlier, the literature identifies internalizing problems and social problems as being particularly linked to social withdrawal, so another logistic binomial regression was run to test the direction of this relationship and whether alexithymia influenced it. To be more specific, we were interested in observing whether internalizing problems, social problems, and the global level of alexithymia could significantly predict social withdrawal. Consequently, the presence or absence of social withdrawal was input in the model as the dependent variable, with the scales for internalizing problems and social problems on the YSR, and the total score on the TAS-20 as predictors.

In both binomial logistic regressions, gender, age, diagnosis, and personality organization were input as factors to control for their effects.

Finally, we calculated Pearson's r correlations—considering both the whole sample and cases and controls separately—between the social withdrawal scale of the YSR and (i) the GAF; (ii) the scales for anxiety–depression, social problems, internalizing problems, and total problems in the YSR; and (iii) the scales in the TAS-20.

The level of statistical significance was set at $p < 0.05$.

3. Results
3.1. Comparability between the Two Groups

No statistically significant association emerged from the χ^2 test between the two groups (with versus without social withdrawal) and gender (χ^2 (1, n = 80) = 2.45, p = 0.117); age (χ^2 (1, n = 80) = 0.238, p = 0.626); diagnosis (χ^2 (1, n = 80) = 0.503, p = 0.478); or personality organization (χ^2 (2, n = 80) = 0.468, p = 0.791). This means that the variables considered were not influential in defining the groups, which could therefore be compared in terms of the presence or absence of social withdrawal alone.

3.2. Social Withdrawal and Alexithymia

The t-test for independent samples, with scores on the TAS-20 scales as the dependent variables, identified a statistically significant difference between the two groups on all the scales, with the group of adolescents with social withdrawal always obtaining higher scores (Table 2).

Table 2. Means and results of the t-tests, with scores in the Toronto Alexithymia Scale (TAS-20) as the dependent variables and group (with vs without social withdrawal) as the independent variable.

TAS-20 Scales	Group	M (SE)	t	df	p
DDF	with social withdrawal (n = 40)	18.0 (0.59)	5.43	78	<0.001
	without social withdrawal (n = 40)	13.3 (0.65)			
DIF	with social withdrawal (n = 40)	23.0 (1.03)	4.00	78	<0.001
	without social withdrawal (n = 40)	16.9 (1.13)			
EOT	with social withdrawal (n = 40)	23.6 (0.69)	2.36	78	0.021
	without social withdrawal (n = 40)	21.4 (0.63)			
TOT	with social withdrawal (n = 40)	64.7 (1.57)	5.65	78	<0.001
	without social withdrawal (n = 40)	51.6 (1.69)			

Notes: DDF = difficulty describing feelings; DIF = difficulty identifying feelings; EOT = externally-oriented thinking; TOT = total score; M = mean; SE = standard error.

Pearson's r correlations between the TAS-20 scales, calculated before running the binomial logistic regression, are shown in Table 3. They were all positive; more specifically, the correlations between DDF and the other TAS-20 subscales were all moderate, while the correlation between DIF and EOT was small.

Table 3. Pearson's r correlations between the TAS-20 values and the social withdrawal scale of the Youth Self-Report 11–18 (YSR), considering the sample as a whole.

	DDF	DIF	EOT	TOT
DDF	-	0.47	0.36	0.79
DIF	0.47	-	0.13	0.83
EOT	0.36	0.13	-	0.57
Withdrawal	0.59	0.40	0.38	0.60

Notes: DDF = difficulty describing feelings; DIF = difficulty identifying feelings; EOT = externally-oriented thinking; TOT = total score of the TAS-20; Withdrawal = social withdrawal scale of the YSR.

Then, from the binomial logistic regression, conducted to see which specific factor of alexithymia was most impaired in the group of socially-withdrawn adolescents, the significant predictor emerged as just the TAS-20 scale for DDF ($\beta = 0.26$, $z = 2.84$, $p = 0.005$, OR = 1.279, 95% CI: 1.08–1.55). Variables input in the model as factors (i.e., gender, age, diagnosis, and personality organization) did not show any statistically significant effect. McFadden's R^2 for the model overall was 0.36.

Lastly, Pearson's r correlations, calculated considering the whole sample, showed that the scale for withdrawal in the YSR correlated significantly and positively with all the TAS-20 scales. Specifically, its strongest associations were with DDF and the TAS-20 total score, while the lowest was with EOT (Table 3). These correlations did not significantly differ considering cases and controls separately (see Appendix A, Table A1).

3.3. Social Withdrawal, Adaptability, and Psychological Disorders

When the t-test for independent samples was run with the scores on the YSR scales as the dependent variables, statistically significant differences emerged between the groups with and without social withdrawal on all the scales considered (the group with social withdrawal is indicated with the subscript "yes", while the group without social withdrawal is indicated with the subscript "no"): anxiety–depression ($t_{78} = 1.45$, $p < 0.001$; $M_{yes} = 73.7$, SE = 1.76; $M_{no} = 61.9$, SE = 1.88); social problems ($t_{78} = 3.51$, $p < 0.001$; $M_{yes} = 66.3$, SE = 1.46; $M_{no} = 59.9$, SE = 1.11); internalizing problems ($t_{78} = 6.63$, $p < 0.001$; $M_{yes} = 72.8$, SE = 1.11; $M_{no} = 58.9$, SE = 1.79); and total problems ($t_{78} = 4.21$, $p < 0.001$; $M_{yes} = 67.8$, SE = 1.21; $M_{no} = 58.8$, SE = 1.77). The group with social withdrawal always scored higher. No significant differences emerged for the GAF.

Finally, Pearson's r correlations, calculated considering the whole sample, showed statistically significant associations between the scale for social withdrawal and all the other scales considered in the YSR (Table 4). The correlations were all positive and strong, ranging from 0.52 (with social problems) to 0.74 (with internalizing problems). The correlation with the score in the GAF was also significant, but low and negative. These correlations did not significantly differ when considering cases and controls separately (see Appendix A, Table A1).

Table 4. Pearson's r correlations between the social withdrawal scale of the YSR, the other YSR scales, and the Global Assessment of Functioning (GAF), considering the sample as a whole.

	Anx-Dep	Int. Prob	Soc. Prob	YSR TOT	GAF
Withdrawal	0.62	0.74	0.52	0.56	−0.21

Notes: Withdrawal = social withdrawal scale; Anx-Dep = anxiety–depression scale; Int. Prob = internalizing problems scale; Soc. Prob = social problems scale; YSR TOT = total problems scale.

3.4. Predictors of Social Withdrawal in Adolescents

Pearson's r correlations between the predictors included in the binomial logistic regression (i.e., the TAS-20 total score, as well as the social problems and internalizing problems scales of the YSR) were all statistically significant, positive, and strong (Table 5).

Subsequently, from the binomial logistic regression, it emerged that the predictors of social withdrawal in the model were the scores for internalizing problems on the YSR ($\beta = 0.16$, $z = 2.89$, $p = 0.004$, OR = 1.18, 95% CI: 1.05–1.32) and the total scores on the TAS-20 ($\beta = 0.11$, $z = 2.42$, $p = 0.015$, OR = 1.12, 95% CI: 1.02–1.23), while social problems were not significant. Moreover, gender was also a significant factor in the model ($\beta = -2.17$, $z = -2.41$, $p = 0.016$, OR = 0.11, 95% CI: 0.02–0.67), with a higher probability (Pr) for males ($Pr = 0.04$) of being in the group of socially-withdrawn adolescents compared to females ($Pr = 0.006$). The McFadden R^2 for the overall model was 0.48.

Table 5. Pearson's r correlations between the TAS-20 total score and the social problems and internalizing problems scales of the YSR.

	Soc. Prob	Int. Prob	TAS TOT
Soc. Prob	-	0.66	0.46
Int. Prob	0.66	-	0.63

Notes: Soc. Prob = social problems scale; Int. Prob = internalizing problems scale; TAS TOT = total score of the TAS-20.

4. Discussion

Our first aim in this study was to investigate the direct relationship between social withdrawal and alexithymia. Significant differences emerged between our two groups with and without social withdrawal in every dimension of alexithymia, with socially-withdrawn adolescents scoring higher on all the scales. Our findings thus confirm that socially-withdrawn adolescents are more impaired in terms of emotional competence, expanding on what emerged from the study by Hattori [2] on emotional problems in socially-withdrawn individuals. Our data also show that difficulty describing feelings (DDF) is the only alexithymia factor influential on social withdrawal. Moreover, DDF is the TAS-20 subscale most correlated to the social withdrawal scale on the YSR. In other words, socially-withdrawn adolescents have a general difficulty with managing their emotions, and are specifically poor at communicating their feelings. This finding confirms Piotti's report, based on clinical experience, that socially-withdrawn adolescents find it difficult to put their feelings and experiences of suffering into words [52].

Some published studies regarding adolescents have associated alexithymia with various psychopathological conditions [43,44,47], because it has been found to be related to an emotional dysregulation acquired already in infancy, and transmissible from one generation to the next [34–36]. The adolescents in the present study had a psychiatric diagnosis with which alexithymia may be associated. Judging from the mean total scores in the TAS-20, the individuals in our group with social withdrawal were alexithymic, while those in the group without social withdrawal were borderline for alexithymia. This would indicate that our whole sample had emotional problems, but what distinguished the socially withdrawn was a greater difficulty in verbalizing their suffering. The inability to ask for help may induce these adolescents to identify withdrawal within their own private worlds and self-exclusion from any form of social interaction as the only strategies able to alleviate their underlying discomfort.

As for the second aim of this study, to establish the psycho-behavioral profile of socially-withdrawn adolescents, our data confirm the reports of an association between social withdrawal and internalizing problems, including anxiety–depression and social problems [22]. In fact, our group with social withdrawal scored significantly higher on the YSR scales measuring these constructs, as well as for total problems. In other words, they showed a greater degree of psycho-emotional suffering, even though there was no significant difference between the two groups with regard to global functioning (GAF). This would suggest that social withdrawal does not compound the contribution of other psychopathological elements to an individual's social, occupational, and psychological functioning in response to the various problems encountered in life.

Since several published studies have considered the relationship between internalizing problems, social problems, and social withdrawal, we tried to examine the direction of this relationship, and to investigate the role of alexithymia. Our data indicate that internalizing problems and alexithymia have a bearing on social withdrawal, while social problems did not emerge as a significant predictor of this type of behavior. We surmise that difficulties with managing emotions (and particularly with communicating them), and internalizing symptoms may be antecedents of social withdrawal, and risk factors for its onset. Social problems, on the other hand, could develop as a consequence of social withdrawal, further trapping the adolescent in a vicious cycle of exclusion from relationships. Another possible explanation is that social problems are not directly linked to social withdrawal, but they may precede internalizing problems. These in turn, along with the presence of alexithymic traits, may encourage withdrawal behaviors.

Moreover, gender also has a significant effect in the model, with a higher probability for males to be in the group of socially-withdrawn adolescents. This would indicate that males with internalizing problems and alexithymia are more at risk of developing social withdrawal compared to females with the same difficulties. Previous studies have shown a higher prevalence of socially-withdrawn adolescents among males [2,3,28]. Our findings thus are in line with those in the literature, and add information about the individual characteristics of boys at risk for withdrawal. Nevertheless, the relationship between gender and social withdrawal should be better investigated in future research.

Although the findings of this study are intriguing, there are some limitations that need to be mentioned, which could also serve as a starting point for future studies. First of all, there is the relatively small size of our sample, and the fact that it only included adolescents in northern Italy. Moreover, another limitation is linked to the retrospective nature of the investigation, which did not allow us to obtain all the information of interest for some participants. Then there is the fact that we used self-report questionnaires: although they have demonstrated their clinical value and are quick to administer, they can suffer from a bias relating to social desirability. Subsequently, the EOT scale of the TAS-20 showed a low reliability in our sample ($\alpha = 0.50$). This result is consistent with previous studies with adolescents (e.g., [46,62–65]), which have reported low Cronbach's alpha values for such scales, ranging from 0.29 to 0.56. Consequently, the EOT scale seems problematic in the adolescent population in general, and not just in our sample. A possible explanation is that externally-oriented thinking does not represent a core feature of alexithymia in adolescents, but it may be more suitable just for adults. La Ferlita et al. [64] stated that this difference between adults and adolescents might be linked to the different strategies used to face emotional difficulties, according to the specific developmental age. Nevertheless, considering that the TAS-20 is widely used, further studies are needed to better investigate the factorial structure of the overall measure and the reliability of the EOT scale in community and clinical adolescent samples. Another shortcoming of the present study is that we considered social withdrawal as a unidimensional construct, so we did not analyze the different components of the phenomenon. This certainly is a limitation of the present study, but it may also be a starting point for future research. In fact, it would be useful to better investigate such a construct on the basis of Asendorpf's model [13,14]. Furthermore, future studies should include other individual and social variables that may constitute risk factors for adolescent social withdrawal (e.g., attachment, relationships with peers and family, specific traumas, social support). Lastly, since the association between social problems and social withdrawal is still not clear, it would be interesting to deepen the knowledge of both this relationship and the role that variables involved play in it.

In conclusion, even with these limitations, our research adds a novel contribution to the still-limited literature on social withdrawal in adolescence. Our focus on the alexithymic traits of socially-withdrawn adolescents could be particularly helpful for the purposes of treatment and prevention. Intervention to improve these teenagers' emotional competence could be a useful way to help them verbalize their psycho-emotional unease, and find more functional ways to deal with it. Understanding the features of social withdrawal in adolescence may be important in the scholastic context, too. In fact, one of the early signs of possible withdrawal is dropping out of school, which represents a risk for adolescents' mental health. Therefore, teachers should be able to recognize adolescents at risk in advance, in order to avoid negative outcomes. Knowledge about the alexithymic traits of socially-withdrawn adolescents could be relevant for both teachers and clinicians. In fact, they could cooperate in the implementation of prevention programs at school, with activities based on students' emotions, dialing in on the best strategies to turn those emotions into words.

Given the increasing frequency with which we are seeing social withdrawal in adolescence, it is hugely important to develop ways to prevent it in order to reduce the risks inherent both in social withdrawal per se, and in the psychopathological conditions that may be associated with it.

Author Contributions: Conceptualization, study design, and supervision, M.G.; formal analysis, S.I. and M.M.; writing—original draft preparation, S.I. and M.M.; writing—review and editing, S.I., M.M., A.R. and M.G.; data curation, S.I. and M.G.; discussion of the data, S.I., M.M., A.R. and M.G. All authors have read and agreed to the published version of the manuscript.

Funding: This research received no external funding.

Institutional Review Board Statement: The present study was part of a broader research project on developmental psychopathologies, conducted according to the guidelines of the Declaration of Helsinki and approved by the local ethical committee (CESC, May 2017, prot.95006).

Informed Consent Statement: Informed consent was obtained from all subjects involved in the study.

Data Availability Statement: The data presented in this study are available on request from the corresponding author. The data are not publicly available because they report private information about participants.

Conflicts of Interest: The authors declare no conflict of interest.

Appendix A

Table A1. Pearson's r correlations between the social withdrawal scale of the YSR and the other scales of the YSR, the TAS-20, and the GAF, considering cases and controls separately.

	Group	
	Cases Withdrawal Scale	Controls Withdrawal Scale
DDF	0.33	0.31
DIF	0.07	0.15
EOT	0.33	0.22
TAS TOT	0.31	0.30
Anx-Dep	0.47	0.55
Soc. Prob	0.33	0.50
Int. Prob	0.57	0.66
YSR TOT	0.36	0.55
GAF	−0.20	−0.19

Notes: Withdrawal = social withdrawal scale; Anx-Dep = anxiety-depression scale; Soc. Prob = social problems scale; Int. Prob = internalizing problems scale; YSR TOT = total problems scale of the YSR; GAF = Global Assessment of Functioning; DDF = difficulty describing feelings; DIF = difficulty identifying feelings; EOT = externally-oriented thinking; TAS TOT = total score of the TAS-20.

References

1. Saito, T. *Hikikomori. Adolescence without End*; Angles, J., Translator; University of Minnesota Press: Minneapolis, MN, USA, 2013.
2. Hattori, Y. Social withdrawal in Japanese youth: A case study of thirty-five hikikomori clients. *J. Trauma Pract.* **2005**, *4*, 181–201. [CrossRef]
3. Aguglia, E.; Signorelli, M.S.; Pollicino, C.; Arcidiacono, E.; Petralia, A. Il fenomeno dell'hikikomori: Cultural bound o quadro psicopatologico emergente? *Petralia Giorn. Ital. Psicopat* **2010**, *16*, 157–164.
4. Toivonen, T.; Norasakkunkit, V.; Uchida, Y. Unable to conform, unwilling to rebel? Youth, culture, and motivation in globalizing Japan. *Front. Psychol.* **2011**, *2*, 207. [CrossRef]
5. ANSA Lifestyle Società e Diritti. Available online: https://www.ansa.it/canale_lifestyle/notizie/societa_diritti/2018/05/24/hikikomori-giovani-in-ritiro-sociale.-la-rete-dei-genitori-per-aiutarli_472b714d-c9c4-47b2-bdae-e83c9403e59d.html (accessed on 24 September 2020).
6. Ministero dell'Istruzione Ufficio Scolastico Regionale per l'Emilia-Romagna. Available online: http://istruzioneer.gov.it/2018/11/06/adolescenti-eremiti-sociali-esiti-e-prime-valutazioni/ (accessed on 1 October 2020).
7. Ranieri, F. Adolescenti tra abbandono scolastico e ritiro sociale: Il fenomeno degli "hikikomori". *Psicol. Clin. Svilupp.* **2016**, *2*, 319–326. [CrossRef]
8. Li, T.M.; Wong, P.W. Editorial Perspective. Pathological social withdrawal during adolescence: A culture-specific or a global phenomenon? *J. Child Psychol. Psychiatry* **2015**, *56*, 1039–1041. [CrossRef]

9. Li, T.M.; Wong, P.W. Youth social withdrawal behavior (hikikomori): A systematic review of qualitative and quantitative studies. *Aust. N. Z. J. Psychiatry* **2015**, *49*, 595–609. [CrossRef] [PubMed]
10. Chan, G.H.Y.; Lo, T.W. Hidden youth services: What Hong Kong can learn from Japan. *Child Youth Serv. Rev.* **2014**, *42*, 118–126. [CrossRef]
11. Procacci, M.; Semerari, A. *Ritiro Sociale. Psicologia e Clinica*; Edizioni Centro Studi Erickson: Trento, Italy, 2019.
12. Rubin, K.H.; Coplan, R.J.; Bowker, J.C. Social withdrawal in childhood. *Annu. Rev. Psychol.* **2009**, *60*, 141–171. [CrossRef] [PubMed]
13. Asendorpf, J.B. Beyond social withdrawal: Shyness, unsociability and peer avoidance. *Hum. Dev.* **1990**, *34*, 259–269. [CrossRef]
14. Asendorpf, J.B. Abnormal shyness in children. *J. Child Psychol. Psychiatry* **1993**, *34*, 1069–1083. [CrossRef]
15. American Psychiatric Association. *Diagnostic and Statistical Manual of Mental Disorders*, 4th ed.; American Psychiatric Association: Washington, DC, USA, 2000.
16. American Psychiatric Association. *Diagnostic and Statistical Manual of Mental Disorders (DSM-5)*; American Psychiatric Association: Arlington, VA, USA, 2013.
17. World Health Organization. *The ICD-11 Classification of Mental Disorders and Behavioral Disorders: Clinical Descriptions and Diagnostic Guidelines*; WHO: Geneva, Switzerland, 2018; Available online: https://icd.who.int/browse11/l-m/en. (accessed on 15 October 2020).
18. World Health Organization. *The ICD-10 Classification of Mental Disorders and Behavioral Disorders: Clinical Descriptions and Diagnostic Guidelines*; WHO: Geneva, Switzerland, 1992.
19. Schneider, B.H.; Younger, A.J.; Smith, T.; Freeman, P.A. Longitudinal exploration of the cross-contextual stability of social withdrawal in early adolescence. *J. Early Adolesc.* **1998**, *18*, 374–396. [CrossRef]
20. Koyoama, A.; Miyake, Y.; Kawakami, N.; Tsuchiya, M.; Tachimori, H.; Takeshima, T.; World Mental Health Japan Survey Group. Lifetime prevalence, psychiatry comorbidity and demographic correlates of hikikomori in a community population in Japan. *Psychiatry Res.* **2010**, *176*, 69–74. [CrossRef]
21. Burgess, K.B.; Younger, A.J. Self-schemas, anxiety, somatic and depressive symptoms in socially withdrawn children and adolescents. *J. Res. Child Educ.* **2006**, *20*, 175–187. [CrossRef]
22. Coplan, R.J.; Rose-Krasnor, L.; Weeks, M.; Kingsbury, A.; Kingsbury, M.; Bullock, A. Alone is a crowd: Social motivations, social withdrawal, and socioemotional functioning in later childhood. *Dev. Psychol.* **2013**, *49*, 861. [CrossRef] [PubMed]
23. Katz, S.J.; Conway, C.C.; Hammen, C.L.; Brennan, P.A.; Najman, J.M. Childhood social withdrawal, interpersonal impairment, and young adult depression: A mediational model. *J. Abnorm. Child Psychol.* **2011**, *39*, 1227–1238. [CrossRef]
24. Rubin, K.H.; Mills, R.S. Conceptualizing developmental pathways to internalizing disorders in childhood. *Can. J. Behav.* **1991**, *23*, 300–317. [CrossRef]
25. Oh, W.; Rubin, K.H.; Bowker, J.C.; Booth-LaForce, C.; Rose-Krasnor, L.; Laursen, B. Trajectories of social withdrawal from middle childhood to early adolescence. *J. Abnorm. Child Psychol.* **2008**, *36*, 553–566. [CrossRef] [PubMed]
26. Spiniello, R.; Piotti, A.; Comazzi, C. *Il Corpo in una Stanza. Adolescenti Ritirati che Vivono di Computer*; Franco Angeli: Milano, Italy, 2015.
27. Rubin, K.H.; Burgess, K.B. Social withdrawal and anxiety. In *The Developmental Psychopathology of Anxiety*; Vasey, M.W., Dadds, M.R., Eds.; Oxford University Press: New York, NY, USA, 2001; pp. 407–434.
28. Malagón-Amor, A.; Martin-López, L.M.; Córcoles, D.; González, A.; Bellsolà, M.; Teo, A.R.; Bulbena, A.; Pérez, V.; Bergé, D. A 12-month study of the hikikomori syndrome of social withdrawal: Clinical characterization and different subtypes proposal. *Psychiatry Res.* **2018**, *270*, 1039–1046. [CrossRef]
29. Frankova, I. Similar but different: Psychological and psychopathological features of primary and secondary hikikomori. *Front. Psychiatry* **2019**, *10*, 558. [CrossRef]
30. Teo, A.R.; Gaw, A.C. Hikikomori, a Japanese culture-bound syndrome of social withdrawal? A proposal for DSM-5. *J. Nerv. Ment. Dis.* **2010**, *198*, 444–449. [CrossRef]
31. Suwa, M.; Suzuki, K. The phenomenon of "hikikomori" (social withdrawal) and the socio-cultural situation in Japan today. *J. Psychopathol.* **2013**, *19*, 191–198.
32. Lancini, M. *Il Ritiro Sociale NEGLI adolescenti. La Solitudine di una Generazione Iperconnessa*; Raffaello Cortina Editore: Milano, Italy, 2019.
33. Sifneos, P.E. The prevalence of 'alexithymic' characteristics in psychosomatic patients. *Psychother. Psychosom.* **1973**, *22*, 255–262. [CrossRef]
34. Taylor, G.J.; Bagby, R.M.; Parker, J.D.A. *Disorder of Affect Regulation. Alexithymia in Medical and Psychiatric Illness*; Cambridge University Press: Cambridge, UK, 1997.
35. Mannarini, S.; Balottin, L.; Toldo, I.; Gatta, M. Alexithymia and psychosocial problems among Italian preadolescents. A latent class analysis approach. *Scand. J. Psychol.* **2016**, *57*, 473–481. [CrossRef]
36. Gatta, M.; Balottin, L.; Mannarini, S.; Chesani, G.; Del Col, L.; Spoto, A.; Battistella, P.A. Familial factors relating to alexithymic traits in adolescents with psychiatric disorders. *Clin. Psychol.* **2017**, *21*, 252–262. [CrossRef]
37. Manninen, M.; Therman, S.; Suvisaari, J.; Ebeling, H.; Moilanen, I.; Huttunen, M.; Joukamaa, M. Alexithymia is common among adolescents with severe disruptive behaviour. *J. Nerv. Ment. Dis.* **2011**, *199*, 506–509. [CrossRef]

38. Karukivi, M.; Vahlberg, T.; Polonen, T.; Filppu, T.; Saarijarvi, S. Does alexithymia expose to mental disorder symptoms in late adolescence? A 4-year follow-up study. *Gen. Hosp. Psychiatry* **2014**, *36*, 748–752. [CrossRef] [PubMed]
39. Muzi, S.; Pace, C.S. Relazioni tra sintomi internalizzanti ed esternalizzanti, attaccamento, regolazione emotiva e alessitimia in adolescenti in comunità residenziale. *Psic. Clin. Svilupp.* **2020**, *1*, 117–126. [CrossRef]
40. Balottin, L.; Nacinovich, R.; Bomba, M.; Mannarini, S. Alexithymia in parents and adolescent anorexic daughters: Comparing the responses to TSIA and TAS-20 scales. *Neuropsychiatr. Dis. Treat.* **2014**, *10*, 1941–1951. [CrossRef]
41. Berger, S.; Elliott, C.; Ranzenhofer, L.M.; Shomaker, L.B.; Hannallah, L.; Field, S.E.; Young, J.F.; Sbrocco, T.; Wilfley, D.E.; Yanovski, J.A.; et al. Interpersonal problem areas and alexithymia in adolescent girls with loss of control eating. *Compr. Psychiatry* **2014**, *55*, 170–178. [CrossRef] [PubMed]
42. Honkalampi, K.; Tolmunen, T.; Hintikka, J.; Rissanen, M.L.; Kylmä, J.; Laukkanen, E. The prevalence of alexithymia and its relationship with Youth Self-Report problem scales among Finnish adolescents. *Compr. Psychiatry* **2009**, *50*, 263–268. [CrossRef]
43. Gatta, M.; Dal Santo, F.; Rago, A.; Spoto, A.; Battistella, P.A. Alexithymia, impulsiveness and psychopathology in non-suicidal self-injured adolescents. *Neuropsychiatr. Dis. Treat.* **2016**, *12*, 2307–2317. [CrossRef] [PubMed]
44. Raffagnato, A.; Angelico, C.; Valentini, P.; Miscioscia, M.; Gatta, M. Using the body when there are no words for feelings: Alexithymia and somatization in self-harming adolescents. *Front. Psychiatry* **2020**, *11*, 262. [CrossRef]
45. Scimeca, G.; Bruno, A.; Cava, L.; Pandolfo, G.; Muscatello, M.R.A.; Zoccali, R. The relationship between alexithymia, anxiety, depression, and internet addiction severity in a sample of Italian high school students. *Sci. World J.* **2014**, *2014*, 1–8. [CrossRef]
46. Loas, G.; Speranza, M.; Pham-Scottez, A.; Perez-Diaz, F.; Corcos, M. Alexithymia in adolescents with borderline personality disorder. *J. Psychosom. Res.* **2012**, *72*, 147–152. [CrossRef]
47. Parolin, M.; Miscioscia, M.; De Carli, P.; Cristofalo, P.; Gatta, M.; Simonelli, A. Alexithymia in young adults with substance use disorders: Critical issues about specificity and treatment predictivity. *Front. Psychol.* **2018**, *9*, 645. [CrossRef]
48. Gatta, M.; Canetta, E.; Zordan, M.; Spoto, A.; Ferruzza, E.; Manco, I.; Addis, A.; Dal Zotto, L.; Toldo, I.; Sartori, S.; et al. Alexithymia in juvenile primary headache sufferers: A pilot study. *J. Headache Pain* **2011**, *12*, 71–80. [CrossRef] [PubMed]
49. Gatta, M.; Spitaleri, C.; Balottin, U.; Spoto, A.; Balottin, L.; Manganoand, S.; Battistella, P.A. Alexithymic characteristics in pediatric patients with primary headache: A comparison between migraine and tension-type headache. *J. Headache Pain* **2015**, *16*, 1–7. [CrossRef] [PubMed]
50. Bagby, R.M.; Parker, J.D.; Taylor, G.J. The twenty-item Toronto Alexithymia Scale—I. Item selection and cross-validation of the factor structure. *J. Psychosom. Res.* **1994**, *38*, 23–32. [CrossRef]
51. Achenbach, T.M.; Rescorla, L.A. *Manual for the ASEBA School-Age Forms and Profiles*; Research Center for Children, University of Vermont: Burlington, NJ, USA, 2001.
52. Piotti, A. *Il Banco Vuoto. Diario di un Adolescente in Estrema Reclusione*; Franco Angeli: Milano, Italy, 2012.
53. Vanheule, S.; Desmet, M.; Meganck, R.; Bogaerts, S. Alexithymia and interpersonal problems. *J. Clin. Psychol.* **2007**, *63*, 109–117. [CrossRef]
54. Qualter, P.; Wagner, H.; Quinton, S.J.; Brown, S. Loneliness, interpersonal distrust, and alexithymia in university students. *J. Appl. Soc. Psychol.* **2009**, *39*, 1461–1479. [CrossRef]
55. Sette, S.; Baumgartner, E.; Laghi, F.; Coplan, R.J. The role of emotion knowledge in the links between shyness and children's socio-emotional functioning at preschool. *Br. J. Dev. Psychol.* **2016**, *34*, 471–488. [CrossRef] [PubMed]
56. Erdfelder, E.; Faul, F.; Buchner, A. GPOWER: A general power analysis program. *Behav. Res. Methods Instrum. Comput.* **1996**, *28*, 1–11. [CrossRef]
57. Kernberg, O.F. *Disturbi Gravi della Personalità*; Bollati Boringhieri: Torino, Italy, 1987.
58. Startup, M.; Jackson, M.C.; Bedix, S. The concurrent validity of the Global Assessment of Functioning (GAF). *Br. J. Clin. Psychol.* **2002**, *41*, 417–422. [CrossRef] [PubMed]
59. Frigerio, A.; Vanzin, L.; Pastore, V. The Italian preadolescent mental health project (PrISMA): Rationale and methods. *Int. J. Methods Psychiatr. Res.* **2006**, *15*, 22–35. [CrossRef] [PubMed]
60. Bressi, C.; Taylor, G.; Parker, J.; Bressi, S.; Brambilla, V.; Aguglia, E.; Allegranti, I.; Buongiorno, A.; Giberti, F.; Bucca, M.; et al. Cross validation of the factor structure of the Twenty-item Toronto Alexithymia Scale: An Italian multicenter study. *J. Psychosom. Res.* **1996**, *41*, 551–559. [CrossRef]
61. The Jamovi Project Jamovi. (Version 1.2) [Computer Software]. 2020. Available online: https://www.jamovi.org.
62. Craparo, G.; Faraci, P.; Gori, A. Psychometric properties of the 20-Item Toronto Alexithymia Scale in a group of Italian Younger Adolescents. *Psychiatry Investig.* **2015**, *12*, 500–507. [CrossRef]
63. Loas, G.; Braun, S.; Delhaye, M.; Linkowski, P. The measurement of alexithymia in children and adolescents: Psychometric properties of the Alexithymia Questionnaire for Children and the twenty-item Toronto Alexithymia Scale in different non-clinical and clinical samples of children and adolescents. *PLoS ONE* **2017**, *12*, e0177982. [CrossRef]
64. La Ferlita, V.; Bonadies, M.; Solano, L.; De Gennaro, L.; Gonini, P. Alessitimia e adolescenza: Studio preliminare di validazione della TAS-20 su un campione di 360 adolescenti italiani. *Infanz. Adolesc.* **2007**, *6*, 131–144.
65. Muzi, S. A narrative review on alexithymia in adolescents with previous adverse experiences placed for adoption, in foster care, or institutions. Prevalence, gender differences, and relations with internalizing and externalizing symptoms. *Mediterr. J. Clin. Psychol.* **2020**, *8*. [CrossRef]

MDPI
St. Alban-Anlage 66
4052 Basel
Switzerland
Tel. +41 61 683 77 34
Fax +41 61 302 89 18
www.mdpi.com

Children Editorial Office
E-mail: children@mdpi.com
www.mdpi.com/journal/children

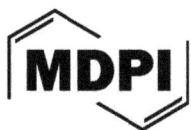

www.ingramcontent.com/pod-product-compliance
Lightning Source LLC
LaVergne TN
LVHW070507100526
838202LV00014B/1807